Grant's
Anatomy Coloring Book

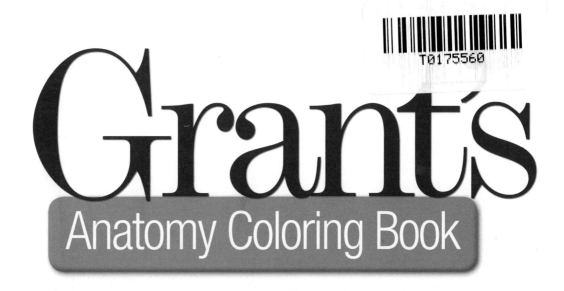

Nicole R. Herring, PhD

Assistant Professor
Department of Anatomical Sciences and Neurobiology
Director, Willed Body Program and Robert Acland Fresh Tissue Dissection Laboratory
University of Louisville
Louisville, Kentucky

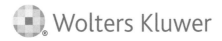 Wolters Kluwer

Philadelphia • Baltimore • New York • London
Buenos Aires • Hong Kong • Sydney • Tokyo

T0175560

Acquisitions Editor: Crystal Taylor
In-House Development Editor: Andrea Vosburgh
Freelance Development Editor: Kathleen Scogna
Editorial Coordinator: Emily Buccieri
Marketing Manager: Michael McMahon
Senior *Production Project Manager:* Alicia Jackson
Creative Director: Larry Pezzato
Art Director: Jennifer Clements
Artist: JDimes MediVisual Communications
Manufacturing Coordinator: Margie Orzech
Prepress Vendor: S4Carlisle Publishing Services

Copyright © 2019 Wolters Kluwer.

All rights reserved. This book is protected by copyright. No part of this book may be reproduced or transmitted in any form or by any means, including as photocopies or scanned-in or other electronic copies, or utilized by any information storage and retrieval system without written permission from the copyright owner, except for brief quotations embodied in critical articles and reviews. Materials appearing in this book prepared by individuals as part of their official duties as U.S. government employees are not covered by the above-mentioned copyright. To request permission, please contact Wolters Kluwer at Two Commerce Square, 2001 Market Street, Philadelphia, PA 19103, via email at permissions@lww .com, or via our website at lww.com (products and services).

9 8 7 6 5 4 3 2 1

Printed in China

Library of Congress Cataloging-in-Publication Data

Names: Herring, Nicole R., author.
Title: Grant's anatomy coloring book / Nicole R. Herring, Ph.D., Assistant
    Professor, Department of Anatomical Sciences and Neurobiology, Director,
    Willed Body Program and Robert Acland Fresh Tissue Dissection Laboratory,
    University of Louisville, Louisville, Kentucky.
Other titles: Anatomy coloring book
Description: Philadelphia : Wolters Kluwer Heath, [2019] | Includes index.
Identifiers: LCCN 2017056796 | ISBN 9781496351258
Subjects: LCSH: Human anatomy—Atlases.
Classification: LCC QM25 .H48 2019 | DDC 612.0022/2—dc23 LC record available at https://lccn.loc
    .gov/2017056796

This work is provided "as is," and the publisher disclaims any and all warranties, express or implied, including any warranties as to accuracy, comprehensiveness, or currency of the content of this work.

This work is no substitute for individual patient assessment based upon healthcare professionals' examination of each patient and consideration of, among other things, age, weight, gender, current or prior medical conditions, medication history, laboratory data, and other factors unique to the patient. The publisher does not provide medical advice or guidance and this work is merely a reference tool. Healthcare professionals, and not the publisher, are solely responsible for the use of this work including all medical judgments and for any resulting diagnosis and treatments.

Given continuous, rapid advances in medical science and health information, independent professional verification of medical diagnoses, indications, appropriate pharmaceutical selections and dosages, and treatment options should be made and healthcare professionals should consult a variety of sources. When prescribing medication, healthcare professionals are advised to consult the product information sheet (the manufacturer's package insert) accompanying each drug to verify, among other things, conditions of use, warnings and side effects and identify any changes in dosage schedule or contrain-dications, particularly if the medication to be administered is new, infrequently used or has a narrow therapeutic range. To the maximum extent permitted under applicable law, no responsibility is assumed by the publisher for any injury and/or damage to persons or property, as a matter of products liability, negligence law or otherwise, or from any reference to or use by any person of this work.

LWW.com

RRS1802

To my love, Michael, for the bountiful supply of patience, joy, and laughter

To Gabriel, for proving that love has no biological boundaries

To my parents, Dan and Joanna, and my brother, Matt, for the heaps of encouragement and support

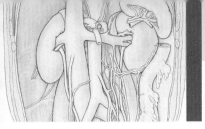

Preface: How to Use This Book

The purpose of this coloring book is to help students develop their understanding of clinical anatomy. This book takes an integrated approach to anatomy by combining illustrations with fill-in-the-blank, numbered structures and descriptive text highlighting key features (attachments, innervation, or relationships). The images are based on the detailed and beautiful dissection-based illustrations from *Grant's Atlas of Anatomy* by Drs. Anne M. R. Agur and Arthur F. Dalley. Because the original illustrations were drawn from cadaveric dissections prepared by Dr. J. C. Boileau Grant, they achieve a realism and precision not found in idealized drawings. By comparing the anatomic relationships depicted in the book with dissections in the lab, students are able to formulate an accurate mental picture of the three-dimensional organization of each region. Additional schematic and orientation figures are provided to supplement the dissection-based illustrations to clarify and reinforce anatomic concepts.

The coloring book follows the layout of *Grant's Atlas of Anatomy* and thus presents the structures regionally in the sequence in which they are revealed during dissection. This book can be utilized independently or in conjunction with *Grant's Atlas of Anatomy* or *Grant's Dissector*. Either way, the primary goal of this book is to be an active learning resource, providing a means of both visual and kinesthetic learning by engaging the motor movements and visual stimulation of coloring with simultaneous presentation of high-yield, essential information.

Based on the feedback provided by more than 20 student reviewers, the book's teaching approach has been carefully crafted and refined. In each coloring book illustration, important and relevant structures are numbered and given a fill-in-the-blank space, allowing the user an opportunity to engage with the image and the learning process. Additional structures have been prelabeled to provide orientation or to highlight key relationships. The text that explains each image is provided on the opposite page and has been developed with students ease of use as the primary focus. Essential material has been provided in bullet point or table format and the numbering of structures chosen to guide the user through the coloring exercise of each image.

How to Use this Book

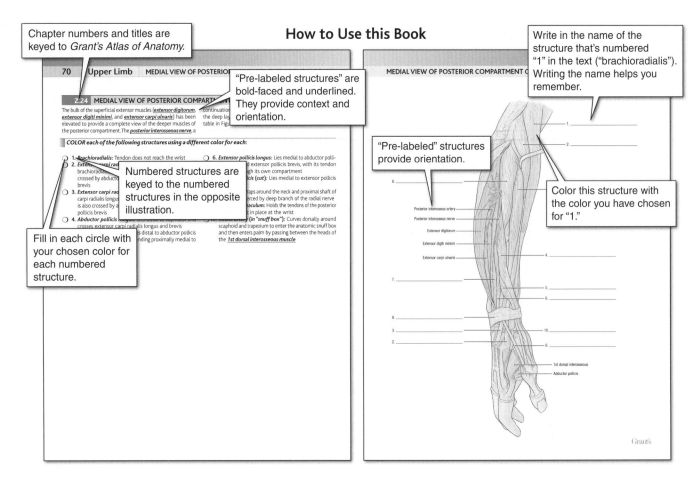

Chapter numbers and titles are keyed to *Grant's Atlas of Anatomy.*

"Pre-labeled structures" are bold-faced and underlined. They provide context and orientation.

Numbered structures are keyed to the numbered structures in the opposite illustration.

Fill in each circle with your chosen color for each numbered structure.

Write in the name of the structure that's numbered "1" in the text ("brachioradialis"). Writing the name helps you remember.

"Pre-labeled" structures provide orientation.

Color this structure with the color you have chosen for "1."

Coloring pencils are the ideal coloring medium for this book; coloring pencils will not bleed through the pages and will provide a range of color options. You are free to color structures as you wish; however, suggested colors are shades of red for arteries, blue for veins, brown for muscles, yellow for nerves, and green for lymphatics and ducts. You are also free and encouraged to color unlabeled structures, add line drawings of nerve and arterial pathways, write in additional information pertinent to your study, and make this coloring book your own personalized study aid.

I hope you enjoy using this coloring book and find it not only a fun method to prepare for class or to review material but also a beneficial exercise that helps build your foundation of anatomic structures and their relationships.

Sincere thanks to my skillful editor, Kathleen Scogna, along with the efforts of Crystal Taylor of Wolters Kluwer. I would also like to thank Jonathan Dimes of JDimes MediVisual Communications for his tireless work with not only developing the style but also final production of the images. I would be remiss if I did not recognize the enormous impact of my mentors: Drs. Art Dalley and Robert Acland for instilling a love for the art of dissection and Dr. Jennifer Brueckner-Collins for showing me the true heart of an educator. Lastly, sincere appreciation for the anatomic donors who make our studies possible.

Nicole R. Herring, PhD

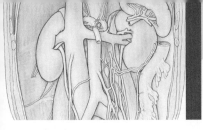

Table of Contents

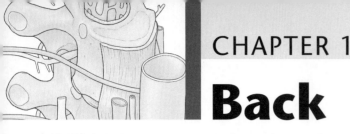

CHAPTER 1

Back

1.1A OSTEOLOGY OF THE VERTEBRAL COLUMN

The vertebrae and the **_intervertebral (IV) discs_** comprise the vertebral column (spine) that extends from the base of the cranium (skull) to the tip of the coccyx. The vertebral column typically consists of a total of 33 vertebrae: 24 separate pre-sacral vertebrae and 9 additional fused vertebrae.

COLOR each of the following using a different color for each region:

○ 1. **_Seven cervical vertebrae_**, with **_C1_** referred to as the atlas and **_C2_** referred to as the axis
○ 2. **_Twelve thoracic vertebrae_**, each articulating with a pair of ribs
○ 3. **_Five lumbar vertebrae_**

The additional vertebrae are located in the sacrum and coccyx:
○ 4. **_Five sacral vertebrae_**, fused
○ 5. **_Four coccygeal vertebrae_**, variably fused or separated

IV foramina are formed laterally on the right and left sides of the vertebral column from the superior and inferior notches of adjacent vertebrae to permit the exit of spinal nerves.

1.1B and C PARTS OF THE TYPICAL VERTEBRA

The basic structure of each vertebra is the same. Each vertebra is composed of a vertebral body, a vertebral arch, and seven processes. Within each region of the vertebral column, vertebrae share similar characteristics that accommodate the different demands of each region. For example, the thoracic vertebrae display costal facets for articulation with the ribs.

COLOR each of the following using a different color for each part of the typical vertebra:

○ 6. **_Vertebral body:_** Anteriorly placed, mostly cylindrical portion that increases in size as the vertebral column descends to support progressively greater body weight

Vertebral arch: Formation posterior to the vertebral body that consists of two pedicles and laminae

○ 7. **_Pedicles:_** Two (right and left) short pillars projecting posteriorly from the vertebral body
○ 8. **_Laminae:_** Two (right and left) plates extending medially from the pedicles to meet in the midline

Vertebral foramen: Space formed by the vertebral arch and posterior aspect of the vertebral body that contains the spinal cord, roots of spinal nerves, meninges, blood vessels, and fat.

Collectively, the vertebral foramina form the vertebral canal in which the spinal cord is housed.

○ 9. **_Transverse processes:_** Two (right and left) posterolateral projections from the junction of the pedicle and lamina
○10. **_Spinous process:_** One median posterior (and often inferior) projection from the junction of the laminae

Articular processes: Four (two **_superior_** and two **_inferior_**) processes that arise at the junction of the pedicle and lamina

○11. **_Superior articular facet:_** One articulating surface on each of the superior articular processes
○12. **_Inferior articular facet:_** One articulating surface on each of the inferior articular processes

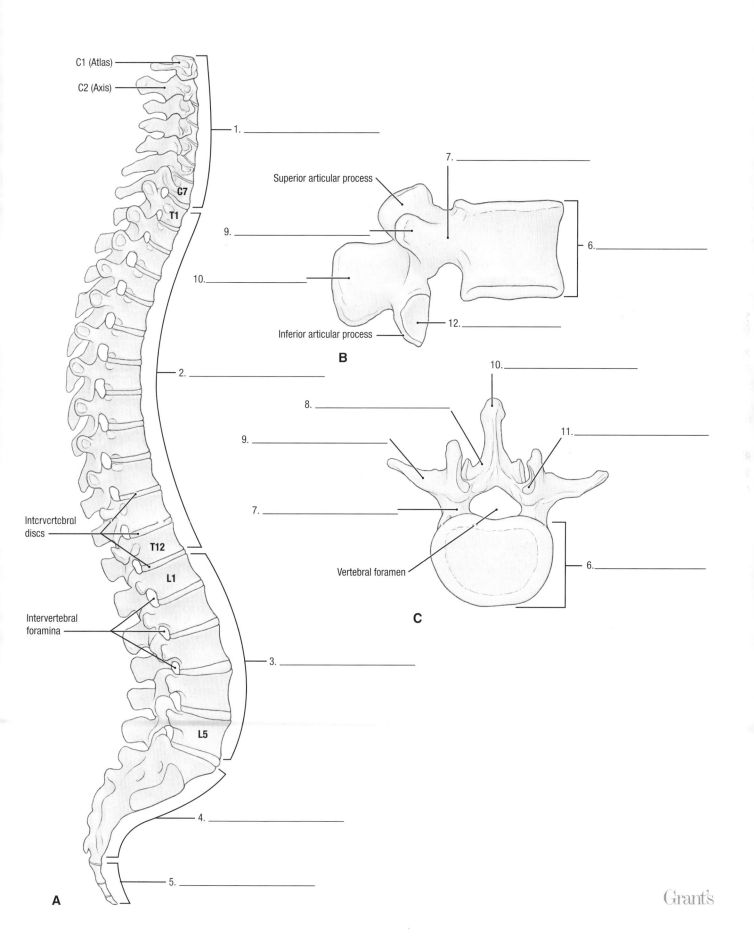

C1 (Atlas)

C2 (Axis)

1. _____

C7

T1

Superior articular process

7. _____

9. _____

6. _____

10. _____

12. _____

Inferior articular process

B

2. _____

10. _____

8. _____

9. _____

11. _____

7. _____

6. _____

Vertebral foramen

C

Intervertebral discs

T12

L1

Intervertebral foramina

3. _____

L5

4. _____

5. _____

A

Grant's

1.2 JOINTS OF THE VERTEBRAL COLUMN

In this image, a midsagittal cut has been performed to demonstrate the joints of the vertebral column, particularly the IV discs and ligaments. The spinal cord has been removed from the *vertebral canal*.

The joints of the *vertebral bodies* are composed of the *IV discs* and ligaments. An IV disc is located between each vertebra, except between C1 and C2 and between sacral and coccygeal vertebra. Each IV disc is composed of an annulus fibrosus and a nucleus pulposus.

COLOR each of the following using a different color for each structure:

⭘ 1. *Annulus fibrosus:* Outer fibrous ring that is thinner posteriorly
⭘ 2. Cavity for *nucleus pulposus:* Semifluid center that permits the flexibility of the vertebral column

The joints of the vertebral bodies are further supported by two ligaments connecting the bodies and IV discs:
⭘ 3. *Anterior longitudinal ligament:* Strong, broad fibrous membrane that connects the anterolateral aspects of the vertebral bodies and IV discs from the pelvic surface of the sacrum to the occipital bone. This is the only ligament that resists hyperextension of the vertebral column.
⭘ 4. *Posterior longitudinal ligament:* Weaker, narrower band that runs within the *vertebral canal* along the posterior aspect of the vertebral bodies from the sacrum to C2. It weakly resists hyperflexion of the vertebral column.

The joints of the vertebral arches are supported by accessory ligaments:
⭘ 5. *Ligamentum flavum:* Broad, elastic membrane that joins the laminae of adjacent vertebral arches only
⭘ 6. *Interspinous ligament:* Thin fibrous membrane that connects adjoining *spinous processes* only
⭘ 7. *Supraspinous ligament:* Cordlike band that connects the tips of the spinous processes from C7 to the sacrum

CLINICAL NOTE: DEGENERATIVE CHANGES

Two degenerative changes are demonstrated:

1. *Nucleus pulposus herniated into vertebral bodies:* The nucleus pulposus of the IV disc between L3 and L4 has herniated into the bodies of the vertebrae superiorly and inferiorly.
2. *Nucleus pulposus herniated posteriorly (herniated disc):* The nucleus pulposus of the IV disc between L1 and L2 has herniated posteriorly through the annulus fibrosus (slipped disc), which can potentially affect *spinal nerves* exiting via the **IV** *foramen*.

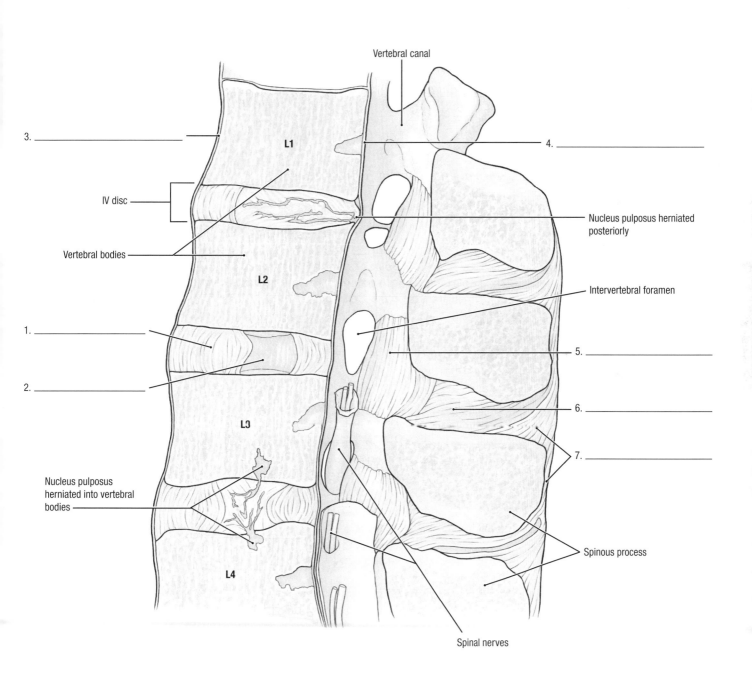

Vertebral canal

3. _____

L1

IV disc

Vertebral bodies

L2

4. _____

Nucleus pulposus herniated posteriorly

Intervertebral foramen

1. _____

2. _____

5. _____

6. _____

L3

7. _____

Nucleus pulposus herniated into vertebral bodies

L4

Spinous process

Spinal nerves

Grant's

1.3 SUPERFICIAL MUSCLES OF THE BACK

The superficial muscles of the back, or axio-appendicular muscles, help attach the upper limb to the trunk and to move the upper limb by acting primarily on the scapula. The superficial muscles of the back are located in two layers: the larger trapezius and latissimus dorsi muscles superficially located and the levator scapulae, rhomboid major, and rhomboid minor located deep to the trapezius. In this image, the trapezius muscle has been reflected on the left side to demonstrate the levator scapulae, rhomboid major, and rhomboid minor. **_Cutaneous nerves of the posterior rami_** of the spinal nerves will pierce through, but not innervate, the superficial muscles of the back to supply the overlying skin of the back.

CLINICAL NOTE: TRIANGLE OF AUSCULTATION

The **_triangle of auscultation_** is an area near the inferior angle of the scapula where a gap in the musculature occurs. The boundaries of the triangle are formed by the superior border of the latissimus dorsi, the inferior border of the trapezius, and the medial border of the scapula. The thinner layer of musculature allows for greater clarity of respiratory sounds during auscultation, especially when the patient draws the scapula anteriorly and thus enlarges the triangle of auscultation.

**COLOR** each of the following using a different color for each muscle:

Superficial Muscles of Back

Muscle	Proximal Attachment	Distal Attachment	Innervation	Action
◯ 1. *Trapezius*	Spinous processes of C7-T12 vertebrae, nuchal ligament, external occipital protuberance, medial third of superior nuchal line of cranium	_**Spine of scapula**_ and acromion; lateral third of clavicle	(Spinal) accessory nerve (CN XI)	Descending fibers: elevate Ascending fibers: depress Middle: retract scapula
◯ 2. *Latissimus dorsi*	◯ 3. _**Thoracolumbar fascia**_, spinous processes of inferior six thoracic vertebrae, _**iliac crest**_, inferior three to four ribs	Floor of intertubercular sulcus of humerus	Thoracodorsal nerve (C6, C7, C8)	Extends, adducts, and medially rotates humerus
◯ 4. *Levator scapulae*	Transverse processes of C1-C4 vertebrae	_**Medial border of scapula**_ superior to the scapular spine	Dorsal scapular (C5) nerve	Elevates scapula and tilts glenoid cavity inferiorly by rotating the scapula
◯ 5. *Rhomboid minor*	Nuchal ligament, spinous processes of C7 and T1 vertebrae	_**Medial border of scapula**_ at the level of the scapular spine		Retracts scapula, rotates scapula to depress glenoid cavity, stabilizes the scapula to the thoracic wall
◯ 6. *Rhomboid major*	Spinous processes of T2-T5 vertebrae	_**Medial border of scapula**_ from scapular spine to inferior angle		

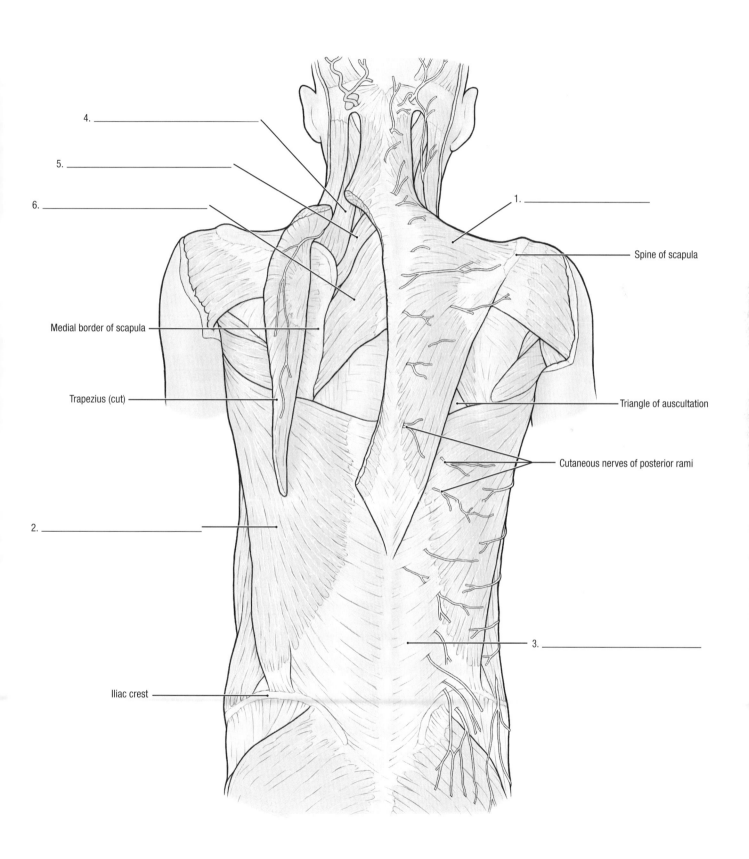

4. _____

5. _____

6. _____

1. _____

Spine of scapula

Medial border of scapula

Trapezius (cut)

Triangle of auscultation

Cutaneous nerves of posterior rami

2. _____

3. _____

Iliac crest

1.4 INTERMEDIATE MUSCLES OF BACK

The intermediate muscles of the back are located deep to the superficial muscles. The serratus posterior superior is located deep to the rhomboids, whereas the serratus posterior inferior is located deep to the latissimus dorsi. In this image, the *trapezius*, *rhomboid major*, and *rhomboid minor* muscles have been cut and the *scapula* pulled away from the thoracic wall to demonstrate the serratus posterior superior muscle. The *latissimus dorsi* and *thoracolumbar fascia* have been cut on both sides to demonstrate the serratus posterior inferior muscle. The *lumbar triangle*, bounded by the iliac crest, inferior border of the latissimus dorsi, and the inferior border of the external oblique, is an anatomic space through which inferior lumbar hernias can occur.

COLOR each of the following superficial muscles of the back using the same colors used for each muscle in the figure in Section 1.3:

○ 1. *Levator scapulae*
○ 2. *Rhomboid minor*

○ 3. *Rhomboid major*
○ 4. *Latissimus dorsi* (cut)

COLOR each of the following using a different color for each muscle:

Intermediate Muscles of the Back

Muscle	Proximal Attachment	Distal Attachment	Innervation	Action
○ 5. **Serratus posterior superior**	Nuchal ligament, spinous processes of C7-T3 vertebrae	Superior borders of the 2nd-4th *ribs*	2nd-5th intercostal nerves	Proprioception; accessory respiration muscles (elevate ribs)
○ 6. **Serratus posterior inferior**	Spinous processes of T11-L2 vertebrae	Inferior borders of the 8th-12th *ribs*	T9-T12 anterior rami of the thoracic spinal nerves	

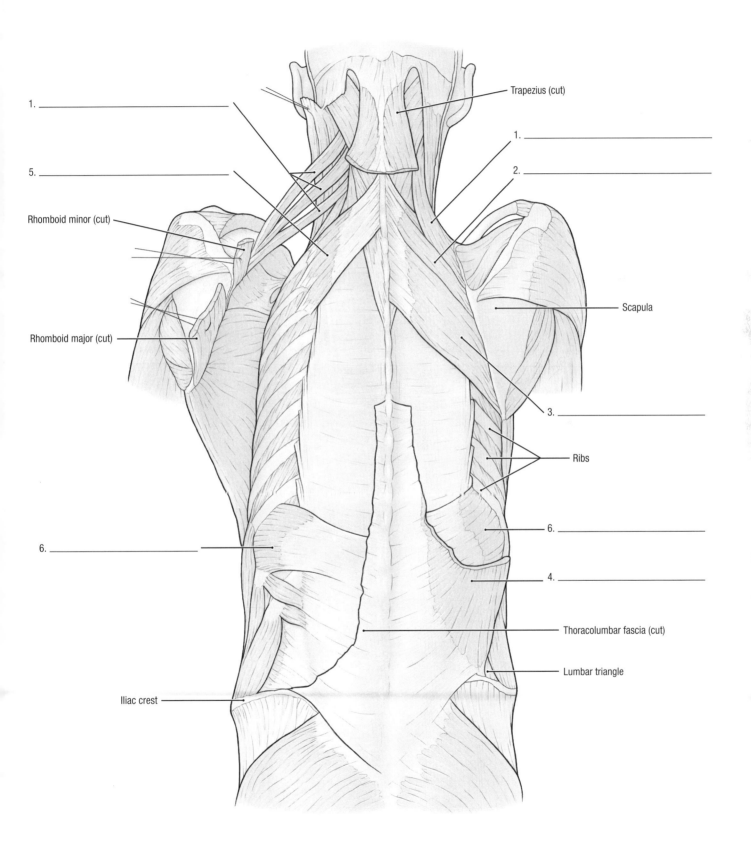

Trapezius (cut)

1. _____

1. _____

5. _____

2. _____

Rhomboid minor (cut)

Scapula

Rhomboid major (cut)

3. _____

Ribs

6. _____

6. _____

4. _____

Thoracolumbar fascia (cut)

Lumbar triangle

Iliac crest

Grant's

1.5   DEEP MUSCLES OF THE BACK (SPLENIUS AND ERECTOR SPINAE)

The deep, or intrinsic, muscles of the back are located deep to the intermediate layer. The deep muscles of the back are involved in postural movements of the vertebral column and movements of the head and neck. They are the only muscles located on the back innervated by **_posterior rami of spinal nerves_**. The deep muscles of the back are located in three layers: the splenius muscles are located in the superficial layer; the **_erector spinae_** (spinalis, longissimus, and iliocostalis) muscles are located in the intermediate layer; and the semispinalis muscles are located in the deep layer.

In the superficial layer, the fibers of the splenius capitus and cervicis often appear blended together until the attachments are visible. The splenius capitus comprises the uppermost fibers and the splenius cervicis the lower fibers.

COLOR each of the following using a different color for each muscle:

Deep Muscles of the Back

Muscle	Proximal Attachment	Distal Attachment	Action
○ 1. *Splenius capitus*	Nuchal ligament, spinous processes of C7-T6 vertebrae	Mastoid process, lateral third superior nuchal line	Unilaterally: Laterally flexes the neck and rotates the head to side of active muscles
○ 2. *Splenius cervicis*		Transverse processes of C1-C3/C4 vertebrae	Bilaterally: Extends the head and neck
○ 3. *Spinalis*	Iliac crest, sacrum, sacroiliac ligaments, sacral and inferior lumbar spinous processes, supraspinous ligament	Spinous processes of upper thoracic vertebrae and cranium	Unilaterally: Laterally flexes vertebral column
○ 4. *Longissimus*		*Ribs* between tubercles and angles, transverse processes of thoracic and cervical vertebrae, mastoid process	Bilaterally: Extends the vertebral column and head
○ 5. *Iliocostalis*		Angles of lower ribs and transverse processes of cervical vertebrae	

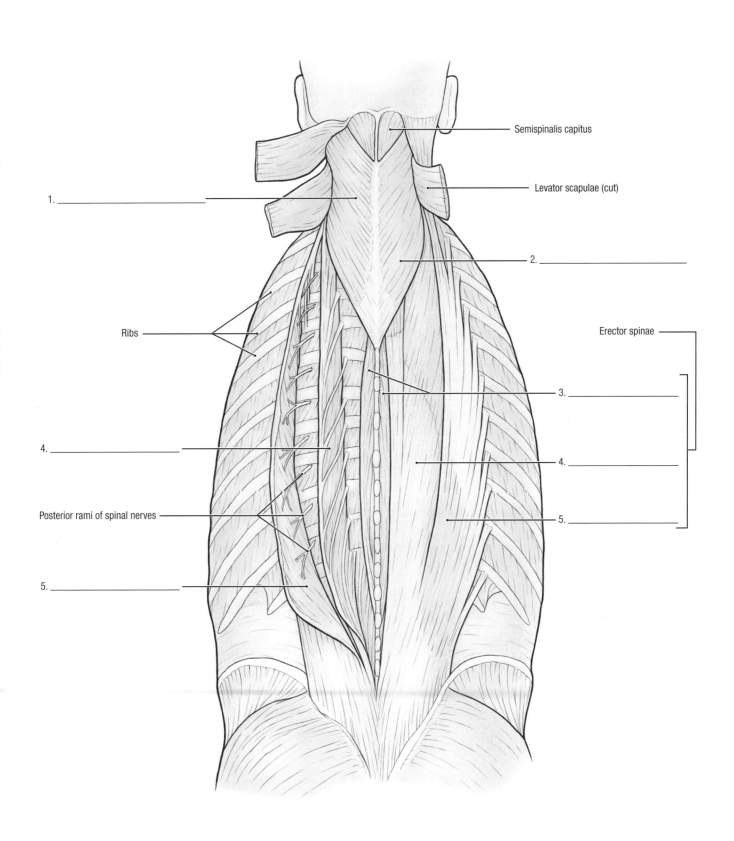

Semispinalis capitus

Levator scapulae (cut)

1.

2.

Ribs

Erector spinae

3.

4.

4.

Posterior rami of spinal nerves

5.

5.

1.6 SEMISPINALIS AND SUBOCCIPITAL REGION MUSCLES

Muscles of the suboccipital region are located deep to the descending fibers of the trapezius, splenius, and semispinalis capitis muscles. The semispinalis muscles are innervated by posterior rami of spinal nerves, whereas all four of the suboccipital muscles (rectus capitis posterior major, rectus capitis posterior minor, obliquus capitis superior, and obliquus capitis inferior) are specifically innervated by the posterior ramus of C1, the suboccipital nerve. Although the splenius capitis and cervicis are located in the same plane (see the figure in Section 1.5), the semispinalis capitis is located superficial to the semispinalis cervicis and suboccipital triangle muscles and is reflected on the right side of this image.

COLOR each of the following using a different color for each muscle:

Suboccipital Muscles				
Muscle	Proximal Attachment	Distal Attachment	Action	Aspect of Suboccipital Triangle
◯ 1. *Semispinalis capitis*	Transverse processes of C4-T6	Between **superior** and inferior **nuchal lines** of occipital bone	Extension of the head and cervical region, rotates the head to the contralateral side	Roof
◯ 2. *Semispinalis cervicis*	Transverse processes of T1-T6	Spinous processes of C2-C5		Inferior to suboccipital muscles (uppermost fibers attach to the spinous process of C2)
◯ 3. *Obliquus capitis inferior*	Posterior arch of C2 vertebra	Transverse process of C1 vertebra	Rotates the head to the ipsilateral side	Inferolateral boundary
◯ 4. *Obliquus capitis superior*	Transverse process of C1 vertebra	Occipital bone between superior and inferior nuchal lines	Extension of the head	Superolateral boundary
◯ 5. *Rectus captitus posterior major*	*Spinous process of axis (C2)*	Lateral part of inferior nuchal line	Rotates the head to the ipsilateral side	Superomedial boundary
◯ 6. *Rectus capitus posterior minor*	Posterior arch of C1 vertebra	Medial part of inferior nuchal line		Superomedial to rectus capitus posterior major

Neurovasculature of the Suboccipital Region

◯ 7. *Greater occipital nerve (C2):* Emerges inferior to the obliquus capitis inferior and then pierces the semispinalis capitis to supply the scalp of the occipital region

◯ 8. *Occipital artery:* Emerges superolateral to the obliquus capitis superior

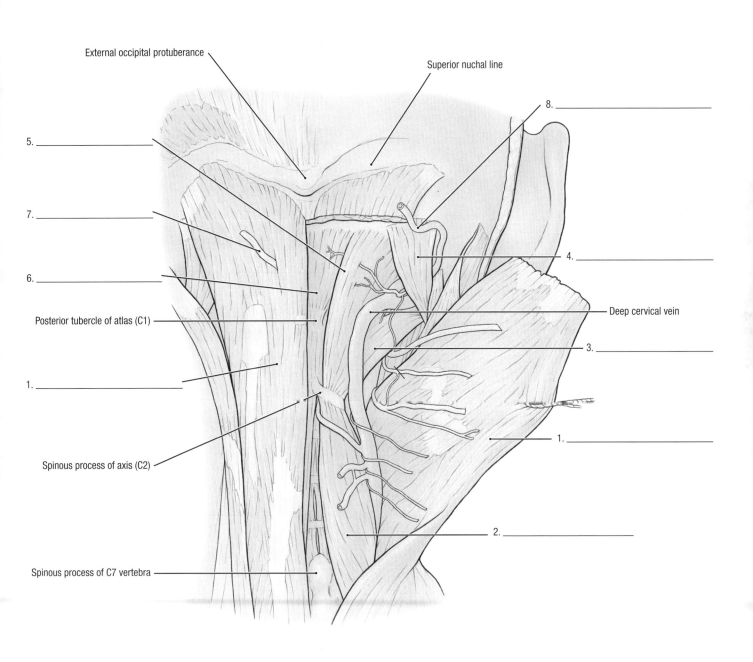

External occipital protuberance

Superior nuchal line

8. _____

5. _____

7. _____

6. _____

Posterior tubercle of atlas (C1)

1. _____

Spinous process of axis (C2)

Spinous process of C7 vertebra

4. _____

Deep cervical vein

3. _____

1. _____

2. _____

Grant's

1.7   SPINAL NERVES AND INFERIOR END OF THE DURAL SAC

All 31 pairs of spinal nerves arise from the spinal cord and exit through the IV foramina. The naming of the spinal nerves is different in the cervical region than in other regions because of the presence of eight cervical nerves and only seven cervical vertebrae. The first seven cervical nerves are named for the cervical vertebrae *inferior* to their exit (eg, **C1 nerve** exits superior to **C1 vertebrae**); however, the eighth cervical nerve (**C8**) exits superior to **T1 vertebrae**. All the remaining spinal nerves arising from the thoracic, lumbar, sacral, and coccygeal levels of the spinal cord are named for the vertebra *superior* to their exit (eg, **T1 nerve** exits inferior to the **T1 vertebra**).

COLOR *each region of the spinal cord and the corresponding spinal nerves using a different color for each:*

◯ 1. *Cervical (8 spinal nerves)*
◯ 2. *Thoracic (12 spinal nerves)*
◯ 3. *Lumbar (5 spinal nerves)*
◯ 4. *Sacral (5 spinal nerves)*
◯ 5. *Coccygeal (1 spinal nerve)*

CLINICAL NOTE: DEVELOPMENT OF THE VERTEBRAL COLUMN AND SPINAL CORD

During development, the growth of the vertebral column and canal outpaces the growth of the spinal cord. There are major anatomic consequences for this developmental phenomenon in the adult:

- The inferior end of the spinal cord typically terminates near the level of the **L1**-L2 IV disc.
- The roots of more inferior spinal nerves have an increasingly longer course to reach the IV foramen for their corresponding exit from the vertebral canal.
- Spinal nerve roots continue to travel within the vertebral canal inferior to the spinal cord to reach their exit, forming the **cauda equina**.

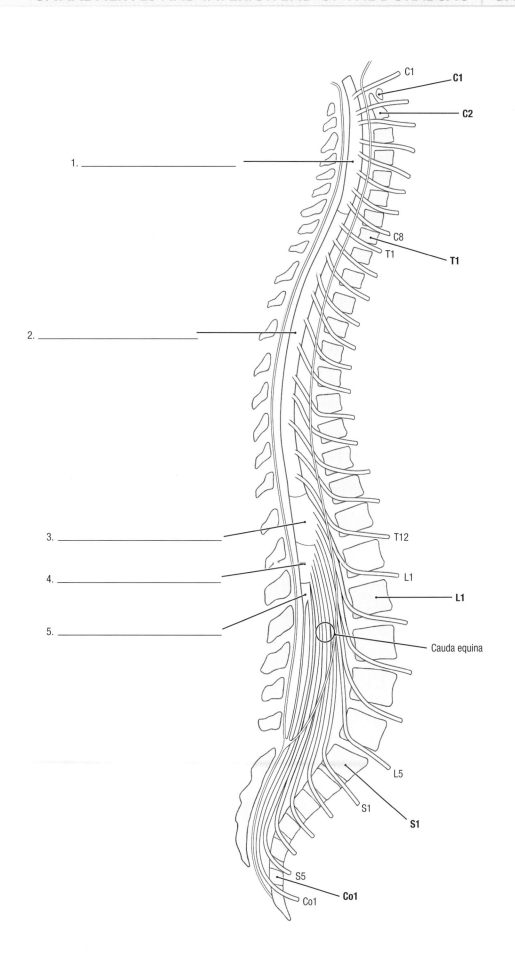

C1
C1
C2

1. _____

C8
T1
T1

2. _____

T12

3. _____

4. _____

L1
L1

5. _____

Cauda equina

L5

S1
S1

S5
Co1
Co1

Grant's

1.8   PARTS OF THE SPINAL NERVE

The gray matter of the spinal cord is organized into an H-shaped area when viewed in transverse sections. The H-shape is subdivided into four horns: a right and left *posterior* (dorsal) *horn* and a right and left *anterior* (ventral) *horn*. The anterior horn is composed of the cell bodies of motor neurons, whereas the posterior horn receives sensory information from cell bodies located in the *spinal (dorsal root) ganglion*.

> **COLOR each of the following using a different color for each part of a spinal nerve:**

◯ 1. *Anterior root and rootlets:* Motor fibers exit the anterior horn of the spinal cord as rootlets, and the root is formed as the rootlets merge together.

◯ 2. *Posterior root and rootlets:* Sensory fibers enter the posterior horn of the spinal cord as rootlets from the root that extends from the spinal ganglion.

◯ 3. *Spinal nerve:* Formed by the union of the anterior and posterior roots within a *dural sleeve* at the *IV foramen* and is composed of both motor and sensory fibers.

◯ 4. *Anterior ramus:* One of the two branches of the spinal nerve. Anterior rami will supply the majority of the structures of the body and can form a plexus (network of nerves). Most anterior rami are named.

◯ 5. *Posterior ramus:* One of the two branches of the spinal nerve. Posterior rami only supply the true back muscles, skin overlying these muscles, and zygapophyseal joints and do not participate in plexus formation.

◯ 6. *White ramus communicans:* Communicating branch conducting presynaptic sympathetic fibers from the spinal nerve to the sympathetic trunk. White rami communicans also include other fibers (visceral afferents).

◯ 7. *Sympathetic trunk:* Paired structure that extends the length of the vertebral column, connects to all 31 pairs of spinal nerves, and is composed of paravertebral ganglia, containing postsympatic sympathetic cell bodies, and interganglionic connections.

◯ 8. *Gray ramus communicans:* Communicating branch conducting postsynaptic sympathetic fibers from the sympathetic trunk to the spinal nerve.

◯ 9. *Intercostal nerve:* This nerve is an example of a named anterior ramus.

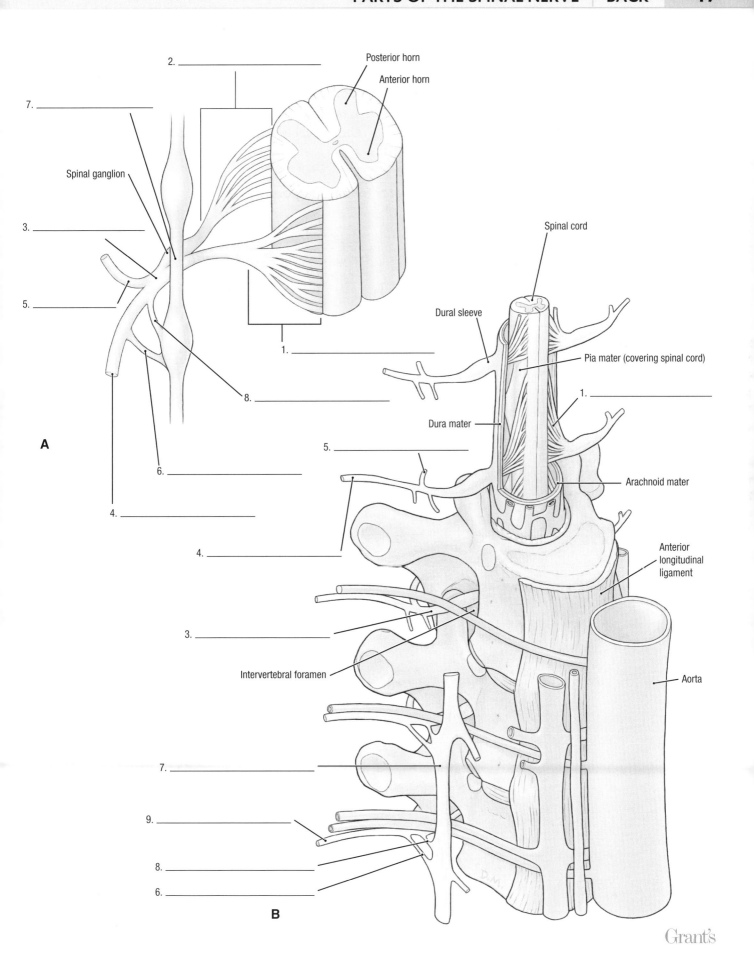

2. _____

Posterior horn

Anterior horn

7. _____

Spinal ganglion

3. _____

5. _____

8. _____

A

6. _____

4. _____

Spinal cord

Dural sleeve

Pia mater (covering spinal cord)

Dura mater

1. _____

5. _____

Arachnoid mater

4. _____

Anterior longitudinal ligament

3. _____

Intervertebral foramen

Aorta

7. _____

9. _____

8. _____

6. _____

B

Grant's

1.9   DERMATOMES

The region of skin innervated by a specific spinal cord level is called a dermatome. Dermatome maps indicate the typical patterns of innervation of the skin by specific spinal cord levels. Spinal nerves do not provide sensory innervation to the anterior head and face.

Dermatome Map

A number of the dermatomes have been labeled for you. For those that have not been labeled, add in the dermatome level.

COLOR each of the following using a different color for each region:

- ⭕ *Cervical dermatomes*
- ⭕ *Thoracic dermatomes*
- ⭕ *Lumbar dermatomes*
- ⭕ *Sacral dermatomes*

CLINICAL NOTE: DERMATOMES

Dermatomes are clinically beneficial in determining nerve damage, especially radiculopathy or conditions affecting the root of a nerve. A compressed nerve (from a herniated disc, tumor, bone spurs, etc.) can cause pain, numbness, tingling, or weakness along the dermatome corresponding to that nerve. Dermatomes are also apparent during some virus infections. Herpes zoster (shingles) is caused by the reactivation of the varicella-zoster virus—which causes chickenpox—that remains dormant (latent) in the dorsal root ganglia. Reactivation commonly results in a painful, itchy, or tingly rash along one or two adjacent dermatomes.

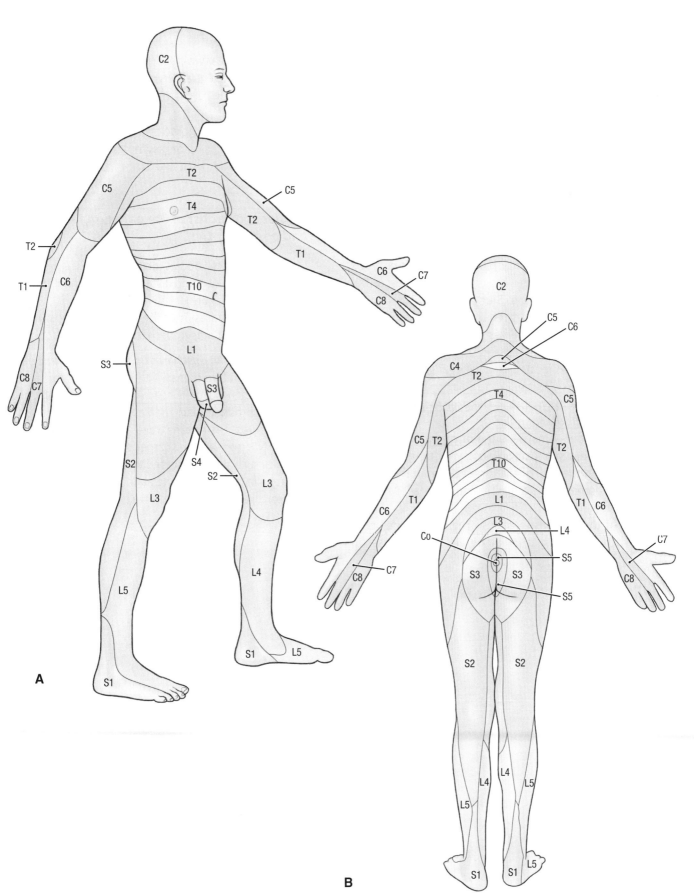

A

B

Grant's

1.10A PARASYMPATHETIC DIVISION OF THE AUTONOMIC NERVOUS SYSTEM

The autonomic nervous system (ANS) is also known as the visceral motor system targeting smooth muscle, cardiac muscle, and glands. The ANS is divided into the sympathetic and parasympathetic divisions. The ANS is a two-neuron system with the presynaptic neuron located in the central nervous system and the postsynaptic neuron located in the peripheral nervous system.

Parasympathetic Division

The parasympathetic division of the ANS is restricted in its distribution to target structures. Parasympathetic innervation will be distributed to specific structures within the head along with the viscera of the thoracic and abdominopelvic cavities. Except for erectile tissue, parasympathetic innervation does not travel to the body wall and is not a component of mixed spinal nerves.

> TRACE *the lines of each of the following components (cell bodies and axons) of the parasympathetic division of the ANS using a different color for presynaptic and postsynaptic:*

○ *Cell bodies of the presynaptic parasympathetic neurons* are located in the brainstem and in the gray matter of the sacral spinal cord from S2 to S4.
  - Axons of the neurons located in the brainstem exit as components of ***cranial nerves (CN) III, VII, IX, and X***.
    - These fibers of CN III, VII, and IX synapse on postsynaptic cell bodies located in specific ganglia in the head.
      - ◆ CN III fibers synapse in the ***ciliary ganglion***.
      - ◆ CN VII fibers synapse in the ***pterygopalatine*** and ***submandibular ganglia***.
      - ◆ CN IX fibers synapse in the ***otic ganglion***.
    - CN X fibers synapse on postsynaptic cell bodies located in the wall of the target organ in the thorax and abdomen (gastrointestinal tract as far as the left colic flexure).
  - Axons of the neurons located in the sacral spinal cord exit within ***pelvic splanchnic nerves*** and synapse on postsynaptic cell bodies located in the wall of the target organ in the pelvis and distal gastrointestinal tract (distal to left colic flexure).
    - Presynaptic parasympathetic axons only synapse on postsynaptic parasympathetic cell bodies.

○ *Cell bodies of the postsynaptic parasympathetic neurons* are located in two areas:
  1. Specific ganglia in the head (ciliary, pterygopalatine, otic, and submandibular) that are located near the target structures. Their axons travel ("hitchhike") via branches of CN V to reach the target structures.
  2. Intramural ganglia located within the wall of the target organ in the thoracic and abdominopelvic cavities. Their axons remain within the wall of the target organ and are very short.

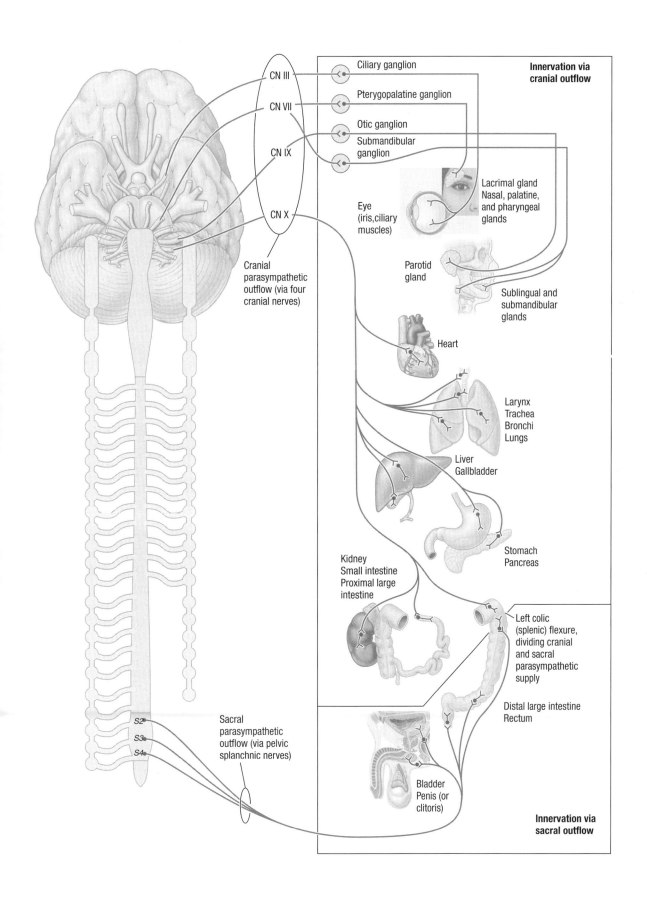

Ciliary ganglion

Pterygopalatine ganglion

Otic ganglion

Submandibular ganglion

CN III

CN VII

CN IX

CN X

Innervation via cranial outflow

Cranial parasympathetic outflow (via four cranial nerves)

Eye (iris, ciliary muscles)

Lacrimal gland Nasal, palatine, and pharyngeal glands

Parotid gland

Sublingual and submandibular glands

Heart

Larynx Trachea Bronchi Lungs

Liver Gallbladder

Stomach Pancreas

Kidney Small intestine Proximal large intestine

Left colic (splenic) flexure, dividing cranial and sacral parasympathetic supply

Distal large intestine Rectum

S2
S3
S4

Sacral parasympathetic outflow (via pelvic splanchnic nerves)

Bladder Penis (or clitoris)

Innervation via sacral outflow

1.10B SYMPATHETIC DIVISION OF THE AUTONOMIC NERVOUS SYSTEM

Sympathetic Division

The sympathetic division differs from the parasympathetic division in that it is widely distributed throughout the body; however, the presynaptic cell bodies are located only in one region of the spinal cord (T1-L2). To reach all areas of the body, the sympathetic division contains multiple pathways to reach its targets. Similar to a subway map, the necessary route is dependent on where the final destination is located.

> *TRACE the lines of each of the following components (cell bodies and axons) of the sympathetic division of the ANS using a different color for presynaptic and postsynaptic:*

○ *Cell bodies of the presynaptic sympathetic neurons* are located in the gray matter of the spinal cord from *T1 to L2* forming a column of neurons referred to as the intermediolateral cell column.
  - Axons of the presynaptic sympathetic neurons exit the spinal cord via the anterior root and enter the spinal nerve briefly before exiting via a white ramus communicans (*WRC*) to the sympathetic trunk. WRC only arise from T1-L2 spinal nerves. This portion of the pathway is the same for all the targets of the sympathetic division.
  - Once in the sympathetic trunk, presynaptic sympathetic axons take one of three possible routes:
    1. Synapse within the sympathetic trunk at the same level they entered the sympathetic trunk. This occurs if the target is located in the body wall at the same level or is located within the thoracic cavity.
    2. Ascend or descend to synapse within the sympathetic trunk at higher or lower levels. Axons ascend in the sympathetic trunk if the target is located in the body wall above T1 (i.e., upper limb and neck) or located in the head. Axons descend in the sympathetic trunk if the target is located in the lower body wall or lower limb.
    Via (1) & (2), the fibers reach the level of all 31 pairs of spinal nerves to synapse with postsynaptic neurons.
    3. Pass through the sympathetic trunk without synapsing, forming *abdominopelvic splanchnic nerves* to synapse on prevertebral ganglia that are primarily located along major branches of the abdominal aorta. Occurs if the target is located within the abdominopelvic cavity.

○ *Cell bodies of the postsynaptic sympathetic neurons* are located in two sites:
  1. Paravertebral ganglia of the sympathetic trunk
    - If the target is located in the body wall (including limbs), postsynaptic sympathetic axons exit the sympathetic trunk via a *gray ramus communicans* to reach the spinal nerve. Postganglionic sympathetic axons then travel as part of both the anterior and posterior rami to their target structures. Gray rami communicantes extend to all 31 spinal nerve pairs.
    - If the target is located within the thoracic cavity (heart, lungs, esophagus), postsynaptic sympathetic axons exit the sympathetic trunk via *cardiopulmonary splanchnic nerves*.
    - If the target is located within the head, axons exit the sympathetic trunk via *cephalic arterial rami* to travel on arteries to target structures of the head
  2. Prevertebral ganglia (*celiac, aorticorenal, superior mesenteric, inferior mesenteric* and pelvic ganglia) if the target is located in the abdominopelvic cavity:
    - Presynaptic sympathetic axons to these ganglia pass through the sympathetic trunk without synapsing.
    - They synapse within the prevertebral ganglia.
    - Postsynaptic sympathetic axons exit the prevertebral ganglia to travel on arteries or form plexuses to target structures of the abdomen and pelvis.

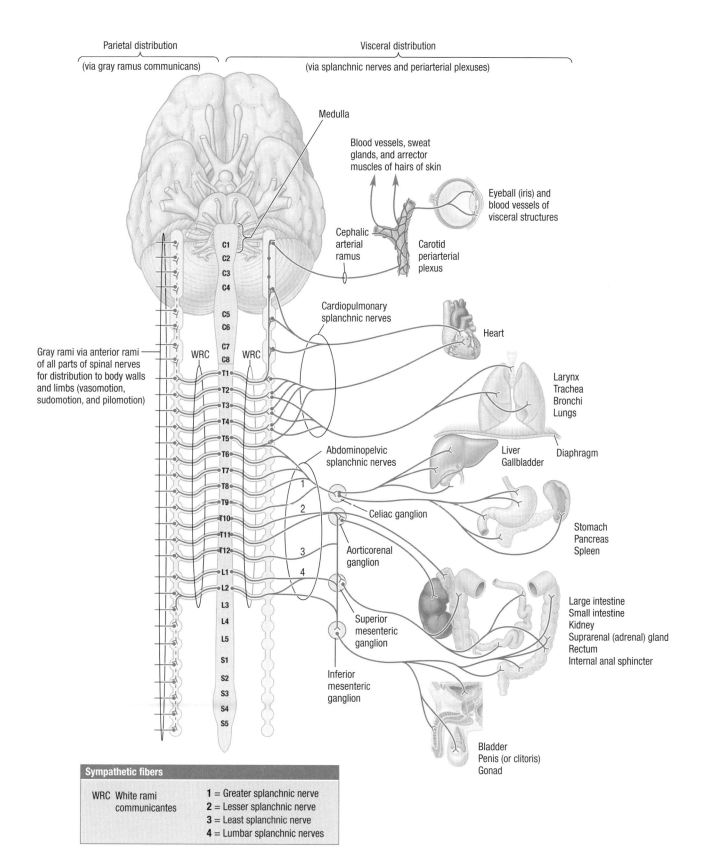

Parietal distribution
(via gray ramus communicans)

Visceral distribution
(via splanchnic nerves and periarterial plexuses)

Medulla

Blood vessels, sweat glands, and arrector muscles of hairs of skin

Eyeball (iris) and blood vessels of visceral structures

Cephalic arterial ramus

Carotid periarterial plexus

Cardiopulmonary splanchnic nerves

Heart

Gray rami via anterior rami of all parts of spinal nerves for distribution to body walls and limbs (vasomotion, sudomotion, and pilomotion)

WRC   WRC

Larynx
Trachea
Bronchi
Lungs

Diaphragm

Abdominopelvic splanchnic nerves

Liver
Gallbladder

Celiac ganglion

Stomach
Pancreas
Spleen

Aorticorenal ganglion

Large intestine
Small intestine
Kidney
Suprarenal (adrenal) gland
Rectum
Internal anal sphincter

Superior mesenteric ganglion

Inferior mesenteric ganglion

Bladder
Penis (or clitoris)
Gonad

Sympathetic fibers

WRC White rami communicantes

1 = Greater splanchnic nerve
2 = Lesser splanchnic nerve
3 = Least splanchnic nerve
4 = Lumbar splanchnic nerves

Grant's

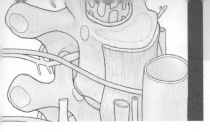

CHAPTER 2

Upper Limb

2.1 ANTERIOR ASPECT OF UPPER LIMB OSTEOLOGY

The upper limb consists of four major regions: shoulder, arm, forearm, and hand.

COLOR each of the following structures using a different color for each:

The only direct articulation between the upper limb and the thoracic wall is between the medial end of the **_clavicle_** and the sternum. The clavicle articulates laterally with the scapula. The **_scapula_** is a triangular flat bone that lies on the posterolateral aspect of the thoracic wall. In anatomic position, the **_medial border_** lies parallel to the vertebral column, whereas the **_lateral border_** runs in a superolateral direction toward the axilla.

○ 1. **_Acromion:_** Anterior projection that forms the point of the shoulder and articulates with lateral end of clavicle
○ 2. **_Coracoid process;_** Beak-like process that projects anterolaterally
○ 3. **_Subscapular fossa:_** Large anterior depression

The **_humerus_** is the largest bone of the upper limb. The humerus articulates proximally with the scapula, forming the shoulder joint. Distally, the humerus articulates with the **_radius_** and **_ulna_**, forming the elbow joint.

○ 4. **_Greater tubercle:_** Lateral projection superior to the **_surgical neck_** of the humerus
○ 5. **_Lesser tubercle:_** Anterior projection superior to the surgical neck of the humerus
○ 6. **_Intertubercular sulcus:_** Depression that separates the greater and lesser tubercles in which the tendon of long head of the biceps brachii lies
○ 7. **_Deltoid tuberosity:_** Lateral projection along the shaft of the humerus for attachment of the deltoid muscle
○ 8. **_Lateral epicondyle:_** Distal lateral end
○ 9. **_Medial epicondyle:_** Distal medial end

○10. **_Capitulum:_** Inferior surface that articulates with the head of the radius
○11. **_Trochlea:_** Spool-shaped surface that articulates with trochlear notch of ulna
○12. **_Coronoid fossa:_** Anterior depression that receives the coronoid process of ulna during full flexion of the elbow

The ulna is medially located, longer than the radius, and is the stabilizing bone of the forearm. The ulna does not participate in the wrist joint.

○13. **_Coronoid process:_** Proximal anterior projection that articulates with the humerus

The radius is the lateral and shorter bone of the forearm.

○14. **_Head of the radius:_** Proximal end of the radius that articulates with the capitulum of the humerus
○15. **_Tuberosity of the radius:_** Medial, oval-shaped projection distal to the **_neck of the radius_** for attachment of the biceps brachii tendon
○16. **_Styloid process of the radius:_** Distal, lateral end

The wrist is composed of eight **_carpal bones_** arranged in two rows of four. The distal row of carpal bones articulates with five **_metacarpal bones_**. The distal ends of the metacarpal bones articulate with five **_proximal phalanges_**. In addition, digits 2 to 5 have a **_middle phalanx_** and **_distal phalanx_**, whereas digit 1 (thumb) has only a distal phalanx.

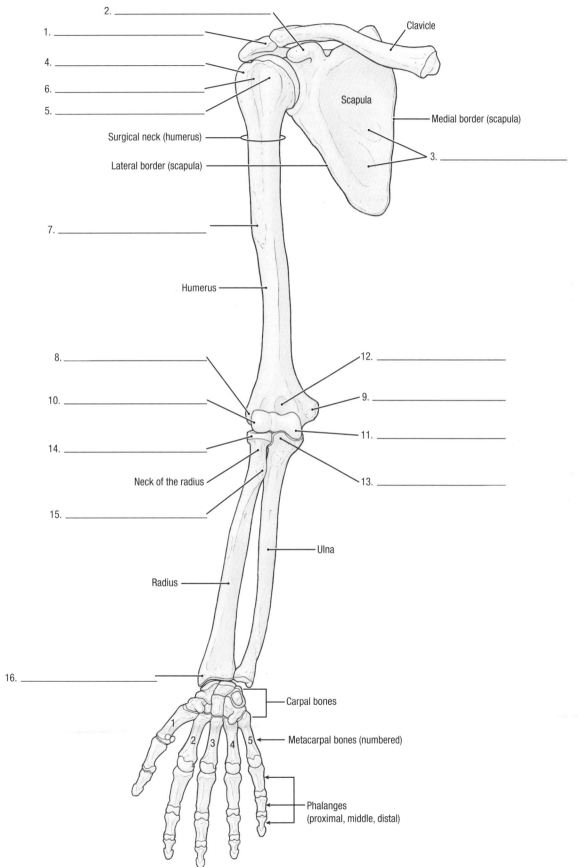

2. _____

1. _____

4. _____

6. _____

5. _____

Clavicle

Scapula

Medial border (scapula)

Surgical neck (humerus) _____

Lateral border (scapula) _____

3. _____

7. _____

Humerus

8. _____

10. _____

12. _____

9. _____

11. _____

14. _____

Neck of the radius _____

13. _____

15. _____

Ulna

Radius

16. _____

Carpal bones

1 2 3 4 5 Metacarpal bones (numbered)

Phalanges
(proximal, middle, distal)

| 2.2 | OSTEOLOGY OF POSTERIOR ASPECT OF UPPER LIMB |

The posterior aspect of the upper limb bones reveals additional key features of the upper limb bones.

COLOR each of the following structures using a different color for each:

Scapula

Superior angle: Superior aspect of the medial border of the scapula

Inferior angle: Inferior aspect of the medial border of the scapula

○ 1. *Spine of scapula:* Projecting ridge of bone that continues laterally to form the *acromion*. The acromion articulates with the clavicle at the *acromioclavicular joint*.

○ 2. *Supraspinous fossa:* Small depression superior to the spine of scapula

○ 3. *Infraspinous fossa:* Larger depression inferior to the spine of scapula

Humerus

○ 4. *Head of humerus:* Spherical, proximal end of the humerus that articulates with the glenoid cavity of the scapula

○ 5. *Anatomic neck:* Groove encircling the head and separating the head from the *greater tubercle* and lesser tubercle

○ 6. *Radial groove:* Oblique depression along the posterior shaft in which the radial nerve and profunda brachii artery lie

○ 7. *Medial supra-epicondylar ridge:* Distal medial widening of the shaft superior to the *medial epicondyle*

○ 8. *Lateral supra-epicondylar ridge:* Distal lateral widening of the shaft superior to the *lateral epicondyle*

Ulna

○ 9. *Olecranon:* Projects proximally forming the point of the elbow and articulates with the olecranon fossa of the humerus during full extension

Radius

Head of Radius
Styloid Process of Radius
Carpal bones

The numbering of the *metacarpal bones* begins again at the thumb (most lateral bone in anatomic position). The arrangement of the *phalanges* remains the same as from the anterior view.

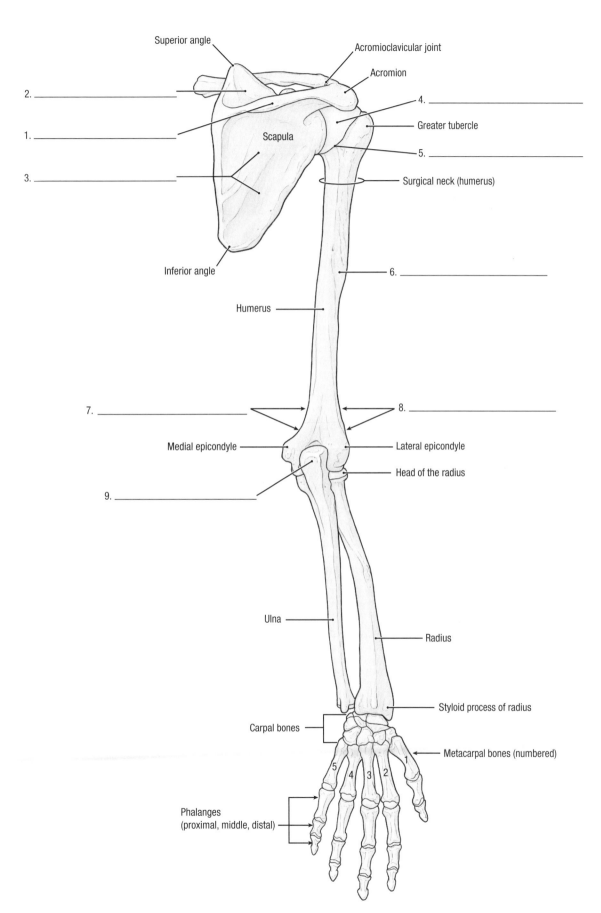

Superior angle

Acromioclavicular joint

Acromion

2. _____

4. _____

Greater tubercle

1. _____

Scapula

5. _____

3. _____

Surgical neck (humerus)

Inferior angle

6. _____

Humerus

7. _____

8. _____

Medial epicondyle

Lateral epicondyle

Head of the radius

9. _____

Ulna

Radius

Styloid process of radius

Carpal bones

Metacarpal bones (numbered)

5 4 3 2 1

Phalanges
(proximal, middle, distal)

Grant's

2.3 PECTORAL REGION

The muscles of the pectoral region, or anterior axio-appendicular muscles, move the pectoral girdle. These muscles include the larger pectoralis major and serratus anterior muscles along with two deeper and smaller muscles, the pectoralis minor and subclavius (see figure in Section 2.6). The **_platysma_** muscle of the neck variably overlies the clavicle and uppermost fibers of the pectoralis major as it inserts into the skin.

COLOR each of the following structures using a different color for each:

Anterior Axio-Appendicular Muscles

Muscle	Proximal Attachment	Distal Attachment	Innervation	Action
○ 1. *Clavicular head of pectoralis major*	Medial half of **_clavicle_**	Lateral lip of intertubercular sulcus of humerus	Lateral and medial pectoral nerves (C5, **C6**, **C7**, **C8**, T1)	Adducts and medially rotates humerus; draws scapula anteriorly and inferiorly
○ 2. *Sternocostal head of pectoralis major*	Sternum, superior six costal cartilages, aponeurosis of external oblique			
○ 3. *Serratus anterior*	Lateral aspect of ribs 1-8	Medial border of scapula	Long thoracic nerve (C5, **C6**, **C7**)	Protracts scapula and holds it against thoracic wall; rotates scapula

The deltoid is the most superficial of the six scapulohumeral muscles that pass from the scapula to the humerus.

Deltoid Muscle

Muscle	Proximal Attachment	Distal Attachment	Innervation	Action
○ 4. *Deltoid*	Lateral third of clavicle, acromion, and spine of scapula	Deltoid tuberosity of humerus	Axillary nerve (**C5**, C6)	• Anterior (clavicular) part: flexes and medially rotates arm • Middle (acromial) part: abducts arm • Posterior (spinal) part: extends and laterally rotates arm

COLOR each of the following structures using a different color for each:

○ 5. *Pectoral fascia:* Invests the pectoralis major and becomes the axillary fascia laterally

○ 6. *Cephalic vein:* Travels between the deltoid and pectoralis major muscle and then enters the **_clavipectoral (deltopectoral) triangle_** to join the axillary vein

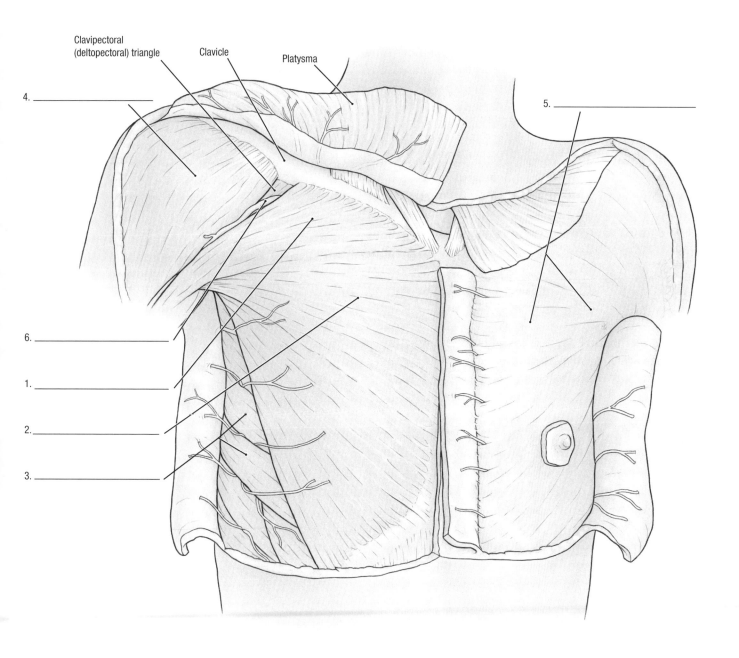

Clavipectoral
(deltopectoral) triangle

Clavicle

Platysma

4. _____

5. _____

6. _____

1. _____

2. _____

3. _____

2.4 WALLS AND CONTENTS OF AXILLA

The axilla is the space inferior to the glenohumeral joint commonly referred to as the "armpit." The axilla provides a passageway for a majority of the neurovascular structures of the upper limb. In this image, the base of the axilla (skin and subcutaneous tissue) has been removed to demonstrate the walls of the axilla. The apex of the axilla, the cervico-axillary canal, is not shown in this image. The cervico-axillary canal is formed by the bony landmarks of the first rib, clavicle, and superior edge of the scapula.

COLOR each of the following structures using a different color for each:

Walls of Axilla	
Walls	**Structure**
Anterior	◯ 1. *Pectoralis major* ◯ 2. *Pectoralis minor*
Posterior	◯ 3. *Subscapularis* ◯ 4. *Latissimus dorsi* ◯ 5. *Teres major*
Medial	◯ 6. *Serratus anterior*
Lateral	Intertubercular sulcus of the humerus. *In this image, concealed by:* ◯ 7. *Biceps brachii, short head* ◯ 8. *Coracobrachialis*

◯ 9. *Axillary sheath:* Encircles the neurovascular structures of the axilla including the axillary vein, axillary artery, and components of the brachial plexus.

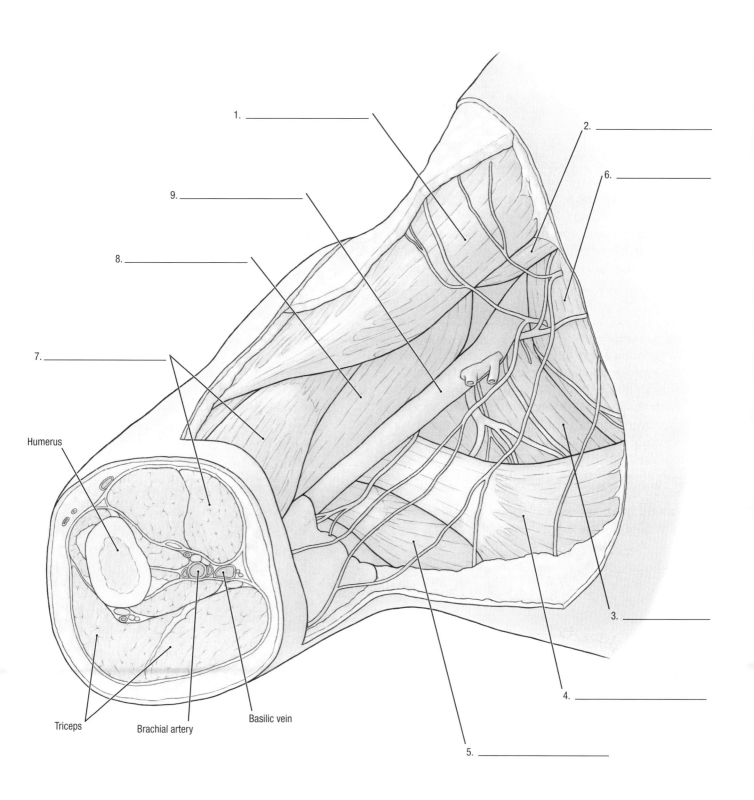

1.

9.

8.

7.

Humerus

2.

6.

3.

4.

5.

Triceps

Brachial artery

Basilic vein

Grant's

2.5 BRACHIAL PLEXUS

The brachial plexus gives rise to most of the nerves of the upper limb beginning in the neck and passing into the axilla. The brachial plexus is composed from the anterior rami of spinal nerves C5-T1. These five rami will combine and divide and then combine and divide again in a specific pattern to give rise to terminal branches.

COLOR each of the following structures using a different color for each:

○ 1. **Roots:** Composed of the anterior rami of **C5**, **C6**, **C7**, **C8**, and **T1**

Above the **clavicle**, the roots of the brachial plexus combine in a specific pattern to form three trunks:

○ 2. **Superior trunk:** Forms from the joining of the anterior rami of C5 and C6
○ 3. **Middle trunk:** Forms from the continuation of the anterior ramus of C7
○ 4. **Inferior trunk:** Forms from the joining of the anterior rami of C8 and T1

Immediately below the clavicle, the three trunks each divide into:

○ 5. **Anterior divisions:** One anterior division from each of the superior, middle, and inferior trunks to total three anterior divisions
○ 6. **Posterior divisions:** One posterior division from each of the superior, middle, and inferior trunks to total three posterior divisions

The six divisions will join in a specific pattern to form three cords:

○ 7. **Lateral cord:** Formed by the joining of the anterior divisions from the superior and middle trunks

○ 8. **Medial cord:** Formed by the continuation of the anterior division of the inferior trunk
○ 9. **Posterior cord:** Formed by the joining of all three posterior divisions

The three cords give rise to terminal branches.

- From the lateral cord:
  ○ 10. **Musculocutaneous nerve**
  ○ 11. **Lateral root of median nerve**

- From the medial cord:
  ○ 12. **Ulnar nerve**
  ○ 13. **Medial root of median nerve**
  ○ 14. **Median nerve:** Forms from the lateral and medial roots from the lateral and medial cords, respectively

- From posterior cord:
  ○ 15. **Axillary nerve**
  ○ 16. **Radial nerve**

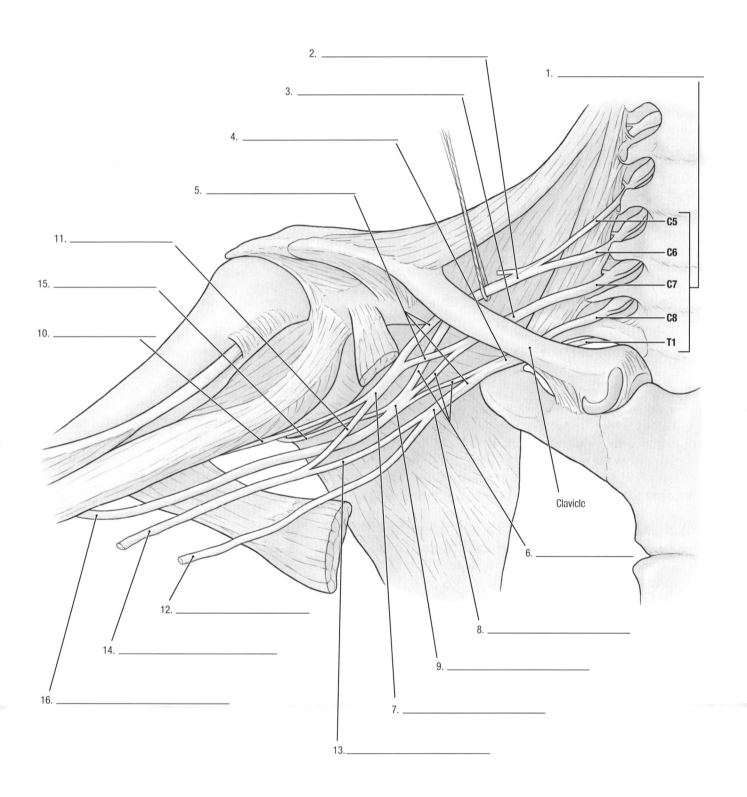

2. _____

3. _____

4. _____

5. _____

11. _____

15. _____

10. _____

1. _____

C5

C6

C7

C8

T1

Clavicle

6. _____

12. _____

14. _____

16. _____

8. _____

9. _____

7. _____

13. _____

Grant's

The axillary sheath has been removed in this image to reveal the contents of the axilla: axillary vein, axillary artery and its branches, and almost all of the branches of the brachial plexus. A small rod has been inserted to elevate the terminal branches of the brachial plexus from the axillary artery. Variations in the typical branching pattern of the brachial plexus often occur, as seen in this image with an additional connection between the medial and lateral roots of the median nerve.

With the **pectoralis major** mostly removed or reflected, the two remaining anterior axio-appendicular muscles are now visible.

COLOR each of the following structures using a different color for each:

Additional Anterior Axio-Appendicular Muscles

Muscle	Proximal Attachment	Distal Attachment	Innervation	Action
○ 1. *Pectoralis minor*	Ribs 3-5 near costal cartilages	Coracoid process of scapula	Medial pectoral nerve (C8, T1)	Stabilizes scapula by drawing it inferiorly and anteriorly against thoracic wall
○ 2. *Subclavius*	Rib 1 near costal cartilage	Middle third of clavicle	Nerve to subclavius (**C5**, C6)	Anchors and depresses clavicle

Neurovasculature of the Axilla

○ 3. *Axillary vein:* In axilla lies anterior to the axillary artery and then medial to the axillary artery in the arm

○ 4. *Axillary artery:* The pectoralis minor muscle divides the axillary artery into three sections with the first part proximal to the pectoralis minor, the second part posterior to the pectoralis minor, and the third part distal to the pectoralis minor. The second part of the axillary artery gives rise to two branches:

○ 5. *Thoraco-acromial artery:* Small trunk that emerges immediately medial to the tendon of pectoralis minor and then branches into deltoid, acromial, clavicular, and pectoral arteries

○ 6. *Lateral thoracic artery:* Descends along the lateral surface of serratus anterior with the **long thoracic nerve**

The first and third parts of the axillary artery, along with their respective 1 and 3 branches, are illustrated in figure in Section 2.7.

○ 7. *Lateral cord of brachial plexus* lies lateral to the axillary artery and gives rise to:

○ 8. *Lateral pectoral nerve (C5, C6, C7):* Side branch of lateral cord proximal to pectoralis minor tendon and supplies pectoralis major

○ 9. *Musculocutaneous nerve (C5-C7):* Terminal branch that pierces the **coracobrachialis muscle** to supply it and the other muscles of the anterior compartment of the arm

○ 10. *Lateral root of the median nerve (C6-C7):* One of two components that join to form the median nerve

○ 11. *Medial cord of brachial plexus* lies medial to the axillary artery and gives rise to:

○ 12. *Medial pectoral nerve (C8-T1):* Side branch of medial cord deep to pectoralis minor, pierces pectoralis minor to reach pectoralis major to supply innervation to both muscles

○ 13. *Medial cutaneous nerve of forearm (C8-T1):* Side branch of medial cord and travels medial to the axillary artery with the ulnar nerve

○ 14. *Ulnar nerve (C8-T1):* Terminal branch that travels medial to axillary artery

○ 15. *Medial root of median nerve (C8-T1):* Joins the lateral root of the median nerve to form the median nerve

○ 16. *Median nerve (C6-T1):* Forms from roots of the medial and lateral cords and travels with the axillary artery

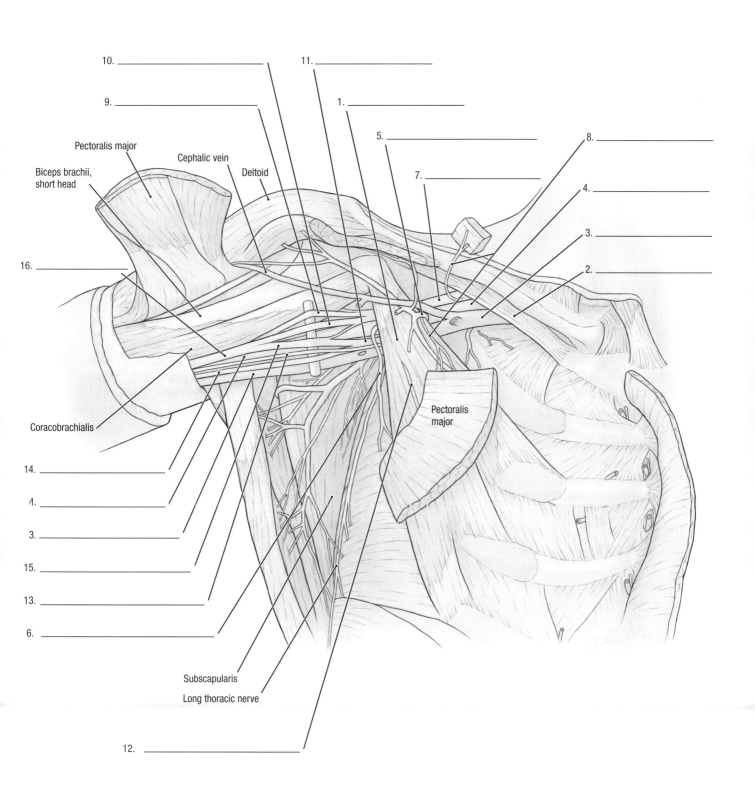

10. _____

11. _____

9. _____

1. _____

Pectoralis major

Cephalic vein

5. _____

8. _____

Biceps brachii,
short head

Deltoid

7. _____

4. _____

3. _____

16. _____

2. _____

Pectoralis
major

Coracobrachialis

14. _____

1. _____

3. _____

15. _____

13. _____

6. _____

Subscapularis

Long thoracic nerve

12. _____

2.7 AXILLA, DEEP DISSECTION II

The *pectoralis major* has been removed and reflected. With the pectoralis minor and axillary vein now removed and the lateral and medial cords and their branches retracted with string, the first and third parts of the axillary artery and the posterior cord are now visible.

COLOR each of the following structures using a different color for each:

○ 1. **Axillary artery**

○ 2. **Superior thoracic artery:** Only branch that arises from the first part of the axillary artery just inferior to subclavius

○ 3. **Subscapular artery** is one of three branches that arise from the third part of the axillary artery; descends along the lateral border of **subscapularis** and terminates into two branches:

   ○ 4. **Circumflex scapular artery:** Turns posteriorly around the lateral border of the scapula between subscapularis and **teres major**

   ○ 5. **Thoracodorsal artery:** Passes inferiorly toward the inferior angle of the scapula and travels with the thoracodorsal nerve

○ 6. **Anterior circumflex humeral artery:** Small branch off the third part of the axillary artery that passes laterally to encircle the surgical neck and anastomose with the posterior circumflex humeral artery

○ 7. **Posterior circumflex humeral artery:** Arises near the anterior circumflex humeral but typically larger in diameter and passes medially through the quadrangular space with the axillary nerve

○ 8. **Long thoracic nerve:** Arises from the anterior rami of C5, C6, C7; descends on the superficial surface of **serratus anterior** with the lateral thoracic artery.

○ 9. **Posterior cord of brachial plexus** lies posterior to the axillary artery and gives rise to:

○ 10. **Upper subscapular nerve (C5):** Side branch that passes posteriorly to supply superior portion of subscapularis

○ 11. **Thoracodorsal nerve (C6, C7, C8):** Side branch that arises in between the upper and lower subscapular nerves and passes inferolaterally with the thoracodorsal artery to supply **latissimus dorsi**

○ 12. **Lower subscapular nerve (C6):** Side branch that passes inferolaterally to supply the inferior portion of subscapularis and teres major

○ 13. **Axillary nerve (C5, C6):** Terminal branch that exits posteriorly through the quadrangular space with the posterior circumflex humeral artery supplying deltoid and teres minor

○ 14. **Radial nerve (C5-T1):** Larger terminal branch that travels posterior to the axillary artery

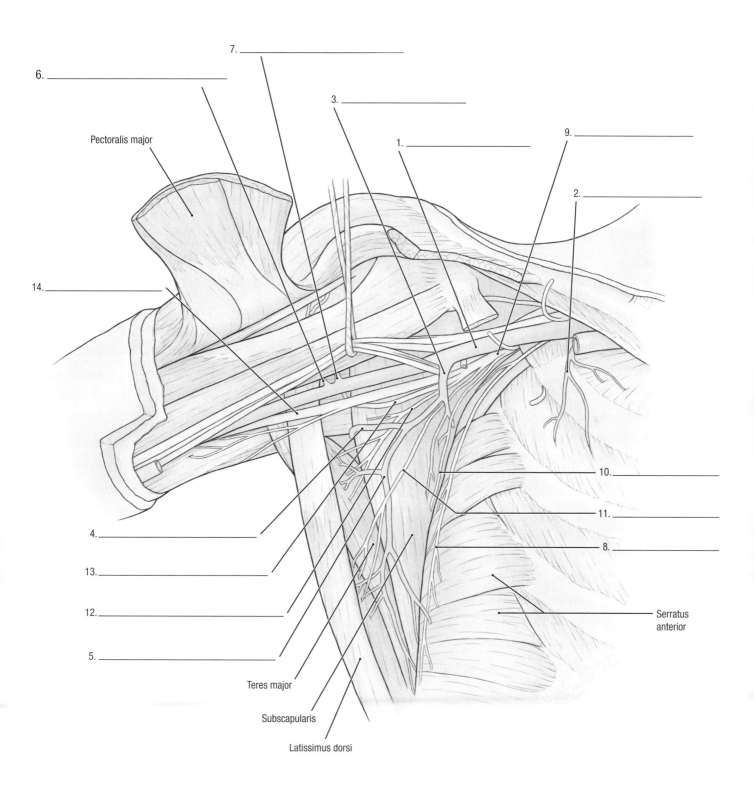

7. _____

6. _____

3. _____

Pectoralis major

9. _____

1. _____

2. _____

14. _____

10. _____

11. _____

4. _____

8. _____

13. _____

Serratus
anterior

12. _____

5. _____

Teres major

Subscapularis

Latissimus dorsi

Grant's

2.8A and B ROTATOR CUFF

Four of the six scapulohumeral muscles are referred to as the rotator cuff muscles because they compose a musculotendinous cuff around the glenohumeral joint. The tendons of these muscles protect the joint and add stability to the joint capsule. Subscapularis, infraspinatus, and teres minor rotate the humerus, whereas supraspinatus initiates abduction of the arm.

CLINICAL NOTE: ROTATOR CUFF INJURY

Damage to one or more of the rotator cuff muscles can occur either because of acute injury or by degenerative damage from repetitive stress, bone spurs, or lack of blood supply as aging progresses. Degenerative damage to the rotator cuff occurs most often with individuals who perform repetitive overhead activities such as carpenters, painters, and baseball or tennis players. The **supraspinatus** tendon is the most commonly damaged of the rotator cuff complex.

COLOR each of the following structures using a different color for each:

Scapulohumeral Muscles

Muscle	Proximal Attachment	Distal Attachment	Innervation	Action
◯ 1. *Subscapularis*	Subscapular fossa of scapula	Lesser tubercle of *humerus*	Upper and lower subscapular nerves (C5, **C6**, C7)	Medially rotates arm
◯ 2. *Supraspinatus*	Supraspinous fossa of scapula	Greater tubercle of humerus	Suprascapular nerve (C4, **C5**, C6)	Initiates (first 15°) abduction and assists deltoid
◯ 3. *Infraspinatus*	Infraspinous fossa of scapula		Suprascapular nerve (**C5**, C6)	Laterally rotates arm
◯ 4. *Teres minor*	Lateral border of scapula		Axillary nerve (**C5**, C6)	

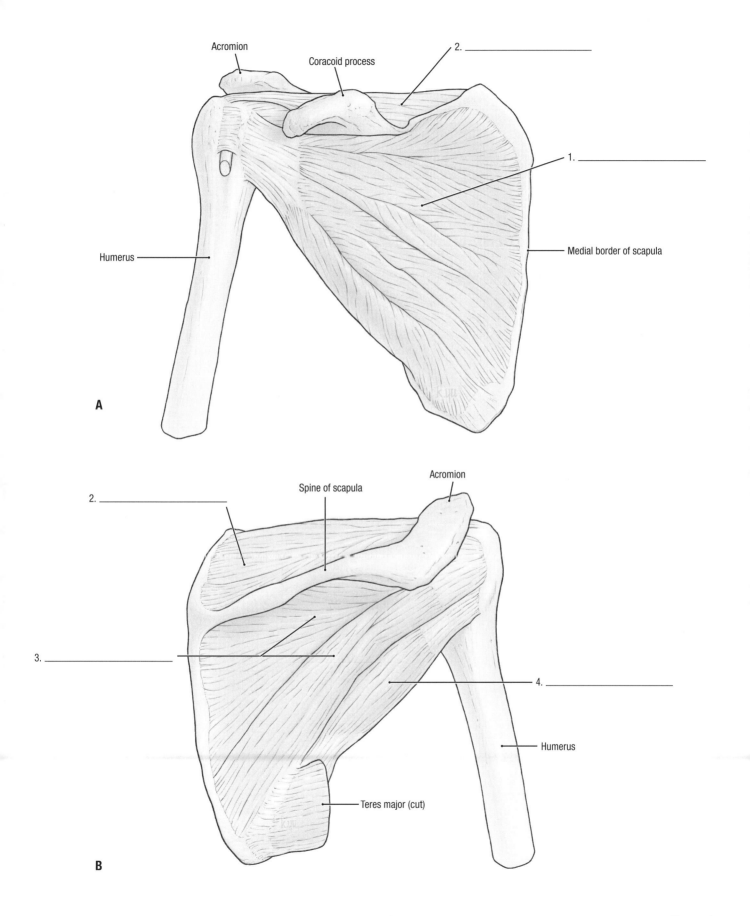

Acromion

Coracoid process

2. _____

1. _____

Humerus

Medial border of scapula

A

Spine of scapula

Acromion

2. _____

3. _____

4. _____

Humerus

Teres major (cut)

B

Grant's

2.9 ANTERIOR ASPECT OF ARM

With the **_deltoid_**, **_pectoralis major_**, and **_pectoralis minor_** reflected or removed, the muscles of the anterior compartment of the arm are visible. All muscles of this compartment act to flex the forearm and are all innervated by the musculocutaneous nerve.

CLINICAL NOTE: INJURY TO THE LONG HEAD OF THE BICEPS BRACHII

Injury to the **_long head of the biceps brachii_** typically presents more commonly than the short head of the biceps brachii. This is due to the relationship of the tendon of the long head passing through the intertubercular sulcus of the humerus deep to the **_transverse humeral ligament_** en route to the supraglenoid tubercle of the scapula. The tendon may become inflamed, dislocated, or ruptured owing to repetitive wear and tear. A ruptured tendon results in a detached muscle belly from the supraglenoid tubercle that forms a bulk of muscle near the center of the anterior aspect of the arm (Popeye deformity).

COLOR each of the following structures using a different color for each:

Muscles of the Anterior Compartment of the Arm

Muscle	Proximal Attachment	Distal Attachment	Innervation	Action
○ 1. *Biceps brachii, short head*	<u>*Coracoid process of scapula*</u>	○ 3. *Biceps tendon* attaches to tuberosity of radius	Musculocutaneous (C5, C6, C7)	1. Supinates forearm 2. Flexes forearm while in the supinated position 3. Resists dislocation of shoulder (short head)
○ 2. *Biceps brachii, long head*	Supraglenoid tubercle of scapula	○ 4. *Bicipital aponeurosis* merges with antebrachial fascia of forearm		
○ 5. *Brachialis*	Distal half of anterior humerus	Coronoid process and tuberosity of ulna		Flexes forearm in all positions
○ 6. *Coracobrachialis*	Coracoid process of scapula	Middle third of medial humerus		1. Assists in flexion and adduction of arm 2. Resists dislocation of shoulder

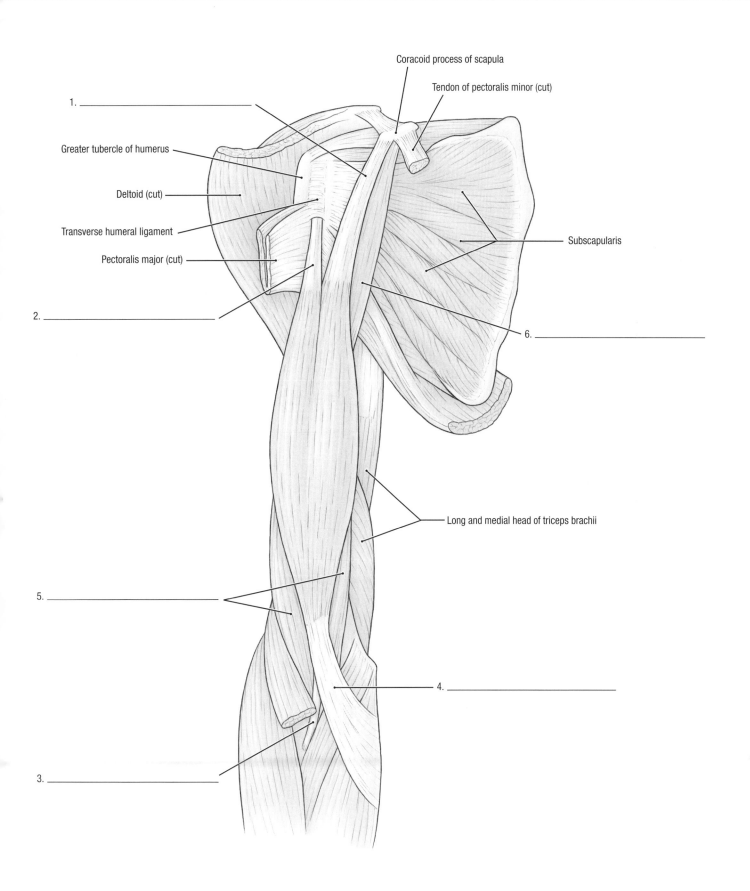

Coracoid process of scapula

Tendon of pectoralis minor (cut)

1. _____

Greater tubercle of humerus _____

Deltoid (cut) _____

Transverse humeral ligament _____

Pectoralis major (cut) _____

2. _____

Subscapularis

6. _____

Long and medial head of triceps brachii

5. _____

4. _____

3. _____

Grant's

2.10 LATERAL ASPECT OF ARM

In the lateral view of the arm, muscles from both the anterior and posterior compartments of the arm, along with two forearm muscles, are visible.

COLOR each of the following structures using a different color for each:

○ 1. *Deltoid:* Forms the rounded contour of the shoulder

○ 2. *Biceps brachii:* Most anterior muscle emerging below the anterior edge of the deltoid muscle

○ 3. *Brachialis:* Immediately deep to biceps brachii

○ 4. *Brachioradialis:* Forearm extensor that originates above the elbow immediately deep to brachialis

○ 5. *Extensor carpi radialis longus:* Forearm extensor immediately deep to brachioradialis originating from the <u>lateral epicondyle</u>

○ 6. *Lateral head of triceps brachii:* Most prominent head of the triceps brachii muscle from the lateral view. Emerges inferior to the postero-inferior edge of the deltoid muscle.

○ 7. *Long head of triceps brachii:* From the lateral view only a small portion is visible medial to the lateral head just inferior to the postero-inferior edge of the deltoid muscle

○ 8. *Triceps tendon:* All three heads of the triceps brachii form the triceps tendon, which inserts into the <u>***olecranon***</u> of the ulna

CLINICAL NOTE: FRACTURES OF THE OLECRANON

Fractures of the olecranon commonly occur because of a direct fall on the elbow or a fall on an outstretched hand with the elbow flexed. Because of the unopposed traction or pull of the *triceps tendon* on the olecranon, the fractured portion of the olecranon is usually widely displaced from the remainder of the ulna. An open reduction-internal fixation (ORIF) procedure, in which the fracture is surgically repaired with screws or pins, is typically required for successful union of the fracture.

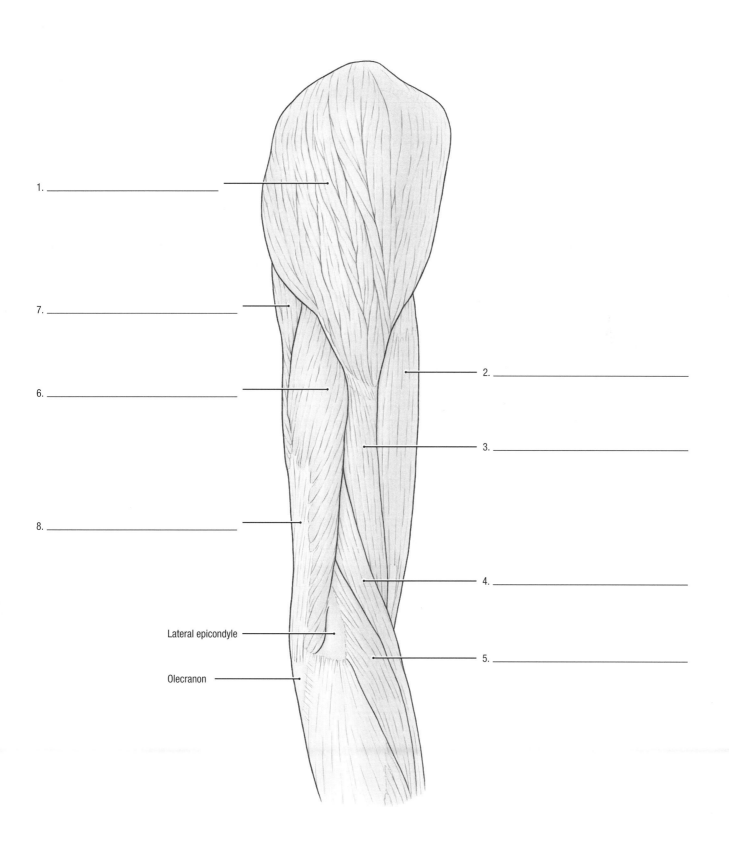

1. _____

7. _____

6. _____

8. _____

Lateral epicondyle

Olecranon

2. _____

3. _____

4. _____

5. _____

Grant's

2.11 MEDIAL ASPECT OF THE ARM

In the medial view of the forearm, muscles of both the anterior and posterior compartments are visible along with the major neurovascular bundle of the arm. The brachial vein has been removed from this image to demonstrate the brachial artery and terminal branches of the brachial plexus in the arm.

COLOR each of the following structures using a different color for each:

○ 1. *Biceps brachii:* Most anterior muscle lying anterior to the brachial artery and median nerve

○ 2. *Brachialis:* Lies in the lower half of the arm, anterior to the *medial intermuscular septum*, and posterior to the brachial artery and median nerve

○ 3. *Coracobrachialis:* Lies in the upper half of the arm, posterior to the short head of biceps brachii, and pierced by the musculocutaneous nerve

○ 4. *Medial head of triceps brachii:* Lies inferior to radial groove, posterior to the medial intermuscular septum

○ 5. *Long head of triceps brachii:* Tendon passes posterior to *teres major* and *latissimus dorsi*, but inserts anterior to teres minor

○ 6. *Brachial artery:* Continuation of the axillary artery at the inferior border of teres major and lies anterior to the brachialis and triceps brachii muscles. In the arm, it gives rise to the profunda brachii, *superior ulnar collateral artery*, and *inferior ulnar collateral artery*.

○ 7. *Median nerve:* In the proximal arm travels lateral to the brachial artery. In the middle of the arm, it crosses the brachial artery anteriorly to the medial side in the middle of the arm. It does not give rise to any branches in the arm.

○ 8. *Ulnar nerve:* In the proximal arm travels anterior to the tendon of teres major and the long head of triceps brachii. In the middle of the arm, it travels with the superior ulnar collateral artery medial to the medial head of the triceps brachii after piercing the medial intermuscular septum. It does not give rise to any branches in the arm.

○ 9. *Musculocutaneous nerve:* Arises from *lateral cord of brachial plexus*, pierces coracobrachialis, and then continues between the biceps brachii and brachialis

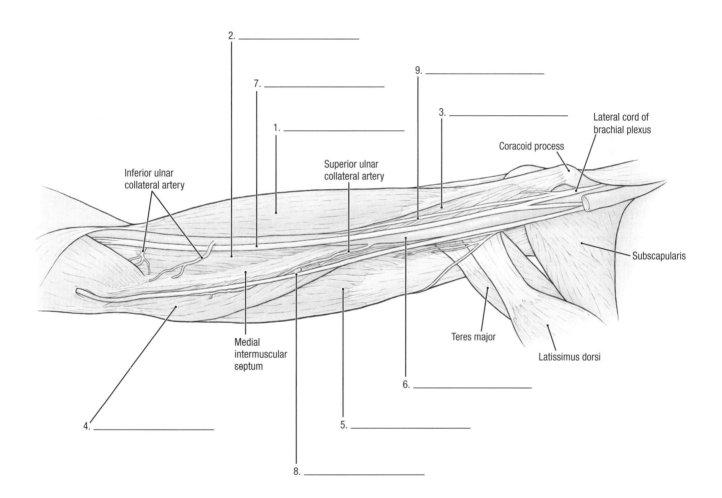

2. _____

7. _____

9. _____

3. _____

1. _____

Lateral cord of
brachial plexus

Coracoid process

Superior ulnar
collateral artery

Inferior ulnar
collateral artery

Subscapularis

Medial
intermuscular
septum

Teres major

Latissimus dorsi

4. _____

6. _____

5. _____

8. _____

Grant's

2.12 POSTERIOR ASPECT OF ARM

With a majority of the deltoid removed and the lateral head of the triceps reflected, the last of the six scapulohumeral muscles, the teres major, along with the muscles and neurovasculature of the posterior compartment of the arm, are observable. The muscles of the posterior compartment are all innervated by the radial nerve and all act as extensors of the forearm.

COLOR each of the following structures using a different color for each:

Teres Major and Muscles of the Posterior Compartment of the Arm

Muscle	Proximal Attachment	Distal Attachment	Innervation	Action
○ 1. *Teres major*	Inferior angle of scapula	Medial lip of inter-tubercular sulcus of humerus	Lower subscapular nerve (C5, **C6**)	Adducts and medially rotates arm
○ 2. *Triceps brachii, long head*	Infraglenoid tubercle of scapula	*Olecranon* of ulna	Radial nerve (C6, **C7**, **C8**)	1. Chief extensor of forearm
○ 3. *Triceps brachii, lateral head*	Posterior humerus, superior to radial groove			2. Long head resists dislocation of humerus
○ 4. *Triceps brachii, medial head*	Posterior humerus, near/inferior to radial groove			

Outline the boundaries:

○ 5. *Quadrangular space:* Bounded superiorly by inferior border of ***teres minor***, inferiorly by the superior border of teres major, laterally by the surgical neck of the humerus, and medially by the lateral border of the long head of triceps

COLOR each of the following structures using a different color for each:

○ 6. *Axillary nerve:* Passes through the quadrangular space with the posterior circumflex humeral artery and then travels around the surgical neck of the humerus deep to the ***deltoid***

○ 7. *Posterior circumflex humeral artery:* Passes through the quadrangular space with the axillary nerve

○ 8. *Profunda brachii (deep brachial) artery:* Largest branch of the brachial artery that accompanies the radial artery within the radial groove and terminates as the middle and radial collateral arteries

○ 9. *Radial nerve:* Enters the posterior compartment of the arm immediately inferior to the tendon of teres major, travels with profunda brachii artery within the radial groove, and then pierces the lateral intermuscular septum to enter the anterior compartment of the arm between the brachialis and brachioradialis to the level of the lateral epicondyle.

○ 10. *Ulnar nerve:* Passes posterior to the ***medial epicondyle*** and medial to olecranon to enter the forearm

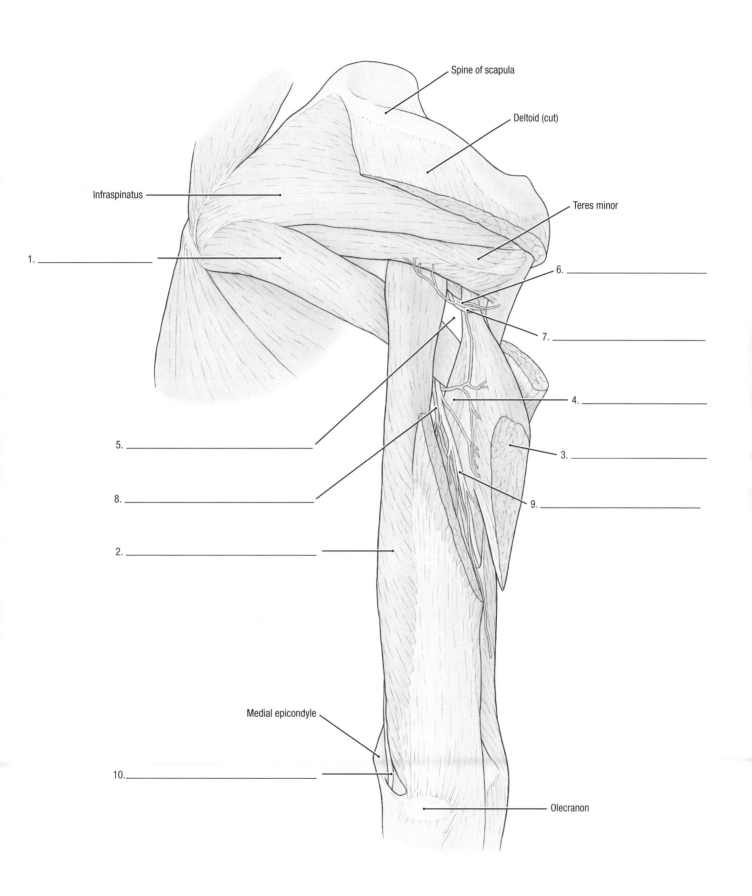

Spine of scapula

Deltoid (cut)

Infraspinatus

Teres minor

1. _____

6. _____

7. _____

4. _____

5. _____

3. _____

8. _____

9. _____

2. _____

Medial epicondyle

10. _____

Olecranon

Grant's

2.13A and B ACROMIOCLAVICULAR AND GLENOHUMERAL JOINTS

The fibrous capsule of the shoulder joint (A) surrounds the glenohumeral joint attaching medially to the margin of the glenoid cavity and laterally to the anatomic neck of the humerus. In B, the fibrous layer of the joint capsule has been removed and the articular cavity has been injected to fully extend the *synovial membrane of the shoulder joint*. The synovial sheath extends along the tendon of the long head of the biceps in the intertubercular sulcus forming the *intertubercular tendon sheath*.

COLOR each of the following structures using a different color for each:

○ **1. Superior acromioclavicular ligament:** Fibrous band extending from clavicle to *acromion process*

The *coracoclavicular ligament* consists of two ligaments that strengthen the acromioclavicular joint superiorly:

  ○ **2. Conoid ligament:** Vertical, inverted triangle that extends from the root of the *coracoid process* to the clavicle

  ○ **3. Trapezoid ligament:** Almost horizontal, extends from superior aspect of coracoid process to clavicle

○ **4. Coraco-acromial ligament:** Extends from coracoid process to acromion process, forming a protective arch over the humeral head and preventing superior displacement from the glenoid cavity

○ **5. Fibrous capsule of shoulder joint:** Contains an opening for the passage of the tendon of the long head of the biceps brachii and an opening for communication to the subscapular bursa

○ **6. Transverse humeral ligament:** Fibrous band that extends from the *greater tubercle* to lesser tubercle of the humerus, forming a bridge over the intertubercular sulcus to hold the tendon of the long head of biceps brachii in place

○ **7. Tendon of long head of biceps brachii:** Crosses the head of the humerus within the glenohumeral joint cavity to travel within the intertubercular sulcus surrounded by the intertubercular tendon sheath

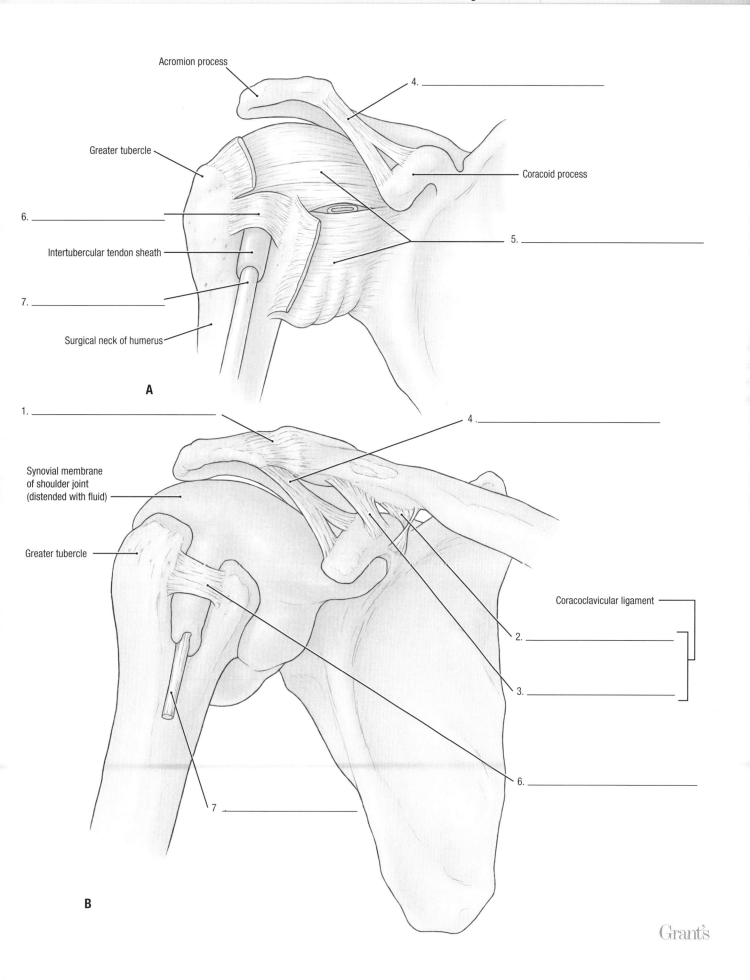

Acromion process

4. _____

Greater tubercle

Coracoid process

6. _____

Intertubercular tendon sheath

5. _____

7. _____

Surgical neck of humerus

A

1. _____

4. _____

Synovial membrane
of shoulder joint
(distended with fluid)

Coracoclavicular ligament

Greater tubercle

2. _____

3. _____

6. _____

7. _____

B

Grant's

2.14 BOUNDARIES AND CONTENTS OF CUBITAL FOSSA

The cubital fossa is a triangular depression on the anterior aspect of the elbow. The superficial veins of the forearm (basilic, cephalic, and *median vein of forearm*) variably form an M-shaped pattern superficially in the cubital fossa (cut and portions removed from this image). The median cubital vein (removed from this image) crosses the cubital fossa superficial to the bicipital aponeurosis joining the *cephalic* and *basilic veins*. The *lateral cutaneous nerve of the forearm* emerges from the lateral aspect of the distal *biceps brachii* muscle coursing superficial and lateral to the boundaries of the cubital fossa to supply the lateral forearm.

COLOR each of the following structures using a different color for each:

Cubital Fossa	
Boundary of Cubital Fossa	**Structure**
Superior	Imaginary line connecting *medial epicondyle* and lateral epicondyle
Medial	◯ 1. *Pronator teres*
Lateral	◯ 2. *Brachioradialis*
Floor	◯ 3. *Brachialis* and supinator
Roof	◯ 4. *Bicipital aponeurosis*

Within the cubital fossa, three structures pass from lateral to medial:

◯ 5. *Biceps brachii tendon:* Most lateral of the cubital fossa contents en route to insert on the radial tuberosity

◯ 6. *Brachial artery:* Lies medial to biceps brachii tendon

◯ 7. *Median nerve:* Lies medial to brachial artery

CLINICAL NOTE: VENIPUNCTURE

Owing to the superficial location of the veins, the cubital fossa is a common site for venipuncture. In addition, the **bicipital aponeurosis** provides some protection by separating the superficial veins from the underlying **brachial artery** and **median nerve**. Presence of a superficial artery in this area is rare; however, an aberrant superficial ulnar artery (branch of the brachial artery) may travel superficial to the flexor muscles of the forearm. Arterial pulsations by palpation and visual observation should be identified when performing phlebotomy procedures in the cubital fossa. Misidentification of an artery for a vein can result in bleeding, and if certain drugs are injected into an artery, it may prove to be fatal.

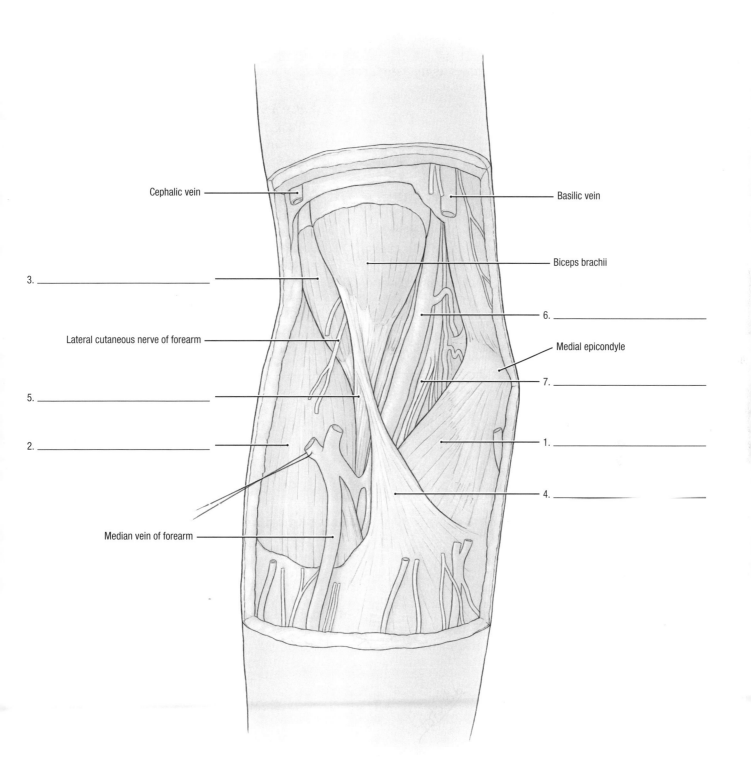

Cephalic vein

Basilic vein

Biceps brachii

3. _____

6. _____

Lateral cutaneous nerve of forearm

Medial epicondyle

7. _____

5. _____

1. _____

2. _____

4. _____

Median vein of forearm

2.15   FLOOR OF CUBITAL FOSSA

With a portion of the ***biceps brachii*** removed along with widely opening the cubital fossa, many of the deeper structures of the cubital fossa are visible. The ***biceps brachii tendon*** remains intact attaching to the radius and lying lateral to the brachial artery.

COLOR each of the following structures using a different color for each:

○ 1. *Brachialis*

○ 2. *Brachioradialis*

○ 3. *Pronator teres*

○ 4. *Supinator:* Lies deep forming the floor of the cubital fossa with brachialis

○ 5. *Brachial artery:* Divides into radial and ulnar arteries in the cubital fossa

○ 6. *Radial artery:* Exits cubital fossa inferolaterally slightly overlapped by brachioradialis and gives rise to the radial recurrent artery before leaving cubital fossa

○ 7. *Ulnar artery:* Descends inferomedially from brachial artery traveling deep to superficial and intermediate muscles of forearm; gives rise to anterior and posterior ulnar recurrent and common interosseous arteries

○ 8. *Median nerve:* Exits cubital fossa by passing between the heads of pronator teres

○ 9. *Radial nerve:* Enters cubital fossa between brachioradialis and brachialis and then divides into superficial and deep radial nerves

○10. *Superficial radial nerve:* Exits cubital fossa deep to brachioradialis to run with the radial artery

○11. *Deep radial nerve:* Exits cubital fossa by piercing supinator muscle to reach posterior compartment of forearm

○12. *Ulnar nerve:* Travels posterior to the medial epicondyle and not through cubital fossa

○13. *Musculocutaneous nerve:* After traveling between *biceps brachii* and brachialis emerges laterally superior to cubital fossa and at this point is referred to as the lateral cutaneous nerve of the forearm

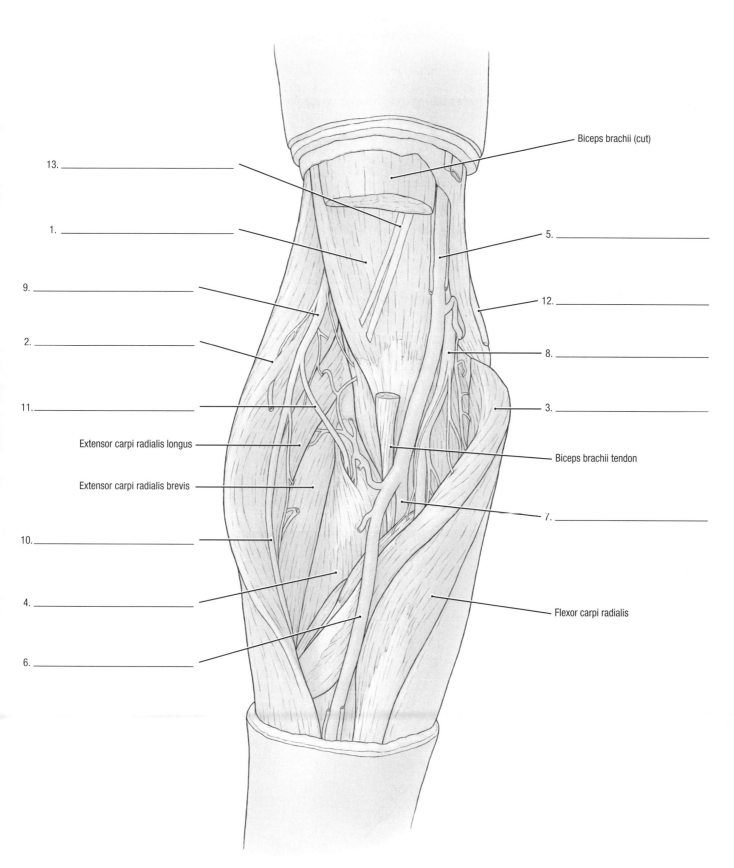

Biceps brachii (cut)

13.

1.

9.

2.

11.

Extensor carpi radialis longus

Extensor carpi radialis brevis

10.

4.

6.

5.

12.

8.

3.

Biceps brachii tendon

7.

Flexor carpi radialis

2.16A and B LIGAMENTS OF THE ELBOW JOINT AND PROXIMAL RADIO-ULNAR JOINT

The elbow joint is a hinge synovial joint. The trochlea and *capitulum* of the humerus articulate with the trochlear notch of the ulna and the head of the radius. The proximal radio-ulnar joint is a pivot synovial joint allowing the head of the radius to move on the ulna.

COLOR each of the following structures using a different color for each:

Elbow Joint

○ 1. *Ulnar collateral ligament:* Medial, triangular ligament extending from *medial epicondyle* of *humerus* to the coronoid process and *olecranon* of *ulna*

○ 2. *Radial collateral ligament:* Lateral, fanlike ligament extending from *lateral epicondyle* of *humerus* to blend with annular ligament of *radius*

Proximal Radio-Ulnar Joint

○ 3. *Anular ligament of radius:* Encircles and holds head of radius in the radial notch of the ulna

Interosseous Membrane

○ 4. *Interosseous membrane:* Connects the interosseous aspects of the radius and ulna forming a syndesmosis between the radius and ulna

CLINICAL NOTE: INJURY TO THE LIGAMENTS OF THE ELBOW

Damage to the *ulnar collateral ligament* and subsequent reconstruction surgical procedures are common in individuals who perform repetitive throwing movements such as baseball pitchers and track and field throwers. Damage to the *radial collateral ligament* is typically associated with trauma such as a fracture or dislocation. The *Anular ligament* can easily be torn away from its distal attachment to the neck of the radius, resulting in subluxation (partial dislocation) of the head of the radius ("nursemaid's elbow"). Subluxation of the radius commonly occurs in young children when the child is suddenly lifted by the upper limb while the forearm is pronated.

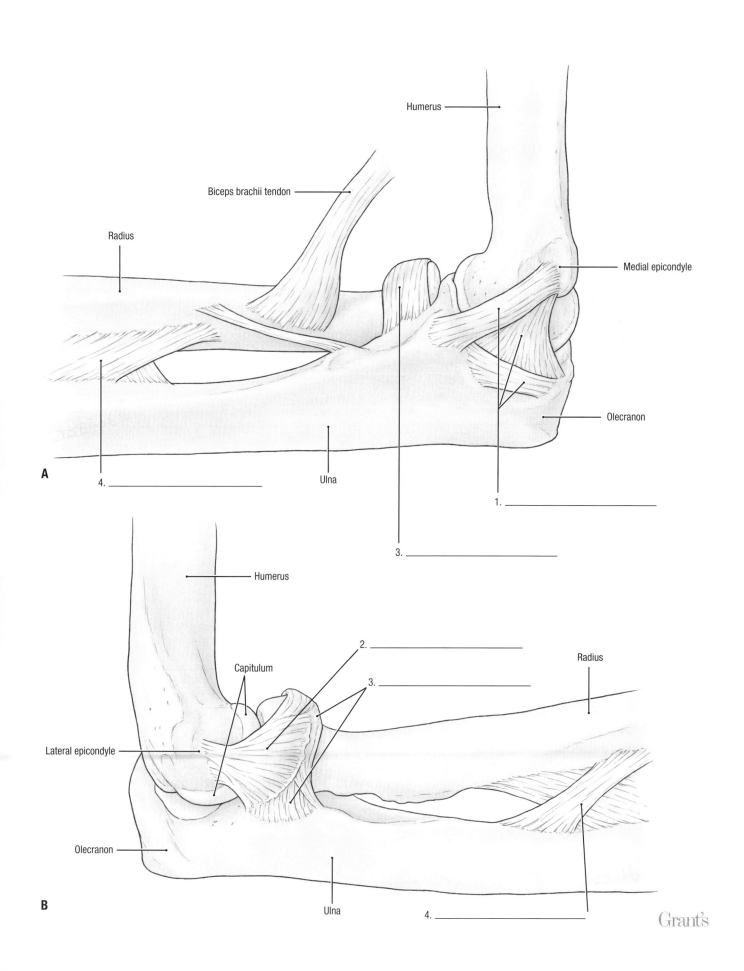

A

Humerus

Biceps brachii tendon

Radius

Medial epicondyle

Olecranon

4. _____

Ulna

1. _____

3. _____

B

Humerus

Capitulum

2. _____

3. _____

Radius

Lateral epicondyle

Olecranon

Ulna

4. _____

Grant's

2.17   SUPERFICIAL LAYER OF ANTERIOR COMPARTMENT OF FOREARM

Similar to the compartments of the arm, the compartments in the forearm contain muscles that share a similar action and innervation. The anterior compartment houses the flexors and pronators of the forearm. The muscles of the anterior compartment are primarily innervated by the median nerve with one and half muscles innervated by the ulnar nerve. The *bicipital aponeurosis* has been cut and reflected with a string in this image.

COLOR each of the following structures using a different color for each:

The muscles of the anterior compartment are arranged in three layers:

1. Superficial layer: four muscles
2. Intermediate layer: one muscle
3. Deep layer: three muscles

Muscles of the Superficial Layer of Anterior Compartment of Forearm

Muscle	Location	Proximal Attachment	Distal Attachment	Innervation	Action
○ 1. *Pronator teres*	Most lateral superficial flexor muscle	Coronoid process of ulna and *__medial epicondyle__* of humerus	Middle convexity of lateral surface of radius	Median nerve (C6, **C7**)	1. Pronates forearm 2. Flexes forearm (at elbow)
○ 2. *Flexor carpi radialis*	Medial to pronator teres	Medial epicondyle of humerus	Base of 2nd metacarpal		1. Flexes hand (at wrist) 2. Abducts hand (at wrist)
○ 3. *Palmaris longus*	Medial to flexor carpi radialis (if present)		Flexor retinaculum and ○ 4. *palmar aponeurosis*	Median nerve (C7, C8)	1. Flexes hand (at wrist) 2. Tenses palmar aponeurosis
○ 5. *Flexor carpi ulnaris*	Most medial superficial flexor muscle	Medial epicondyle of humerus and olecranon of ulna	Pisiform, hook of hamate, 5th metacarpal	Ulnar nerve (C7, **C8**)	1. Flexes hand (at wrist) 2. Adducts hand (at wrist)

○ 6. **Brachioradialis:** Exception to the compartment rule as it functionally acts as a flexor of the forearm, but is located in the posterior compartment

○ 7. **Brachial artery**

○ 8. **Radial artery:** Travels through proximal forearm deep to brachioradialis, lies lateral to flexor carpi radialis tendon in the distal forearm, and exits anterior compartment by winding around lateral aspect of the radius

○ 9. **Superficial branch of radial nerve:** Lies between pronator teres and brachioradialis in proximal forearm, travels with radial artery in the distal forearm, and exits anterior compartment laterally to reach dorsum of hand

○ 10. **Median nerve:** Travels deep to *flexor digitorum superficialis* in the proximal forearm and deep to palmaris longus distally

○ 11. **Ulnar artery:** Travels deep to pronator teres, palmaris longus, and flexor digitorum superficialis in the proximal forearm. In the mid-to-distal forearm, lies deep to flexor carpi ulnaris traveling with ulnar nerve.

○ 12. **Ulnar nerve:** Enters anterior compartment by piercing through the heads of flexor carpi ulnaris and travels through forearm deep to flexor carpi ulnaris with ulnar artery

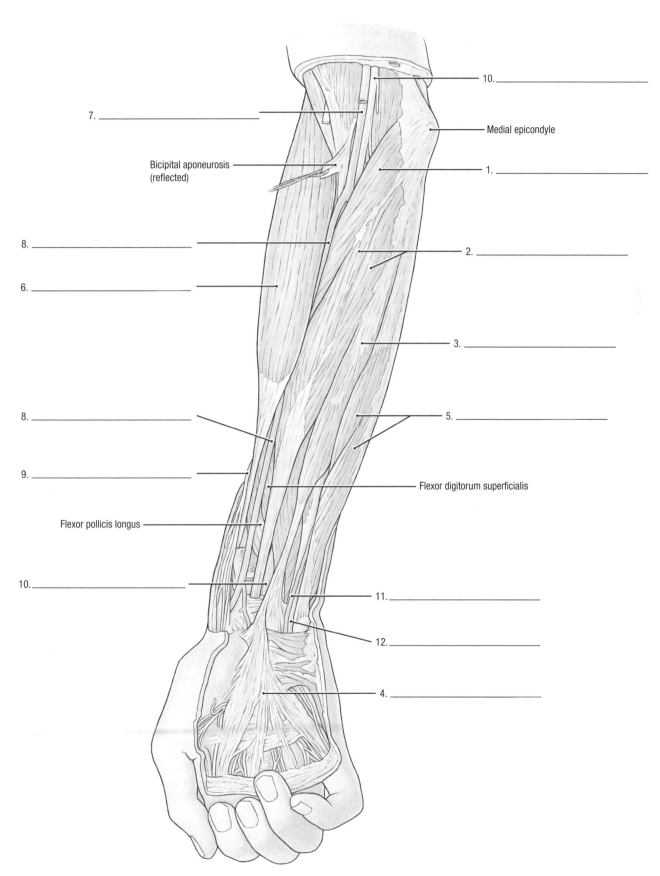

7. _____

10. _____

Medial epicondyle

Bicipital aponeurosis
(reflected)

1. _____

8. _____

2. _____

6. _____

3. _____

8. _____

5. _____

9. _____

Flexor digitorum superficialis

Flexor pollicis longus

10. _____

11. _____

12. _____

4. _____

Grant's

2.18 INTERMEDIATE LAYER OF ANTERIOR COMPARTMENT OF FOREARM

The middle portions of the **_pronator teres_**, **_flexor carpi radialis_**, and **_palmaris longus_** have been removed and the remaining aspects reflected. The **_flexor carpi ulnaris_** and **_brachioradialis_** muscles have been opened widely to reveal the flexor digitorum superficialis and the branching of the **_brachial artery_**.

A small probe has been inserted to elevate the flexor digitorum superficialis along with the median nerve and a persistent median artery (variable presence in the adult). A longer probe has been inserted to elevate the tendons and neurovascular structures at the wrist.

COLOR each of the following structures using a different color for each:

Muscle of the Intermediate Layer of Anterior Compartment of Forearm

Muscle	Proximal Attachment	Distal Attachment	Innervation	Action
⭕ 1. *Flexor digitorum superficialis*	Humero-ulnar head: medial epicondyle of humerus and coronoid process of ulna Radial head: proximal anterior surface of radius	Four tendons course deep to flexor retinaculum to attach to middle phalanges of medial four digits	Median nerve (C7, C8, T1)	Flexes middle phalanges at proximal interphalangeal joints of medial four digits

⭕ 2. *Radial artery:* Travels deep to brachioradialis and exits anterior compartment by winding around lateral aspect of the radius

⭕ 3. *Ulnar artery:* Enters the anterior compartment by passing between the two heads of flexor digitorum superficialis and travels medial to flexor digitorum superficialis through the forearm

⭕ 4. *Median nerve:* Also enters the anterior compartment by passing between the two heads of flexor digitorum

superficialis. At the wrist, it lies lateral to the four tendons of flexor digitorum superficialis passing deep to flexor retinaculum, and in a small percentage of the population it can be accompanied by a persistent median artery.

⭕ 5. *Ulnar nerve:* Travels with ulnar artery medial to flexor digitorum superficialis

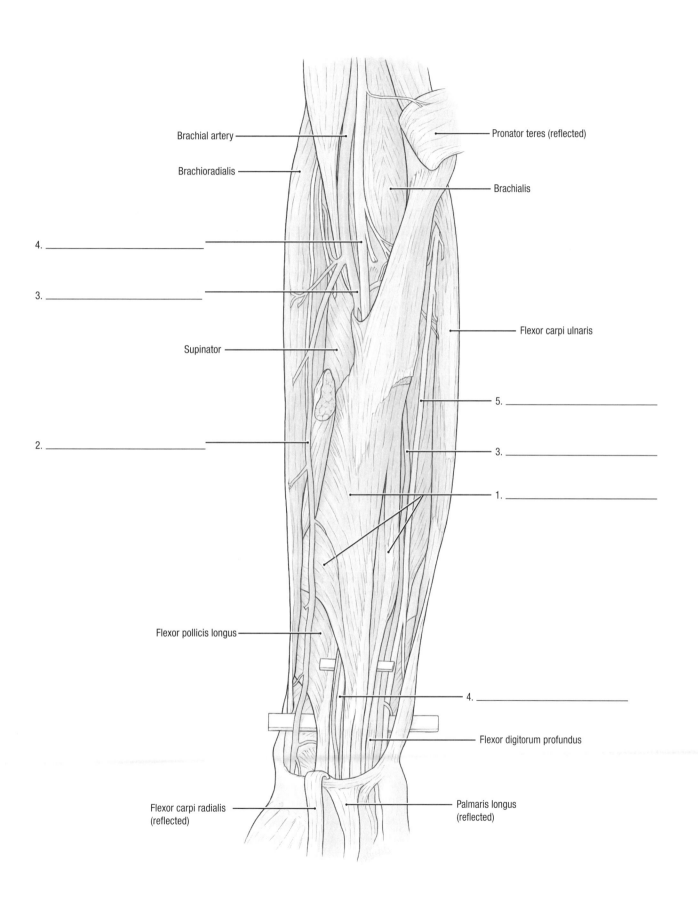

Brachial artery

Brachioradialis

Pronator teres (reflected)

Brachialis

4. _____

3. _____

Supinator

Flexor carpi ulnaris

5. _____

2. _____

3. _____

1. _____

Flexor pollicis longus

4. _____

Flexor digitorum profundus

Flexor carpi radialis
(reflected)

Palmaris longus
(reflected)

Grant's

2.19 DEEP LAYER OF ANTERIOR COMPARTMENT OF FOREARM

Pronator teres, flexor carpi radialis, palmaris longus, *median nerve*, and flexor digitorum superficialis have been removed and/or reflected. The *brachioradialis* and *flexor carpi ulnaris* have been opened widely to not only demonstrate the deep muscles of the anterior compartment, but also the *extensor carpi radialis longus* and *extensor carpi radialis brevis* of the posterior compartment.

COLOR each of the following structures using a different color for each:

Muscles of the Deep Layer of Anterior Compartment of the Forearm

Muscle	Proximal Attachment	Distal Attachment	Innervation	Action
◯ 1. *Flexor digitorum profundus*	Proximal three quarters of the ulna and interosseous membrane	Four tendons course deep to *flexor retinaculum* and deep to flexor digitorum superficialis tendons to attach to distal phalanges of medial four digits	Medial part (digits 4 and 5): Ulnar nerve (C8, **T1**) Lateral part (digits 2 and 3): *Median nerve* (**C8**, T1)	Flexes distal phalanges at distal interphalangeal joints of medial four digits
◯ 2. *Flexor pollicis longus*	Anterior surface of radius and interosseous membrane	Courses deep to flexor retinaculum to attach to the base of distal phalanx of the thumb	Median nerve (**C8**, T1)	Flexes phalanges of the thumb
◯ 3. *Pronator quadratus*	Distal quarter of ulna	Distal quarter of radius		Pronates forearm

◯ 4. *Supinator:* Visible in the deep aspect of the anterior compartment as it wraps around the radius, but is a posterior compartment muscle

COLOR the arterial pathway in the anterior compartment of the forearm, retracing the relationships of the arteries:

◯ 5. *Brachial artery*
◯ 6. *Radial artery*
◯ 7. *Ulnar artery*

COLOR the nerves coursing through the deep aspect of the anterior compartment, retracing the relationships of the nerves:

◯ 8. *Superficial radial nerve*
◯ 9. *Deep radial nerve*
◯10. *Ulnar nerve*

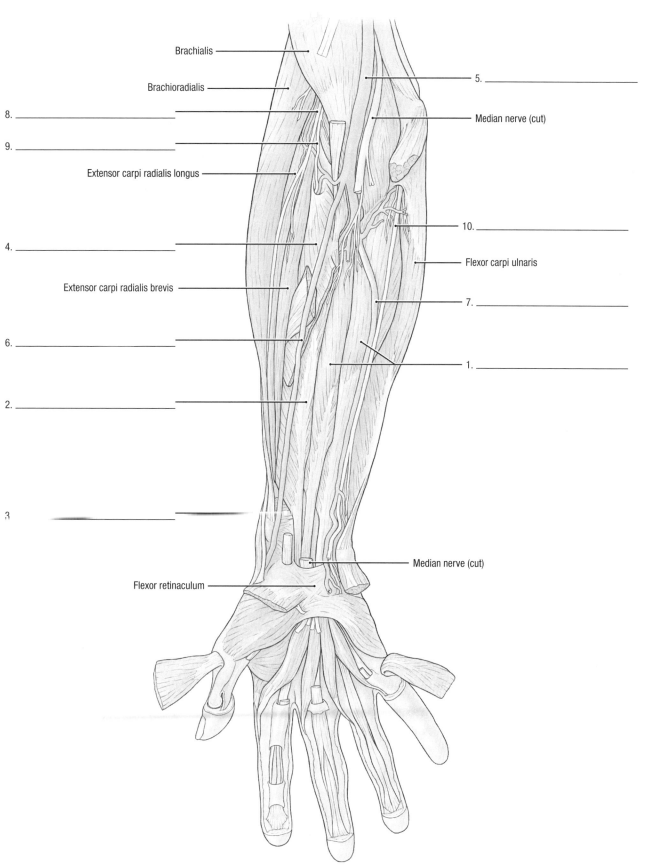

Brachialis

Brachioradialis

8. _____

9. _____

Extensor carpi radialis longus

4. _____

Extensor carpi radialis brevis

6. _____

2. _____

3. _____

Flexor retinaculum

5. _____

Median nerve (cut)

10. _____

Flexor carpi ulnaris

7. _____

1. _____

Median nerve (cut)

Grant's

2.20 SUPERFICIAL PALM

With a majority of the skin and *palmar aponeurosis* removed, the superficial muscles of the thenar and hypothenar compartments can be viewed. In the central palm, the superficial palmar arch and its branches are the most superficial structures lying immediately deep to the palmar aponeurosis. The tendons of flexor digitorum superficialis and profundus, branches of the ulnar and median nerves, and the lumbricals lie deep to the superficial palmar arch.

COLOR each of the following structures using a different color for each:

Superficial Muscles of Palm

Muscle	Proximal Attachment	Distal Attachment	Innervation	Action
◯ 1. *Abductor pollicis brevis*	Flexor retinaculum, scaphoid, and trapezium	Proximal phalanx of the thumb	Recurrent branch of median nerve (**C8**, T1);	Abducts the thumb
◯ 2. *Flexor pollicis brevis*			deep head of flexor pollicis brevis by deep branch of ulnar nerve	Flexes the thumb
◯ 3. *Abductor digiti minimi*	Pisiform	Proximal phalanx of the 5th digit	Deep branch of ulnar nerve (C8, **T1**)	Abducts the 5th digit
◯ 4. *Lumbrical, 1st and 2nd*	Lateral two tendons of flexor digitorum profundus (unipennate muscles)	Lateral sides of extensor expansion of 2nd-5th digits	Median nerve (C8, **T1**)	1. Flex metacarpophalangeal joints
◯ 5. *Lumbrical, 3rd and 4th*	Medial three tendons of flexor digitorum profundus (bipennate muscles)		Deep branch of ulnar nerve (C8, **T1**)	2. Extend interphalangeal joints of 2nd-5th digits

◯ 6. *Flexor digitorum superficialis:* Tendons lie in the central palm with the tendons of flexor digitorum profundus immediately deep to each

◯ 7. *Radial artery:* Passes dorsally to anatomic snuffbox

◯ 8. *Superficial palmar branch of radial artery:* Small branch of radial artery that contributes to the superficial palmar arch

◯ 9. *Ulnar artery:* Courses anterior to flexor retinaculum within the ulnar canal (between *pisiform* and hook of hamate) and divides into two terminal branches: the superficial palmar arch and the deep palmar branch

◯ 10. *Superficial palmar arch:* Main termination of ulnar artery that gives rise to three common palmar digital arteries

◯ 11. *Common palmar digital artery:* Divides into two proper palmar digital arteries

◯ 12. *Proper palmar digital artery:* Course along adjacent sides of 2nd to 4th digits

◯ 13. *Recurrent branch of median nerve:* Arises from median nerve immediately distal to flexor retinaculum supplying abductor pollicis brevis, opponens pollicis, and flexor pollicis brevis (superficial head)

◯ 14. *Ulnar nerve:* Courses anterior to flexor retinaculum within ulnar canal medial to ulnar artery and divides into superficial and deep ulnar nerves

◯ 15. *Common palmar digital nerve:* Arise from superficial branch of ulnar nerve or from median nerve to supply sensory innervation to the medial four digits

◯ 16. *Proper palmar digital nerve:* Arise from common palmar digital nerves

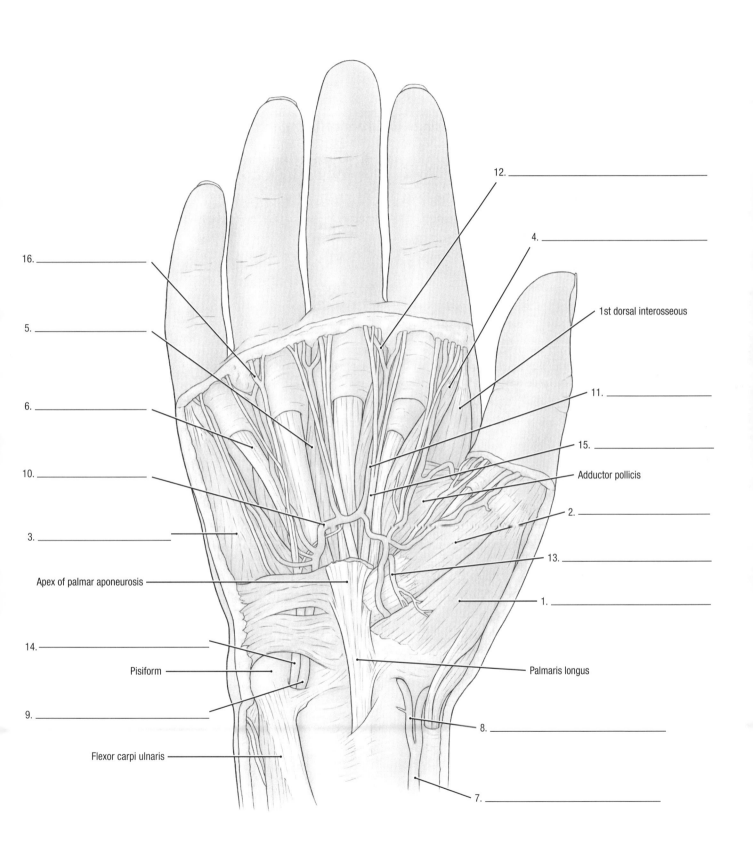

12. _____

4. _____

16. _____

5. _____

6. _____

10. _____

3. _____

Apex of palmar aponeurosis _____

14. _____

Pisiform _____

9. _____

Flexor carpi ulnaris _____

1st dorsal interosseous

11. _____

15. _____

Adductor pollicis

2. _____

13. _____

1. _____

Palmaris longus

8. _____

7. _____

2.21 DEEP PALM

The reflection of the superficial muscles of the thenar and hypothenar compartments, the removal of the **_median nerve_** and its branches, and the removal of the **_tendons of flexor_** **_digitorum superficialis_** and **_flexor digitorum profundus_** from the central palm allow for visualization of the deep muscles of the palm and the deep palmar arch.

COLOR each of the following structures using a different color for each:

Deep Muscles of the Palm

Muscle	Proximal Attachment	Distal Attachment	Innervation	Action
◯ 1. *Opponens pollicis*	Flexor retinaculum, scaphoid, and trapezium	1st metacarpal	Recurrent branch of median nerve (**C8**, T1)	To oppose thumb by drawing 1st metacarpal medially to center of palm and to medially rotate it
◯ 2. *Adductor pollicis, transverse head*	3rd metacarpal	Proximal phalanx of thumb	Deep branch of ulnar (C8, **T1**)	Adducts thumb
◯ 3. *Adductor pollicis, oblique head*	2nd and 3rd metacarpals, capitate, and adjacent carpals			
◯ 4. *Flexor digiti minimi brevis (cut)*	Hook of hamate and flexor retinaculum	Proximal phalanx of the 5th digit		Flexes proximal phalanx of the 5th digit
◯ 5. *Opponens digiti minimi*	Hook of hamate and flexor retinaculum	5th metacarpal		Enables the 5th digit to oppose the thumb by drawing the 5th metacarpal anteriorly and rotating it

◯ 6. *Flexor pollicis longus tendon:* Courses through thenar compartment deep to **_flexor_** and **_abductor pollicis brevis muscles_**

◯ 7. *Deep palmar arch:* Continuation of **_radial artery_** (with small contribution from deep branch of **_ulnar artery_**)

that courses deep to flexor digitorum profundus tendons and gives rise to **_palmar metacarpal arteries_**

◯ 8. *Radialis indicis artery:* Typically arises from radial artery coursing along lateral aspect of the index finger

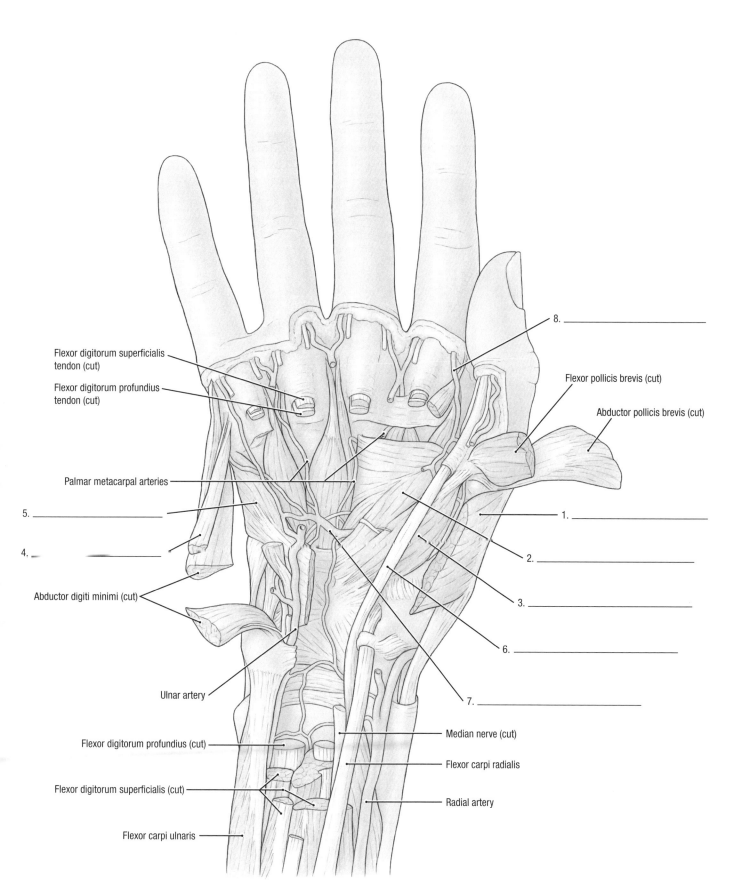

Flexor digitorum superficialis
tendon (cut)

Flexor digitorum profundius
tendon (cut)

Palmar metacarpal arteries

5. _____

4. _____

Abductor digiti minimi (cut)

Ulnar artery

Flexor digitorum profundius (cut)

Flexor digitorum superficialis (cut)

Flexor carpi ulnaris

8. _____

Flexor pollicis brevis (cut)

Abductor pollicis brevis (cut)

1. _____

2. _____

3. _____

6. _____

7. _____

Median nerve (cut)

Flexor carpi radialis

Radial artery

2.22 DEEP PALM AND DIGITS

Muscles of the thenar and hypothenar compartments and the superficial and deep palmar arches have been removed, leaving the cut end of the *radial artery* from the dorsal aspect of the hand. The tendons of the flexor digitorum superficialis and flexor digitorum profundus along with the lumbricals and adductor pollicis muscle have been cut and removed from the palm of the hand.

COLOR each of the following structures using a different color for each:

Muscles of the Deep Palm

Muscle	Proximal Attachment	Distal Attachment	Innervation	Action
○ 1. *Dorsal interossei, 1st-4th (D1-D4)*	Adjacent sides of two meta-carpals (bipennate muscles)	Proximal phalanges and extensor expansions of the 2nd-4th digits	Deep branch of ulnar (C8, **T1**)	1. Abduct the 2nd-4th digits from axial line 2. Assist lumbricals
○ 2. *Palmar interossei, 1st-3rd (P1-P3)*	2nd, 4th, and 5th metacar-pals (unipennate muscles)	Proximal phalanges and extensor expansions of the 2nd, 4th, and 5th digits		1. Adduct the 2nd, 4th, and 5th digits toward axial line 2. Assist lumbricals

○ 3. *Flexor retinaculum:* Forms the roof of the carpal tunnel that lies between the scaphoid and *trapezium* laterally and the *pisiform* and hook of the hamate on the medial side. The median nerve along with the tendons of flexor digitorum superficialis and profundus and flexor pollicis longus travel through the carpal tunnel.

○ 4. *Flexor digitorum superficialis:* Each tendon splits to attach to medial and lateral aspects of middle phalanges of medial four digits

○ 5. *Flexor digitorum profundus:* Attaches to distal phalanges of medial four digits

○ 6. *Ulnar nerve:* Courses superficial to flexor retinaculum dividing into superficial and deep branches

○ 7. *Superficial ulnar nerve (cut):* Supplies sensation to medial one and a half digits and adjacent palm

○ 8. *Deep branch of ulnar nerve:* Supplies hypothenar muscles, 3rd and 4th lumbricals, adductor pollicis, palmar and dorsal interossei, and deep head of flexor pollicis brevis

○ 9. *Median nerve (cut):* Travels deep to flexor retinaculum supplying thenar muscles (except adductor pollicis and deep head of flexor pollicis brevis), 1st and 2nd lumbricals, and sensation to skin of lateral three and a half digits and adjacent palm

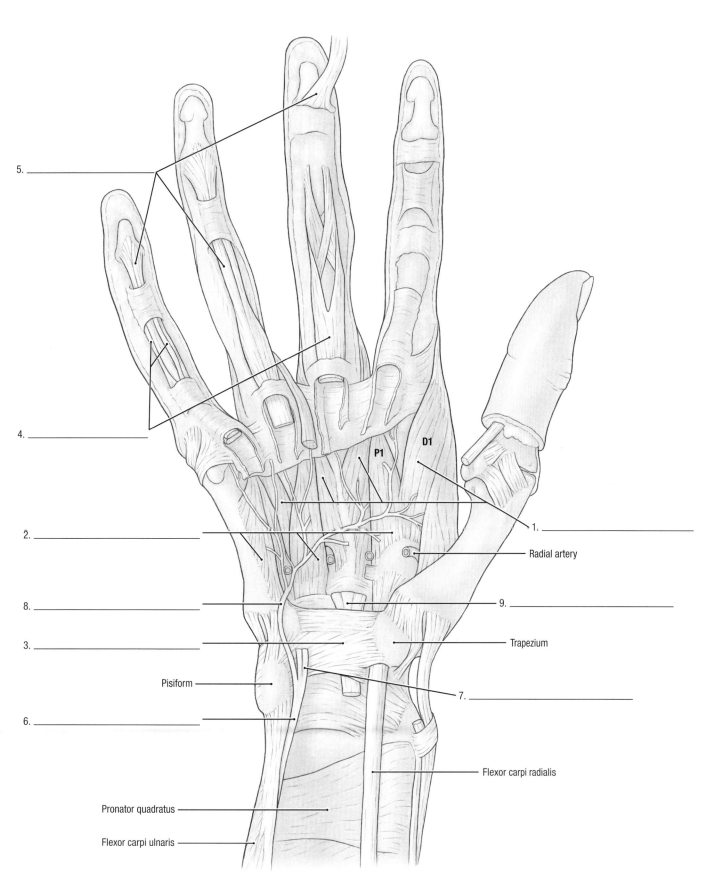

5. _____

4. _____

P1

D1

1. _____

Radial artery

2. _____

8. _____

9. _____

3. _____

Trapezium

Pisiform

7. _____

6. _____

Flexor carpi radialis

Pronator quadratus

Flexor carpi ulnaris

2.23   SUPERFICIAL POSTERIOR COMPARTMENT OF FOREARM

The posterior compartment houses the extensors of the forearm. The muscles of the posterior compartment are primarily innervated by branches of the radial nerve. A majority of the extensors to digits 2 to 4 have been cut at the distal aspect of the extensor retinaculum and reflected in this image to demonstrate the dorsal interossei of the hand.

COLOR each of the following structures using a different color for each:

Muscles of the Superficial Posterior Compartment of the Forearm

Muscle	Proximal Attachment	Distal Attachment	Innervation	Action
○ 1. *Brachioradialis*	Lateral supra-epicondylar ridge of humerus	Radius proximal to styloid process	Radial nerve (C5, **C6**, C7)	Relatively weak flexion of the forearm
○ 2. *Extensor carpi radialis longus*		2nd metacarpal	Radial nerve (C6, C7)	1. Extend hand (at wrist) 2. Abduct hand (at wrist)
○ 3. *Extensor carpi radialis brevis*	Lateral epicondyle of humerus	3rd metacarpal	Deep branch of radial nerve (**C7**, C8)	
○ 4. *Extensor digitorum*		Extensor expansions of medial four digits		Extends medial four digits primarily at the metacarpophalangeal joints
○ 5. *Extensor digiti minimi*		Extensor expansion of the 5th digit		Extends the 5th digit primarily at the metacarpophalangeal joint
○ 6. *Extensor carpi ulnaris*	Lateral epicondyle of humerus and ulna	5th metacarpal		1. Extends hand (at wrist) 2. Adducts hand (at wrist)
○ 7. *Extensor indicis*	Distal third of ulna and interosseous membrane	Extensor expansion of 2nd digit	Posterior interosseous nerve (C7, **C8**), continuation of deep branch of radial nerve	1. Extends the 2nd digit 2. Assists in extending hand (at wrist)
○ 8. *Abductor pollicis longus*	Proximal half of ulna, radius, and interosseous membrane	1st metacarpal		1. Abducts the thumb 2. Extends it at carpometacarpal joint
○ 9. *Extensor pollicis brevis*	Distal third of radius and interosseous membrane	Proximal phalanx of thumb		1. Extends proximal phalanx of the thumb at the metacarpophalangeal joint 2. Extends the carpometacarpal joint
○ 10. *Extensor pollicis longus*	Middle third of ulna and interosseous membrane	Distal phalanx of thumb		1. Extends distal phalanx of the thumb at the interphalangeal joint 2. Extends metacarpophalangeal and carpometacarpal joints

○11. *Extensor retinaculum:* Strong, fibrous band of antebrachial fascia stretching across the posterior aspect of the wrist binding down the extensor tendons of the digits.

○12. *Anconeus:* Small, triangular muscle located along the posterolateral aspect of elbow that usually blends with and assists the triceps brachii

○13. *Dorsal interossei:* Bipennate muscles located between two adjacent metacarpals numbered 1st to 4th (1st located between the thumb and 2nd digit)

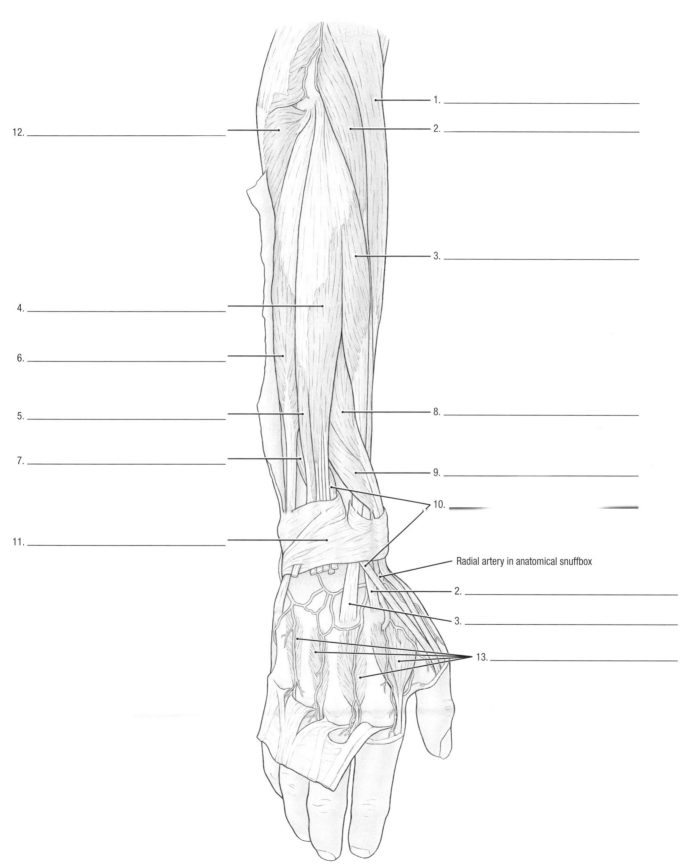

1. _____

2. _____

12. _____

3. _____

4. _____

6. _____

5. _____

8. _____

7. _____

9. _____

10. _____

11. _____

Radial artery in anatomical snuffbox

2. _____

3. _____

13. _____

2.24 MEDIAL VIEW OF POSTERIOR COMPARTMENT OF THE FOREARM

The bulk of the superficial extensor muscles (**_extensor digitorum_**, **_extensor digiti minimi_**, and **_extensor carpi ulnaris_**) has been elevated to provide a complete view of the deeper muscles of the posterior compartment. The **_posterior interosseous nerve_**, a continuation of the deep branch of the radial nerve, innervates the deep layer of muscles in the posterior compartment (see table in Section 2.23).

COLOR each of the following structures using a different color for each:

○ 1. **_Brachioradialis:_** Tendon does not reach the wrist

○ 2. **_Extensor carpi radialis longus:_** Partially overlapped by brachioradialis, and in the distal forearm its tendon is crossed by abductor pollicis longus and extensor pollicis brevis

○ 3. **_Extensor carpi radialis brevis:_** Lies medial to extensor carpi radialis longus, and in the distal forearm its tendon is also crossed by abductor pollicis longus and extensor pollicis brevis

○ 4. **_Abductor pollicis longus:_** Lies distal to supinator and crosses extensor carpi radialis longus and brevis

○ 5. **_Extensor pollicis brevis:_** Lies distal to abductor pollicis longus, with its tendon extending proximally medial to abductor pollicis longus

○ 6. **_Extensor pollicis longus:_** Lies medial to abductor pollicis longus and extensor pollicis brevis, with its tendon passing through its own compartment

○ 7. **_Extensor indicis (cut):_** Lies medial to extensor pollicis longus

○ 8. **_Supinator:_** Wraps around the neck and proximal shaft of radius and pierced by deep branch of the radial nerve

○ 9. **_Extensor retinaculum:_** Holds the tendons of the posterior compartment in place at the wrist

○ 10. **_Radial artery (in "snuff box"):_** Curves dorsally around scaphoid and trapezium to enter the anatomic snuff box and then enters palm by passing between the heads of the **_1st dorsal interosseous muscle_**

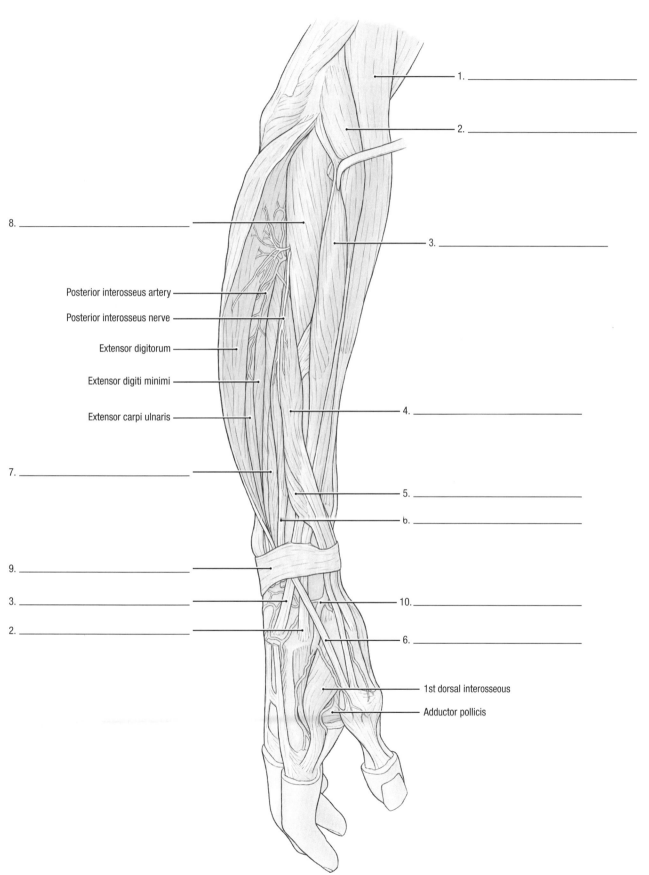

1. _____

2. _____

8. _____

3. _____

Posterior interosseus artery _____

Posterior interosseus nerve _____

Extensor digitorum _____

Extensor digiti minimi _____

Extensor carpi ulnaris _____

4. _____

7. _____

5. _____

6. _____

9. _____

3. _____

10. _____

2. _____

6. _____

1st dorsal interosseous

Adductor pollicis

Grant's

2.25 DORSUM OF HAND

The extensor retinaculum attaches at various points to the radius and ulna creating tunnels for passage of 12 tendons.

A synovial sheath surrounds each tendon as it passes through its tunnel.

COLOR each of the following structures using a different color for each:

○ 1. **Extensor retinaculum:** Attaches to distal radius and ulna and forms six osseofibrous tunnels that extensor muscle tendons pass through

Extensor Retinaculum Tunnels

Tunnel	Structure
1	○ 2. *Abductor pollicis longus* ○ 3. *Extensor pollicis brevis*
2	○ 4. *Extensor carpi radialis longus* ○ 5. *Extensor carpi radialis brevis*
3	○ 6. *Extensor pollicis longus*
4	○ 7. *Extensor digitorum* ○ 8. *Extensor indicis*
5	○ 9. *Extensor digiti mimimi*
6	○ 10. *Extensor carpi ulnaris*

○ 11. **Intertendinous connection:** Proximal to the metacarpophalangeal joints, three oblique bands link adjacent tendons, restricting independent extension of the medial four digits

○ 12. **Extensor (dorsal) expansion:** Tendons of the extensor digitorum flatten and expand along the distal ends of the metacarpals and proximal phalanges of the medial four digits

CLINICAL NOTE: SYNOVIAL CYSTS

Synovial ("ganglion") cysts are benign soft tissue tumors that most commonly occur on the dorsum of the wrist. On examination, the cyst is usually 1-2 cm in size (small grape) and upon palpation feels like a tethered, firm rubber ball to its attachment to the underlying joint capsule of the wrist. Presence of a synovial cyst on the dorsum of the wrist may result in decreased range of motion or strength along with variable compliant of pain.

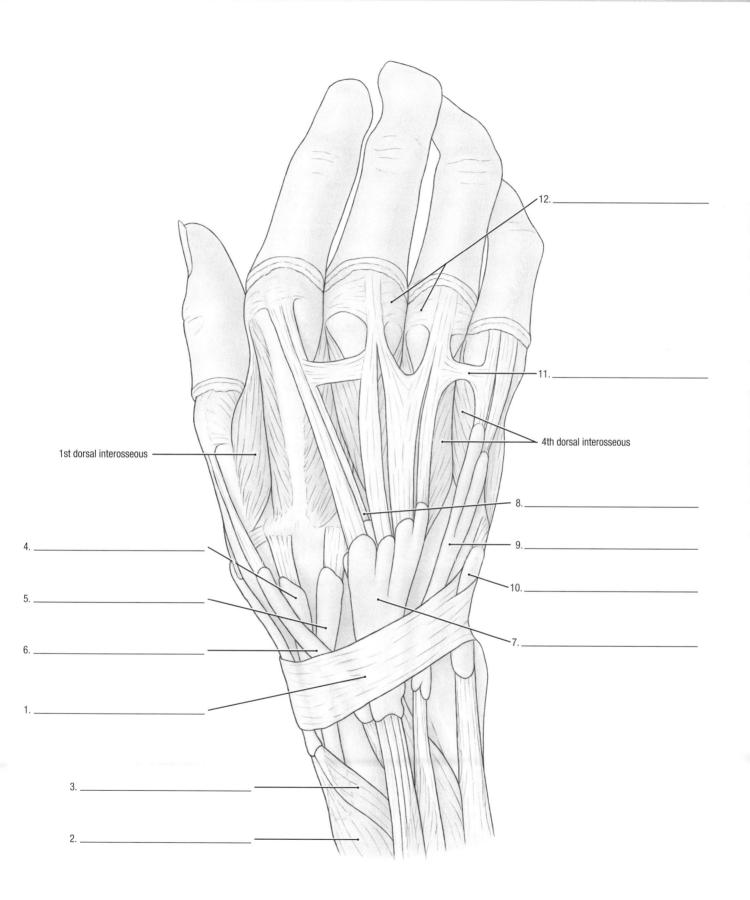

12. _____

11. _____

4th dorsal interosseous

1st dorsal interosseous _____

8. _____

4. _____

9. _____

5. _____

10. _____

6. _____

7. _____

1. _____

3. _____

2. _____

Grant's

2.26 WRIST JOINT

The wrist joint is a condyloid synovial joint. The distal end of the radius and the articular disc of the distal radio-ulnar joint articulate with the proximal row of carpal bones (except *pisiform*). The ulna does not participate in the wrist joint. The hand has been forcibly extended in this image.

COLOR each of the following structures using a different color for each:

○ 1. *Palmar radiocarpal ligaments:* Pass from radius to carpal bones so that the hand follows the radius through supination

○ 2. *Radial collateral ligament:* Laterally placed attached to *styloid process of radius* and *scaphoid*

○ 3. *Ulnar collateral ligament:* Medially placed attached to *styloid process of ulna* and *triquetrum*

CLINICAL NOTE: CARPAL TUNNEL SYNDROME

Carpal tunnel syndrome is a result of damage to the median nerve within the rigid boundaries of the *carpea tunnel*. Lesions that reduce the size of the carpal tunnel or increase the size of the structures passing through the carpal tunnel result in compression of the *median nerve*. Inflammation of the synovial sheaths surrounding the nine tendons (removed in this image) that pass through the carpal tunnel is a common cause of carpal tunnel syndrome. Sensory deficits over the palmar aspect of the lateral 3.5 digits typically present before motor deficits of the thenar compartment. Partial or full surgical release of the *flexor retinaculum* may be necessary to relieve compression of the median nerve.

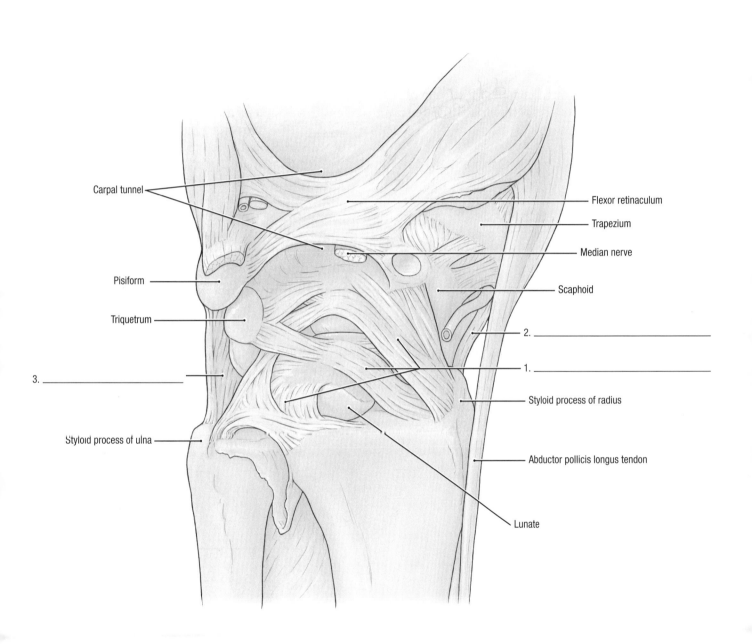

Carpal tunnel

Flexor retinaculum

Trapezium

Median nerve

Pisiform

Scaphoid

Triquetrum

2. _____

1. _____

3. _____

Styloid process of radius

Styloid process of ulna

Abductor pollicis longus tendon

Lunate

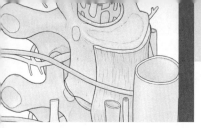

CHAPTER 3

Thorax

The thoracic skeleton is composed of the sternum, 12 pairs of ribs and their costal cartilages, and 12 **_thoracic vertebrae_** and the intervertebral (IV) disk between them.

COLOR each of the following using a different color for each structure:

Sternum

The sternum is a flat, elongated bone in the midline of the anterior thoracic wall and consists of three parts: manubrium, body, and xiphoid process.

○ 1. **_Manubrium:_** Superior portion, primarily trapezoid in shape, and is the widest and thickest part of the sternum

○ 2. **_Body:_** Longer, narrower, and thinner than the manubrium and is located at T5-T9 vertebral levels

The manubrium and body of the sternum lie in slightly different planes as they meet forming a projection referred to as the **_manubriosternal joint (sternal angle)_**.

○ 3. **_Xiphoid process:_** Smallest and most variable part of the sternum. The inferior end lies at the T10 vertebral level.

Junction of the body and xiphoid process creates the **_xiphisternal joint_**, which indicates the inferior limit of the central part of the thoracic cavity.

Ribs

Ribs are curved, flat bones that form the majority of the thoracic cage. Ribs are numbered sequentially from superior to inferior (**_1st-12th_**). There are three classifications of ribs:

○ 4. **_True ribs:_** 1st to 7th ribs, which directly attach to the sternum through costal cartilages

○ 5. **_False ribs:_** 8th and 9th ribs and, usually, the 10th rib

○ 6. **_Floating ribs:_** 11th and 12th ribs and, sometimes, the 10th rib with anterior caps of costal cartilage

○ 7. **_Costal cartilage:_** Articulates with the anterior aspects of each rib, providing a flexible attachment

○ 8. **_Costal margin:_** Formed by the costal cartilages of the false ribs (8th-10th) connecting to the costal cartilages superior to them

Intercostal spaces separate the ribs and their costal cartilages from each other. Each intercostal space is numbered for the rib forming its superior border. For example, the **_8th intercostal space_** is between the 8th and 9th ribs. There are only 11 intercostal spaces; the space below the 12th rib is the subcostal space.

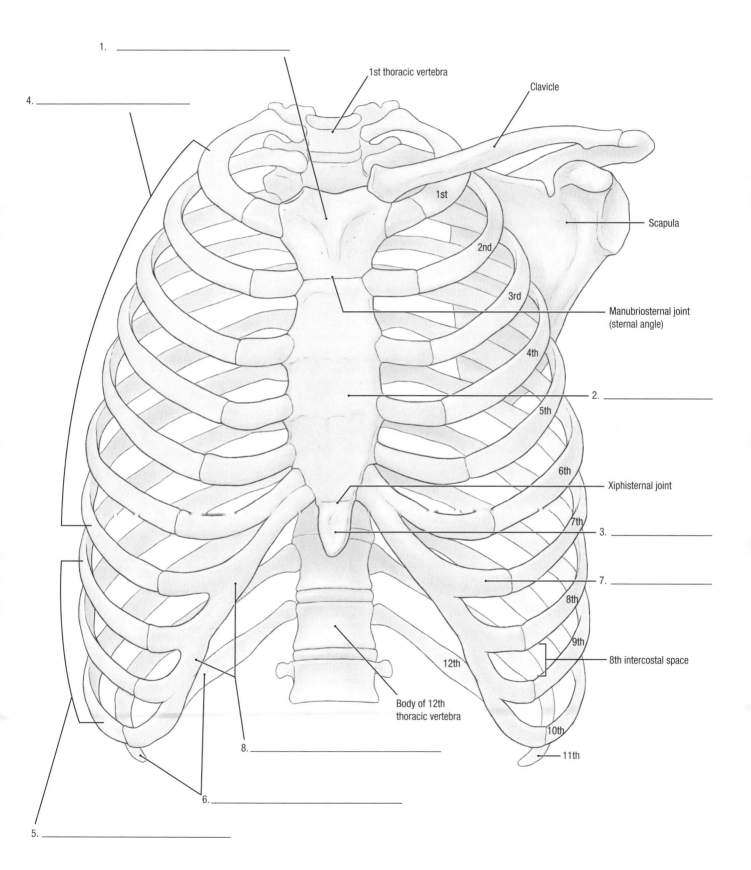

1. _____

4. _____

1st thoracic vertebra

Clavicle

1st

2nd

3rd

Scapula

Manubriosternal joint
(sternal angle)

4th

2. _____

5th

6th

Xiphisternal joint

7th

3. _____

7. _____

8th

9th

8th intercostal space

12th

Body of 12th
thoracic vertebra

10th

8. _____

11th

6. _____

5. _____

3.2A and B   FEATURES OF TYPICAL RIBS

COLOR each of the following using a different color for each structure:

Each typical rib (3rd-9th) has the following features:

○ 1. *Head:* Wedge shaped and marked by a ***crest of head***. The head is demarcated by two facets that articulate with the vertebral bodies:
  ○ 2. *Superior facet*
  ○ 3. *Inferior facet*

The head of each typical rib articulates with the vertebral body of the same number and the vertebral body superior to it, forming the ***joints of the head of the rib***. The head of the ***7th rib***, for example, will articulate with the superior costal facet of the ***T7*** vertebral body and to the inferior costal facet of ***T6***. The heads of the 1st, 11th, and 12th ribs only articulate with the vertebral body of the same number.

○ 4. *Superior costal facet of T6:* Articulates with the inferior facet of the head of the ***6th rib***
○ 5. *Inferior costal facet of T7:* Articulates with the superior facet of the head of the ***8th rib***
○ 6. *Neck:* Connects the head to the body (shaft) of the rib

○ 7. *Tubercle:* Located at the junction of the neck and body (shaft)

The tubercle of each rib will articulate with the transverse process of the vertebra of the same number, forming the ***costotransverse joint***. The tubercle of the 7th rib, for example, articulates with the transverse costal facet of T7.

○ 8. *Transverse costal facet of T6:* Articulates with the tubercle of the 6th rib
○ 9. *Body (shaft):* Thin, flat, and curved component of the rib. The ***costal angle*** occurs where the body turns anterolaterally.
○ 10. *Costal groove:* Slight concave indentation paralleling the inferior border of the body of the rib that protects the intercostal neurovasculature

The anterior blunt end of the rib marks the ***site of articulation with the costal cartilage***.

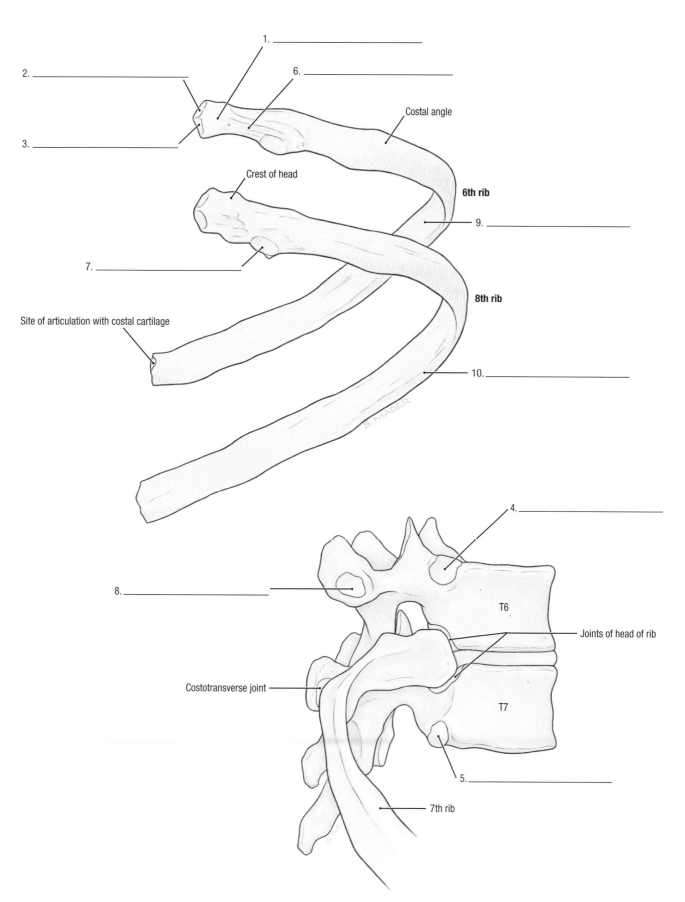

1. _____

2. _____

6. _____

3. _____

Costal angle

Crest of head

6th rib

7. _____

9. _____

8th rib

Site of articulation with costal cartilage

10. _____

4. _____

T6

Joints of head of rib

8. _____

Costotransverse joint

T7

5. _____

7th rib

S. MADER

Grant's

3.3 FEMALE PECTORAL REGION WITH THE BREAST

Breasts consist of glandular tissue surrounded by *__fat__* and are typically more developed in women.

COLOR each of the following using a different color for each structure:

○ 1. *Pectoralis muscle* (and *__pectoral fascia__*): Underlies the majority of the breast. Between the breast and the pectoral fascia is a loose connective tissue plane (potential space), the *__retromammary space__*. This space allows a minor amount of movement of the breast on the pectoral fascia.

○ 2. *Serratus anterior muscle:* Underlies a minor component of the lateral breast

○ 3. *Axillary process (tail):* Portion of the mammary gland extending along the inferolateral margin of the pectoralis major and into the axilla

○ 4. *Suspensory ligaments:* Attach the mammary gland to the dermis of the overlying skin

○ 5. *Lactiferous duct:* Drains each of the 15 to 20 lobules of the mammary gland. The lactiferous ducts dilate peripherally as the lactiferous sinuses as they converge toward the nipple surrounded by the *__areola__*.

CLINICAL NOTE: BREAST CANCER

The breast is divided into four quadrants: superolateral, superomedial, inferolateral, and inferomedial. Most carcinomas of the breast are located in the superolateral quadrant, which is associated with the **axillary tail**. Breast cancer can spread through lymphatic vessels to the axillary lymph nodes.

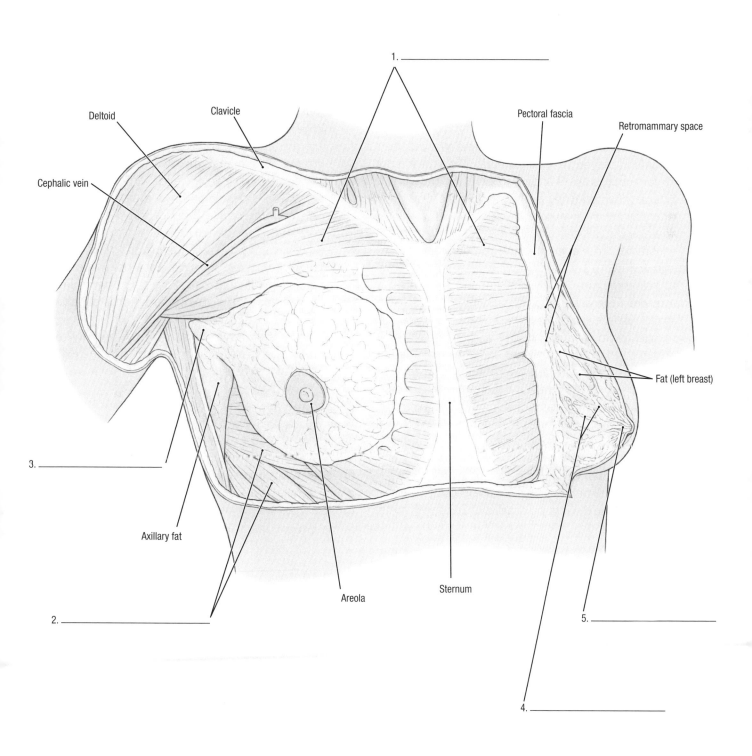

1. _____

Deltoid

Clavicle

Pectoral fascia

Retromammary space

Cephalic vein

3. _____

Axillary fat

2. _____

Areola

Sternum

Fat (left breast)

5. _____

4. _____

3.4   EXTERNAL ASPECT OF ANTERIOR THORACIC WALL

Axioappendicular muscles (**_pectoralis major_** and **_pectoralis minor_**) and anterolateral abdominal muscles (**_external oblique_** and **_rectus abdominis_**) attach to the anterior thoracic wall, but are involved in functions of other regions and have been mostly removed in this figure. The true muscles of the anterior thoracic wall include the external and internal intercostal muscles along with the transversus thoracis muscle.

A small window has been cut into the external intercostal membrane and internal intercostal muscle near the sternum on the right side to reveal the underlying structures.

COLOR each of the following using a different color for each structure:

1. **_External intercostal muscles:_** Fill the intercostal spaces from the tubercles of the ribs posteriorly to the junction of the ribs and the costal cartilages anteriorly. The fibers run inferoanteriorly from the superior rib to the inferior rib (direction is like "hands in a pocket").

2. **_External intercostal membranes:_** Replace the fibers of the external intercostal muscle between the costal cartilages anteriorly to the sternum. The fibers continue to run in an inferoanterior direction, but the membrane is often thin enough to see the underlying internal intercostal muscle through it.

3. **_Internal intercostal muscles:_** Also fill the intercostal spaces, but are located deep to the external intercostal muscles and membranes. The internal intercostal muscles attach to the costal cartilages and bodies of the ribs from the sternum to the angles of the ribs posteriorly. The fibers run at right angles to the external intercostal muscles and membranes in an inferoposterior direction. Posteriorly, from the angles of the ribs to the vertebral column, the muscle fibers are replaced by the internal intercostal membrane.

4. **_Transversus thoracis muscles_**: Composed of four to five slips of muscle that extend from the internal aspect of the sternum to the internal aspects of 2nd to 6th costal cartilages

5. **_Internal thoracic artery_**: Paired arteries that descend on the internal surface of the thoracic wall on either side of the sternum between the internal intercostal and transversus thoracis muscles

6. **_Internal thoracic vein:_** Travels with the internal thoracic artery on each side of the sternum

7. **_Anterior intercostal arteries_** and **_veins:_** Arise from or drain into the internal thoracic artery and vein, respectively, supplying the anterior aspects of the superior nine intercostal spaces. Each anterior intercostal artery and vein will anastomose with a posterior intercostal artery and vein of the same intercostal space in the lateral thoracic wall.

8. **_Intercostal nerve:_** Formed by the anterior ramus of spinal nerves T1-T11 and innervates the extent of a single intercostal space.

Because only one source (the spinal cord) gives rise to the intercostal nerves, anterior/posterior is not utilized in the naming of intercostal nerves. In contrast, anterior/posterior is used in naming the intercostal arteries and veins because there are two sources that give rise to the vascular supply of the intercostal spaces (posterior intercostals from the aorta/to the azygos system of veins and anterior intercostals from/to the internal thoracic artery and vein).

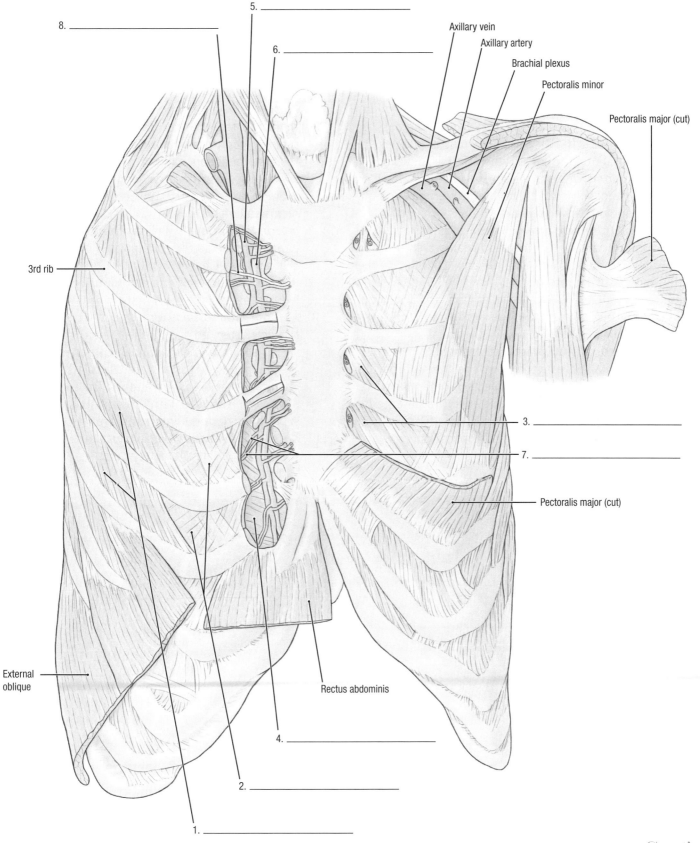

5. _____

8. _____

6. _____

Axillary vein

Axillary artery

Brachial plexus

Pectoralis minor

Pectoralis major (cut)

3rd rib

3. _____

7. _____

Pectoralis major (cut)

External
oblique

Rectus abdominis

4. _____

2. _____

1. _____

Grant's

3.5   INTERNAL ASPECT OF THE ANTERIOR THORACIC WALL

The anterior thoracic wall has been removed and the internal aspect displayed. The endothoracic fascia and costal layer of the parietal pleura have been removed. The diaphragm has been cut and also removed on the right side of the specimen. The arteries from the arch of the aorta and the brachiocephalic veins have also been cut.

COLOR each of the following using a different color for each structure:

○ 1. *Internal intercostal muscles:* Completely fill the inter-costal spaces along the internal view of the anterior thoracic wall. The innermost intercostal muscles are not present on the anterior thoracic wall.

○ 2. *Diaphragm:* Originates from the internal surface of the inferior six costal cartilages, the **_sternum_**, and the superior lumbar vertebrae

○ 3. *Internal thoracic artery:* Paired arteries that arise from the first part of the subclavian artery, descend lateral to the sternum, and then travel anterior to the transversus thoracis muscle

○ 4. *Subclavian artery:* On the right side typically arises from the brachiocephalic trunk, whereas on the left typically arises directly from the arch of the aorta

○ 5. *Transversus thoracis muscle:* Composed of four to five slips of muscle that extend from the internal aspect of the sternum to the internal aspects of 2nd to 6th costal cartilages. The internal thoracic artery travels anterior to the transversus thoracis muscle and terminates in the 6th intercostal space into the musculophrenic and superior epigastric arteries.

○ 6. *Musculophrenic artery:* Terminal branch of internal thoracic artery that courses along the costal margin supplying portions of the diaphragm and muscles of the anterior abdominal wall

○ 7. *Superior epigastric artery:* Terminal branch of internal thoracic artery that continues inferiorly posterior to rectus abdominis muscle

○ 8. *Internal thoracic vein:* Follows the same course as the internal thoracic artery, but typically drains to the bra-chiocephalic veins

○ 9. *Brachiocephalic vein:* Formed by the union of the internal jugular vein and the subclavian on each side

○ 10. *Anterior intercostal artery:* Arises from the internal thoracic artery to supply the 1st to 6th intercostal spaces and from the musculophrenic artery to supply the 7th to 9th intercostal spaces. Each intercostal space is typically supplied by a small pair of anterior intercostal arteries. The 10th to 11th intercostal spaces are only supplied by posterior intercostal arteries.

○ 11. *Anterior intercostal vein:* Follows the same course as the anterior intercostal artery

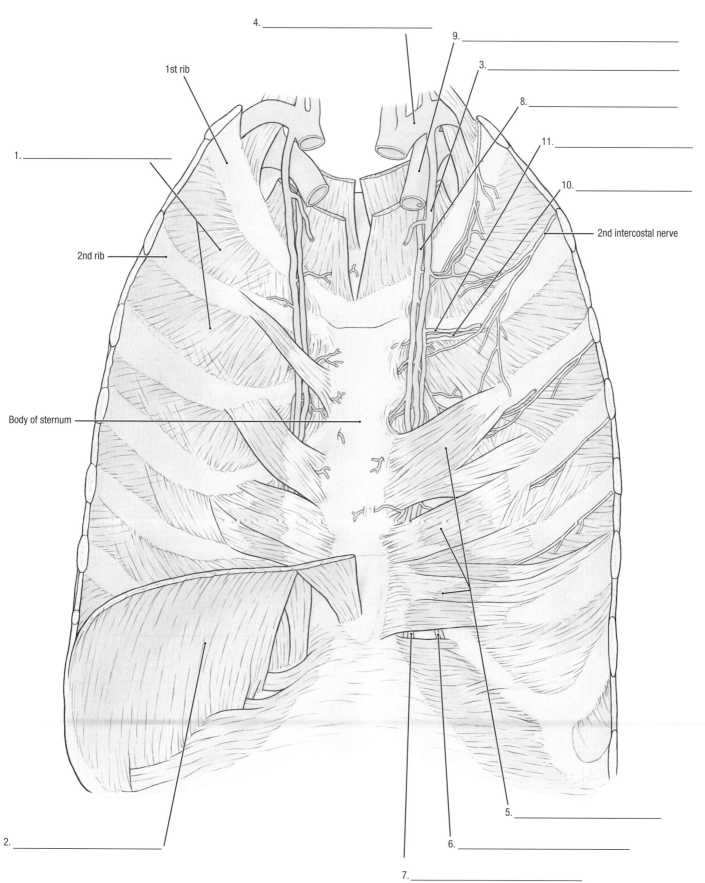

4. _____

9. _____

1st rib

3. _____

8. _____

11. _____

1. _____

10. _____

2nd rib

2nd intercostal nerve

Body of sternum

5. _____

2. _____

6. _____

7. _____

Grant's

3.6A and B   FEATURES OF THE RIGHT AND LEFT LUNGS

The lungs have been removed from the thoracic cavity. A lateral and posterior view is displayed from the right lung (A) and the left lung (B).

COLOR each of the following using a different color for each structure:

Each lung has a superiorly positioned **apex** and a concave, inferiorly positioned base. Each lung also has costal, mediastinal, and diaphragmatic surfaces along with **anterior**, inferior, and **posterior borders**.

Right Lung (A)

Divided into three lobes:

- ◯ 1. *Superior*
- ◯ 2. *Middle*
- ◯ 3. *Inferior*
- ◯ 4. *Oblique fissure:* Separates the inferior lobe from the superior and middle lobes
- ◯ 5. *Horizontal fissure:* Separates the middle and superior lobes

Left Lung (B)

Divided into two lobes:

- ◯ 1. *Superior*
- ◯ 3. *Inferior*
- ◯ 4. *Oblique fissure:* Separates the superior and inferior lobes

The superior lobe of the left lung is demarcated by two features:

- ◯ 6. *Cardiac notch:* Deep indentation along the antero-inferior border
- ◯ 7. *Lingula:* Tongue-like process that extends inferior to the cardiac notch

CLINICAL NOTE: LUNG RESECTIONS

Owing to the branching pattern of the bronchi and pulmonary arteries, the lung is organized not only into lobes but also into smaller bronchopulmonary segments. This anatomic arrangement permits multiple levels of treatment options for various pulmonary diseases, including lung cancer. One or more bronchopulmonary segments (segmentectomy), lobe (lobectomy), or the whole lung (pneumonectomy) can be resected (removed).

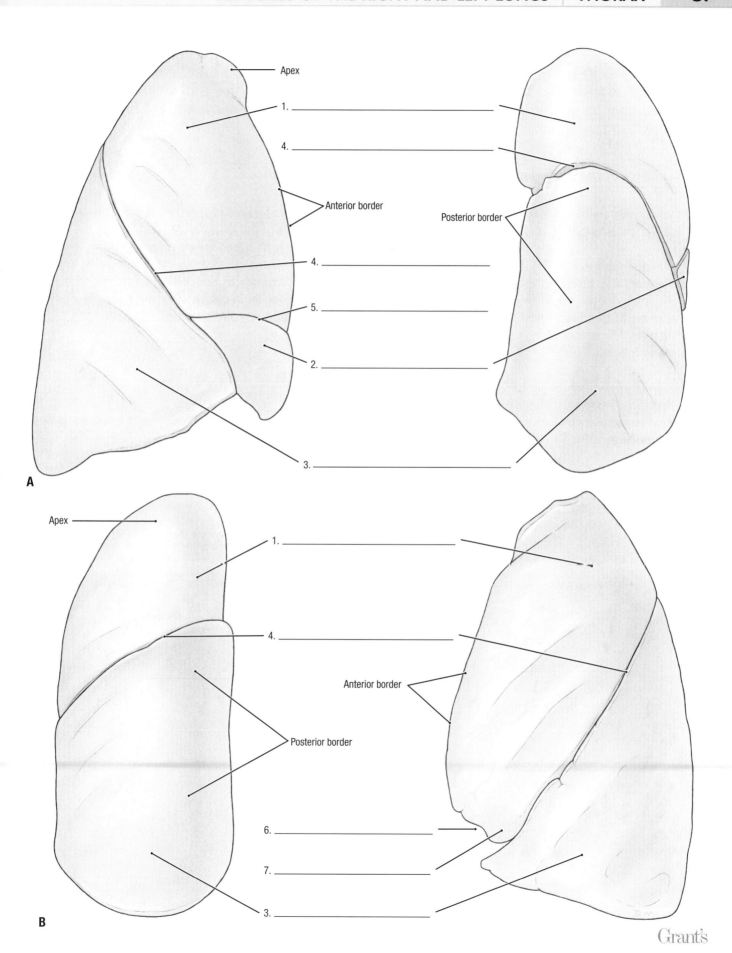

Apex

1. _____

4. _____

Anterior border

Posterior border

4. _____

5. _____

2. _____

3. _____

A

Apex

1. _____

4. _____

Anterior border

Posterior border

6. _____

7. _____

3. _____

B

3.7 MEDIASTINAL SURFACE OF THE RIGHT LUNG

The right lung has been cut at the hilum, removed from the thoracic cavity, and the mediastinal surface displayed. In this image, the cut was performed slightly lateral (closer to the lung) and displays the right main bronchus as it branches into the secondary (lobar) bronchi. The branching of the pulmonary artery and veins is also visible. Impressions of surrounding structures are also present, as is common with embalmed cadavers.

COLOR each of the following using a different color for each structure:

The fissures continue to the mediastinal surface of the right lung dividing it into *superior*, *middle*, and *inferior lobes*.

○ 1. *Oblique fissure*
○ 2. *Horizontal fissure*

The hilum of the lung is penetrated by the root of the lung structures. The structures in the root of the right lung are organized as follows:

○ 3. *Right main bronchus:* Located posteriorly
○ 4. *Bronchial vessels:* Small vessels located immediately next to the bronchus
○ 5. *Pulmonary artery*: Situated anteriorly to the right main bronchus
○ 6. *Pulmonary veins:* Located anteroinferiorly

The mediastinal surface demonstrates impressions made by nearby structures that come into contact with the right lung.

○ 7. *Groove for esophagus:* Lies posterior to the hilum of the lung

○ 8. *Groove for arch of azygos vein:* Passes over the superior aspect of the hilum of the lung
○ 9. *Groove for superior vena cava:* Lies anterior to the hilum of the lung
○ 10. *Cardiac impression:* Lies inferior to the groove for the superior vena cava along the inferior aspect of the superior lobe and the middle lobe

CLINICAL NOTE: PULMONARY EMBOLISM

A pulmonary embolus (blood clot) typically arises from a thrombus that originates in the deep venous system of the lower limb. The thrombus travels through the venous system to the heart and then through one of the pulmonary arteries to either lung. The thrombus then becomes lodged either at the bifurcation of the pulmonary artery or at the further divisions of the lobar arteries. Consequently, blood flow to a lung or a portion of a lung is blocked. Clinical presentation of pulmonary embolism varies greatly. A large thrombus blocking a pulmonary artery may cause sudden and catastrophic hemodynamic (blood flow dynamics) collapse, whereas a small thrombus blocking a bronchopulmonary segment may cause gradually progressive dyspnea (shortness of breath).

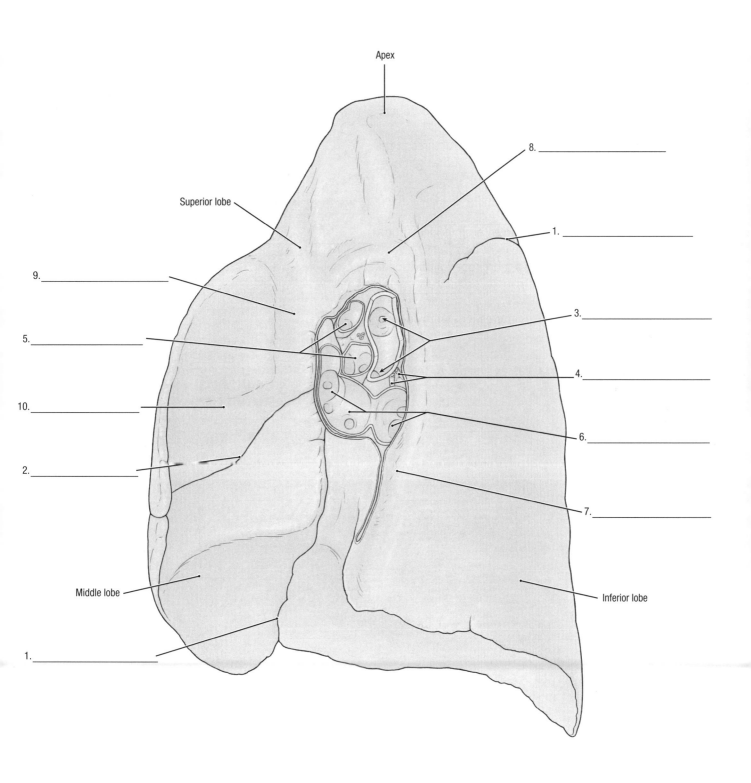

Apex

Superior lobe

8. _____

1. _____

9. _____

5. _____

3. _____

10. _____

4. _____

2. _____

6. _____

7. _____

Middle lobe

Inferior lobe

1. _____

3.8 MEDIASTINAL SURFACE OF THE LEFT LUNG

The left lung has been cut at the hilum, removed from the thoracic cavity, and the mediastinal surface displayed. In this image, the cut was performed medial to the branching of the main bronchus, pulmonary artery, and the left superior and inferior pulmonary veins. Impressions of surrounding structures are also present, as is common with embalmed cadavers.

COLOR each of the following using a different color for each structure:

○ 1. *Oblique fissure:* Continues to the mediastinal surface, dividing the left lung into superior and inferior lobes

The arrangement of the root of the lung structures at the hilum of the left lung differs slightly from that of the right lung.

○ 2. *Left main bronchus:* Located posteriorly, similar in arrangement to the right lung
○ 3. *Pulmonary veins:* Located in an anteroinferior location, similar in arrangement to the right lung
○ 4. *Pulmonary artery:* Shifts to a more superior position in the left lung

The left lung also demonstrates impressions left by nearby structures.

○ 5. *Groove for arch of aorta:* Passes superior to the hilum of the left lung

○ 6. *Groove for the descending aorta:* Passes posteriorly to the hilum of the left lung
○ 7. *Cardiac impression:* Lies along the inferior aspect of the superior lobe and the anteroinferior aspect of the inferior lobe

CLINICAL NOTE: ENLARGEMENT OF BRONCHOPULMONARY LYMPH NODES

<u>Bronchopulmonary (hilar) lymph nodes</u> are located in the region of the hilum and drain the parenchyma (tissue) of the lung and the visceral pleura directly. Bronchopulmonary lymph nodes also indirectly drain the root of the lung structures (bronchi and vascular) via the pulmonary lymph nodes. Lymph from the bronchopulmonary lymph nodes continues to the tracheobronchial lymph nodes located at the bifurcation of the trachea, to bronchomediastinal trunks, and then to the thoracic duct or right lymphatic duct. Enlargement of these nodes can occur with a variety of pathologies including pulmonary manifestations of sarcoidosis, lung cancer, mesothelioma, pulmonary tuberculosis, pulmonary infection, and occupational lung disease such as coal workers' pneumoconiosis.

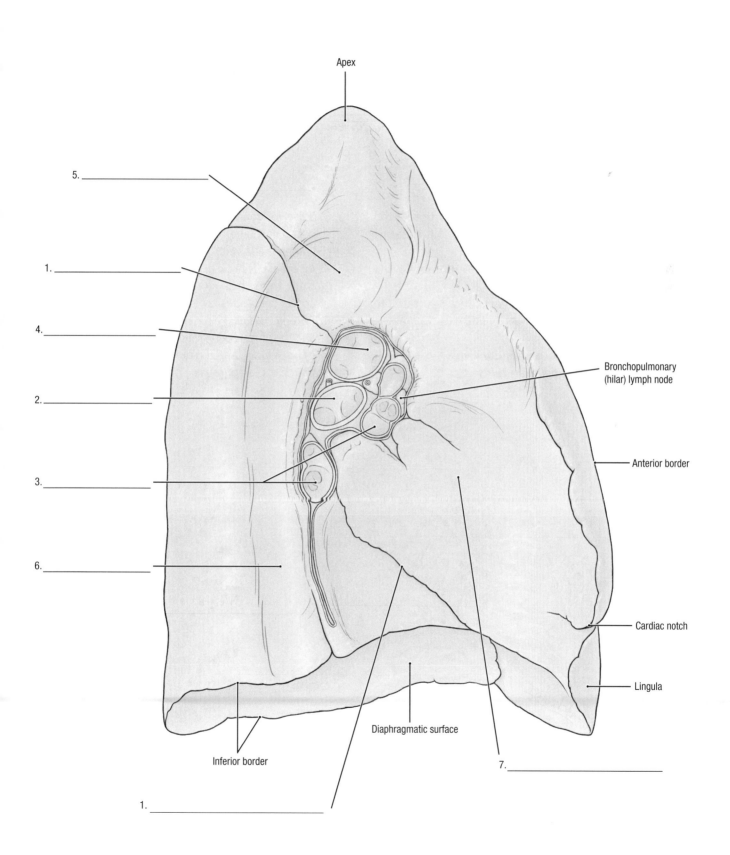

Apex

5. _____

1. _____

4. _____

2. _____

3. _____

6. _____

Bronchopulmonary
(hilar) lymph node

Anterior border

Cardiac notch

Lingula

Inferior border

Diaphragmatic surface

7. _____

1. _____

Grant's

3.9   PERICARDIAL RELATIONSHIPS TO THE STERNUM

The mediastinum is the central component of the thoracic cavity between the two pleural cavities and contains all of the thoracic viscera and structures except for the lungs. The mediastinum is subdivided into the superior and inferior mediastinum by a line passing from the *sternal angle* to the IV disk between T4 and T5. The inferior mediastinum is further subdivided into the anterior, middle, and posterior mediastinum. The heart and the roots of the great vessels contained within the pericardium compose the middle mediastinum.

COLOR each of the following using a different color for each structure:

The majority of the pericardium (and the heart within the pericardial sac) lies to the left of the median plane.

○ 1. *Body of the sternum:* Lies anterior to a portion of the pericardium (and the heart) to the level of the sternal angle

○ 2. *Diaphragm:* The central portion lies inferior to the pericardium

○ 3. *Right and left brachiocephalic veins:* Forms posterior to the sternoclavicular (SC) joints by union of two vessels on each side of the body:

  ○ 4. *Right and left internal jugular veins*
  ○ 5. *Right and left subclavian veins*

○ 6. *Superior vena cava:* Forms at the level of the 1st right costal cartilage by the union of the right and left brachiocephalic veins

○ 7. *Internal thoracic arteries:* Paired arteries that course from the subclavian artery posterior to the first six *costal cartilages* on either side of the sternum

○ 8. *Phrenic nerves:* Paired nerves that supply the diaphragm and the fibrous pericardium; descend anterior to *the root of both lungs* and run along the fibrous *pericardium* to pierce the diaphragm

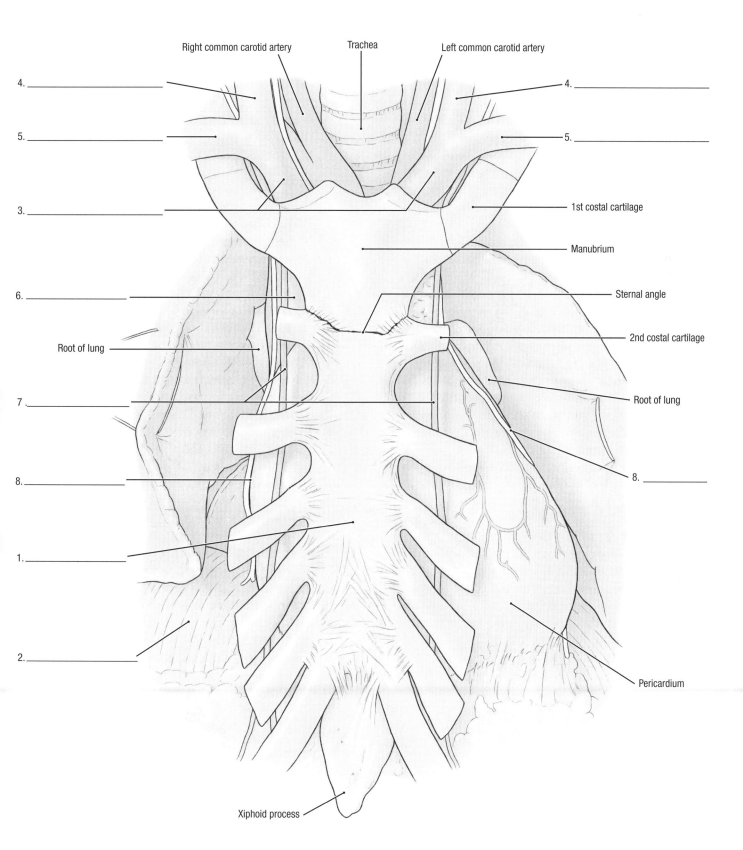

Right common carotid artery

Trachea

Left common carotid artery

4. _____

4. _____

5. _____

5. _____

3. _____

1st costal cartilage

Manubrium

Sternal angle

6. _____

2nd costal cartilage

Root of lung

Root of lung

7. _____

8. _____

8. _____

1. _____

2. _____

Pericardium

Xiphoid process

3.10 STERNOCOSTAL (ANTERIOR) SURFACE OF THE HEART AND GREAT VESSELS

The sternum and *pericardium* (fibrous and parietal layers) have been removed to visualize the anterior (sternocostal) surface of the heart and great vessels intact in the thoracic cavity. The majority of the left brachiocephalic vein has been removed from this image to demonstrate the arch of the aorta and its branches.

COLOR each of the following using a different color for each structure:

○ 1. *Right ventricle:* Comprises a majority of the anterior (sternocostal) surface of the heart

○ 2. *Left ventricle:* Contributes to a minor component of the anterior surface of the heart at the apex of the heart. The right ventricle is separated from the left ventricle by the anterior interventricular groove (sulcus), which is occupied by two vessels:

   ○ 3. *Anterior interventricular branch of left coronary artery* (left anterior descending artery)

   ○ 4. *Great cardiac vein*

○ 5. *Right atrium:* Contributes to the right margin of the heart and is separated from the right ventricle by the atrioventricular groove (coronary sulcus) occupied by the right coronary artery. Each atrium has an anteriorly directed earlike projection called the *auricle*.

○ 6. *Right coronary artery:* Originates from the ascending aorta and travels within the atrioventricular groove between the right atrium and right ventricle

○ 7. *Marginal artery:* Arises from the right coronary artery near the right margin of the heart

○ 8. *Anterior cardiac veins:* Superficially cross over the right coronary artery to drain directly into the right atrium. These veins are unlike the remainder of the venous system of the heart, which drains into the coronary sinus before reaching the right atrium.

○ 9. *Superior vena cava:* Forms by the union of the *brachiocephalic veins* and enters the right atrium superiorly

○10. *Ascending aorta:* Lies to the left of the superior vena cava as it extends from the left ventricle. Two branches, the left and right coronary arteries, arise from the ascending aorta.

○11. *Arch of the aorta:* Curved continuation of the aorta. The arch typically gives rise to three branches:

   ○12. *Brachiocephalic trunk:* First and largest branch arises posterior to the manubrium, anterior to the trachea, and posterior to the left brachiocephalic vein

   ○13. *Left common carotid artery:* Second branch arises posterior to the manubrium and slightly posterior and to the left of the brachiocephalic trunk. Ascends anterior to the trachea initially and then courses along the left side as it enters the neck posterior to the left SC joint.

   ○14. *Left subclavian artery:* Third branch arises posterior to the left common carotid artery. Ascends lateral to the trachea and left common carotid artery and exits the mediastinum posterior to the left SC joint.

○15. *Pulmonary trunk:* Arises anterior to the origin of the ascending aorta to then pass to the left. The pulmonary trunk divides into two branches:

   ○16. *Right pulmonary artery:* Courses posterior to the ascending aorta and superior vena cava to the hilum of the right lung

   ○17. *Left pulmonary artery*: Shorter than the right because of its proximity to the left lung

○18. *Ligamentum arteriosum:* Passes from the origin of the left pulmonary artery to the arch of the aorta and is an embryologic remnant of the ductus arteriosus. The *left recurrent laryngeal nerve* loops under the arch of the aorta in proximity to the ligamentum arteriosum.

○19. *Superior pulmonary veins:* Two veins (right and left) along with two inferior pulmonary veins drain into the left atrium posteriorly

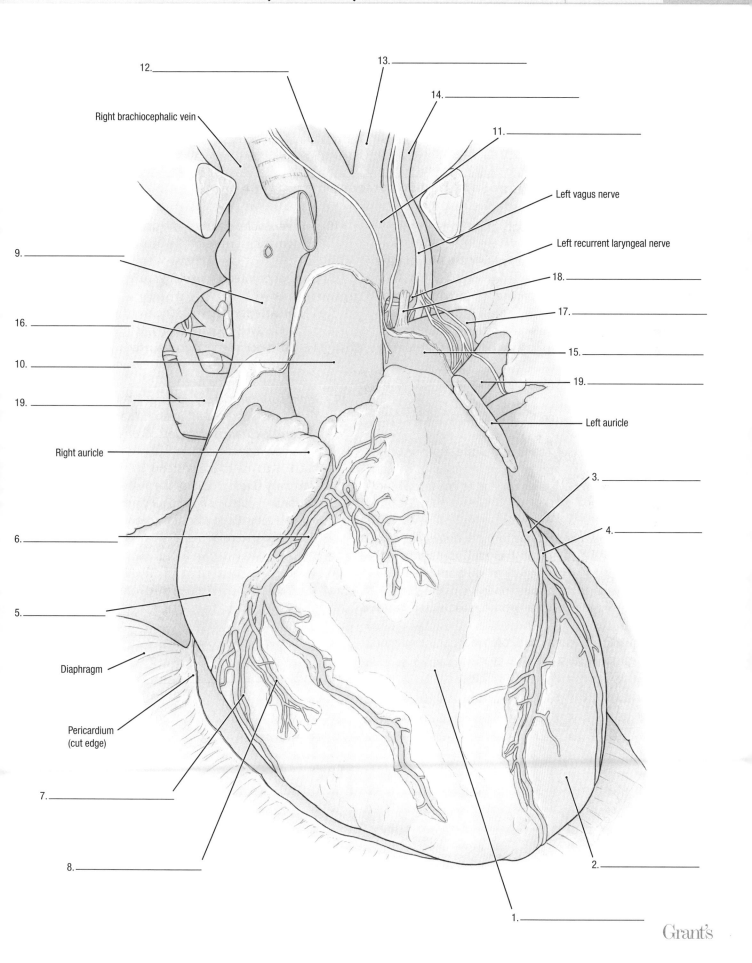

12.

13.

14.

Right brachiocephalic vein

11.

Left vagus nerve

9.

Left recurrent laryngeal nerve

18.

16.

17.

10.

15.

19.

19.

Left auricle

Right auricle

3.

6.

4.

5.

Diaphragm

Pericardium
(cut edge)

7.

2.

8.

1.

Grant's

The heart has been removed from the pericardial sac and the entirety of the posterior surface (base) and a portion of the inferior (diaphragmatic) surface are displayed. The _**visceral pericardium**_ (epicardium) remains adhered to the surface of the heart and proximal portions of the great vessels, except where it has been removed to demonstrate the vasculature of the heart. Visceral pericardium reflects on the great vessels to transition to the parietal pericardium forming the pericardial sac. The lines of reflection can be observed between the pulmonary veins, superior and inferior venae cavae, aorta, and pulmonary trunk.

COLOR each of the following using a different color for each structure:

○ 1. _**Left atrium:**_ Composes a majority of the posterior surface (base) of the heart

○ 2. _**Right pulmonary veins:**_ Enter the left atrium from the right lung

○ 3. _**Left pulmonary veins:**_ Enter the left atrium from the left lung

○ 4. _**Right atrium:**_ Occupies a small portion of the posterior surface (base) and is separated from the left atrium by the _**interatrial sulcus**_

○ 5. _**Superior vena cava:**_ Enters the superior aspect of the right atrium

○ 6. _**Inferior vena cava:**_ Enters the inferior aspect of the right atrium

○ 7. _**Ascending aorta:**_ Lies to the left of the superior vena cava

○ 8. _**Pulmonary trunk:**_ Lies anterior and to the left of the ascending aorta

The _**transverse pericardial sinus**_ forms during embryonic development of the heart and, in the adult, separates the outflow vessels (aorta and pulmonary trunk) from the inflow vessels (superior vena cava and pulmonary veins).

The posterior interventricular groove (sulcus) separates the ventricles:

○ 9. _**Right ventricle**_: Forms a small component of the inferior (diaphragmatic) surface of the heart

○ 10. _**Left ventricle:**_ Forms a majority of the inferior (diaphragmatic) surface of the heart

The posterior interventricular groove (sulcus) is occupied by two vessels:

○ 11. _**Middle cardiac vein:**_ Drains to the coronary sinus and travels with the posterior interventricular artery

○ 12. _**Posterior interventricular artery:**_ Typically originates from the right coronary artery and descends toward the apex of the heart

○ 13. _**Right coronary artery:**_ In a right-dominant heart gives rise to the posterior interventricular artery

○ 14. _**Circumflex branch of the left coronary artery:**_ Travels in the atrioventricular (coronary) sulcus; and in a left-dominant heart gives rise to the posterior interventricular artery

○ 15. _**Coronary sinus:**_ Occupies the posterior atrioventricular (coronary) sulcus and drains to the right atrium. All cardiac veins drain into the coronary sinus, except for the anterior cardiac veins.

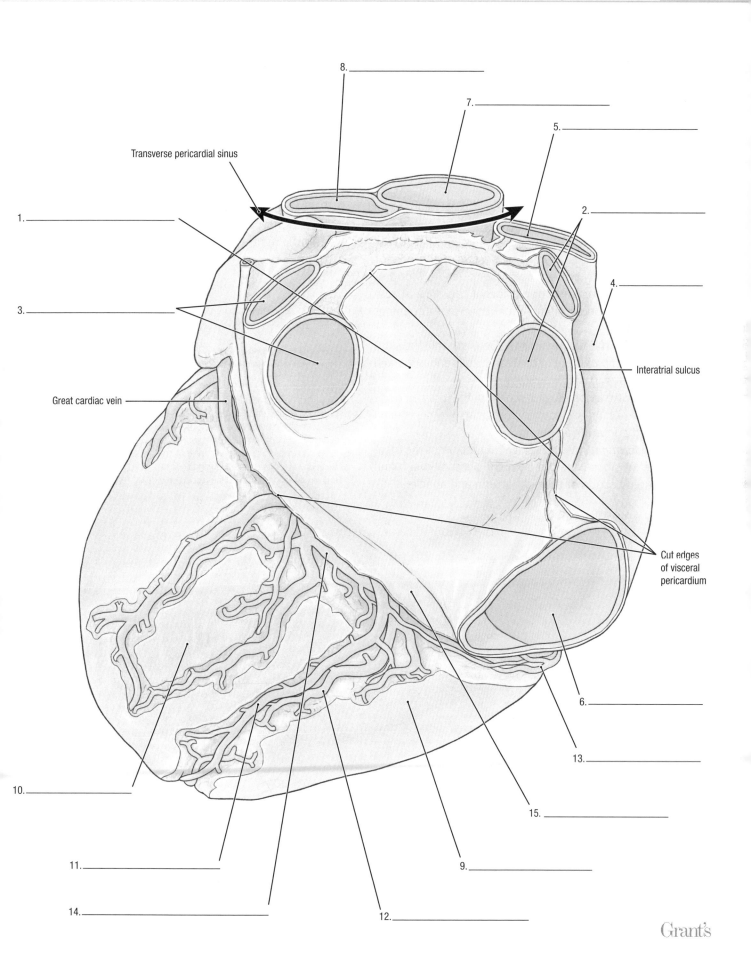

8. _____

7. _____

5. _____

Transverse pericardial sinus

1. _____

2. _____

3. _____

4. _____

Interatrial sulcus

Great cardiac vein

Cut edges
of visceral
pericardium

6. _____

10. _____

13. _____

15. _____

11. _____

9. _____

14. _____

12. _____

Grant's

3.12 | RIGHT ATRIUM

The right margin of the heart is displayed with the anterior wall of the right atrium cut and reflected to reveal the interior structures. The right atrium receives poorly oxygenated blood from the body through the superior and inferior venae cavae and from the heart through the coronary sinus and anterior cardiac veins. Blood exits the right atrium through the tricuspid valve to the right ventricle at the ***right atrioventricular orifice***.

COLOR each of the following using a different color for each structure:

○ 1. **Superior vena cava:** Opens directly into the right atrium superiorly

○ 2. **Inferior vena cava:** Opens into the inferior aspect of the right atrium and is guarded by a ***valve of the inferior cava*** to partially prevent backflow of venous blood

○ 3. **Sinus venarum:** Smooth portion of the right atrium where the superior and inferior venae cavae openings are located

○ 4. **Opening of the coronary sinus:** Occurs within the sinus venarum in proximity to the fossa ovalis and is marked by the ***valve of coronary sinus***

○ 5. **Fossa ovalis:** Embryologic remnant of the foramen ovale located within the sinus venarum as an oval depression along the interatrial septum

○ 6. **Crista terminalis:** Vertical ridge that separates the more posterior sinus venarum from the anterior rough and textured portion of the right atrium and auricle

○ 7. **Pectinate muscles:** Comprise the textured anterior portion of the right atrium and are primarily located in the right auricle

---

CLINICAL NOTE: ATRIAL SEPTAL DEFECTS

Atrial septal defect (ASD) is a congenital cardiac anomaly characterized by a defect in the interatrial septum. Small defects may be present in up to 25% of the adult population and typically do not result in hemodynamic abnormalities or clinical symptoms. Large ASDs may present in infancy and childhood with a heart murmur. Large ASDs allow oxygenated blood from the lungs in the left atrium to be shunted through the defect into the right atrium. Consequently, hypertrophy of the right atrium and ventricle and pulmonary arteries occurs, causing dyspnea (shortness of breath), fatigue, palpitations, atrial arrhythmias, and even heart failure.

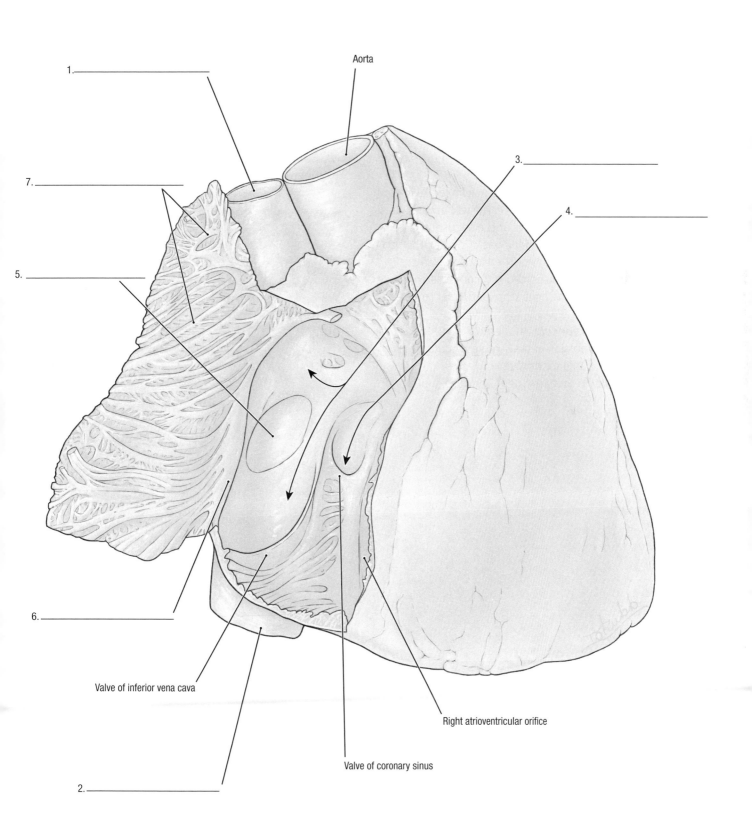

Aorta

1. _____

7. _____

5. _____

3. _____

4. _____

6. _____

Valve of inferior vena cava

2. _____

Valve of coronary sinus

Right atrioventricular orifice

Grant's

3.13 RIGHT VENTRICLE

The anterior (sternocostal) wall of the right ventricle is removed to reveal the interior structures. The right ventricle receives blood from the right atrium through the tricuspid valve and pumps blood through the pulmonary valve to the pulmonary trunk, which leads to the lungs.

COLOR each of the following using a different color for each structure:

○ 1. *Trabeculae carneae:* Numerous irregular muscular ridges that comprise a majority of the internal aspect of the right ventricle giving the walls a rough and textured appearance

○ 2. *Anterior papillary muscle:* One of three fingerlike inward projections from the trabeculae carneae. Each papillary muscle corresponds to a cusp of the tricuspid valve.

○ 3. *Tendinous cords* (chordae tendineae): Connect the papillary muscles to the cusps of the tricuspid valve

○ 4. *Tricuspid valve:* Located posteriorly, composed of three cusps, and occupies the right atrioventricular (tricuspid) orifice

○ 5. *Septomarginal trabecula* (moderator band): Extends from the inferior portion of the *interventricular septum* to the anterior papillary muscle

○ 6. *Pulmonary trunk:* Exits the right ventricle superiorly

○ 7. *Pulmonary valve:* Located superiorly, composed of three cusps, and guards the entrance to the pulmonary trunk

○ 8. *Conus arteriosus* (infundibulum)*:* Smooth area of the right ventricle before the pulmonary valve

---

CLINICAL NOTE: VENTRICULAR SEPTAL DEFECTS

Ventricular septal defect (VSD) is a congenital cardiac anomaly that can occur on its own or with other cardiac anomalies such as tetralogy of Fallot, atrioventricular canal defects, and transposition of great arteries. The defect may occur within the membranous, muscular, or both portions of the interventricular septum. Defects may be small and asymptomatic or large, up to 25 mm, and result in a left-to-right shunt of blood through the defect. A large VSD consequently results in elevated pulmonary blood flow and pulmonary artery pressures, reduced systemic cardiac output, and increased left ventricular volume load. Symptoms in infants include increased respiratory rate and fatigue, especially during feeding because of the increased cardiac output. Consequently, lack of adequate growth is commonly observed. Sweating may also occur because of increased sympathetic response.

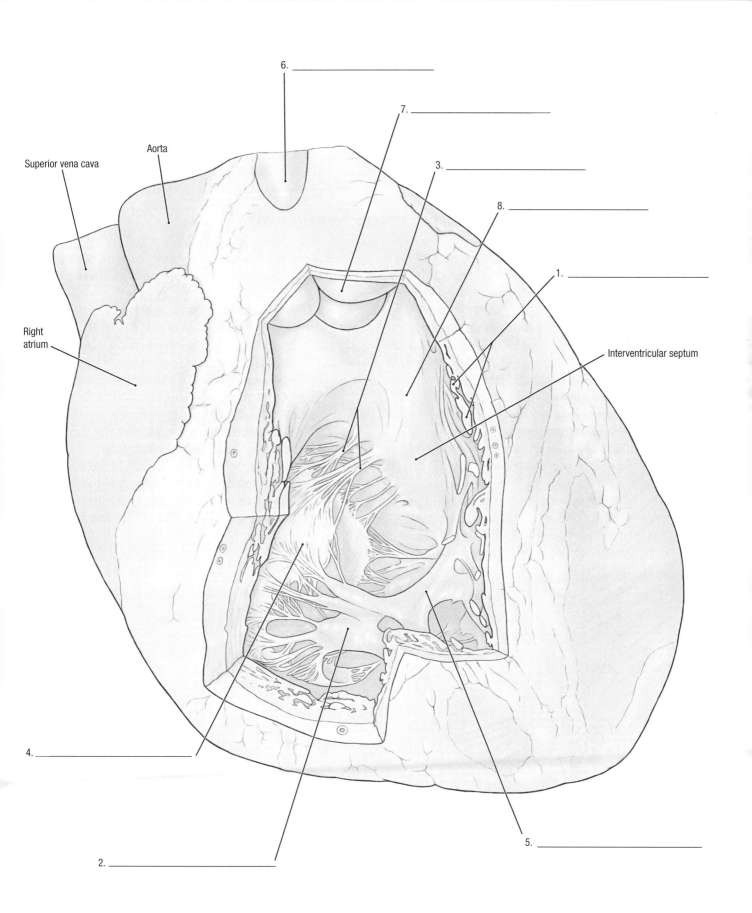

6. _____

7. _____

3. _____

8. _____

1. _____

Aorta

Superior vena cava

Right atrium

Interventricular septum

4. _____

2. _____

5. _____

Grant's

3.14A and B LEFT ATRIUM AND LEFT VENTRICLE

In A, the walls of the **_left ventricle_** and atrium have been opened up from the **_apex_** to the base of the heart by a diagonal cut passing between the left superior and left inferior pulmonary veins and through the posterior aspect of the mitral (bicuspid) valve.

In B, the left ventricle has been opened from the apex along the left margin of the heart continuing superiorly posterior to the **_pulmonary trunk_** to open the ascending aorta.

Oxygenated blood from the lungs is carried to the left atrium by four pulmonary veins. Blood is pumped from the left atrium through the mitral (bicuspid) valve to the left ventricle and then through the aortic valve into the ascending aorta.

COLOR each of the following using a different color for each structure:

○ 1. **_Left atrium:_** Internally composed of a smooth wall except for the internal aspect of the **_left auricle_**, where the wall is composed of pectinate muscles.

There are four pulmonary veins that enter the right atrium posteriorly:

○ 2. **_Left superior pulmonary vein_**
○ 3. **_Left inferior pulmonary vein_**
○ 4. **_Right superior pulmonary vein_**
○ 5. **_Right inferior pulmonary vein_**
○ 6. **_Mitral valve_** (bicuspid valve): Lies between the left atrium and left ventricle, occupying the left atrioventricular orifice
○ 7. **_Trabeculae carneae:_** Irregular, muscular ridges that compose the majority of the walls of the left ventricle (similar to the right ventricle)
○ 8. **_Papillary muscles:_** Two papillary muscles (anterior and posterior) project into the left ventricle

○ 9. **_Tendinous cords:_** Connect the cusps of the mitral valve to the papillary muscles within the left ventricle

The interventricular septum is located between the right and left ventricles and is composed of two parts:

○ 10. **_Muscular part of the interventricular septum:_** Forms the majority of the septum
○ 11. **_Membranous part of the interventricular septum:_** Forms superiorly and posteriorly replacing the muscle with a thin membrane
○ 12. **_Ascending aorta:_** Exits the left ventricle superiorly
○ 13. **_Aortic valve:_** Lies at the beginning of the ascending aorta separating it from the smooth area of the left ventricle, the aortic vestibule. The **_orifices of the left and right coronary arteries_** are visible immediately superior to the left and right cusps of the aortic valve, respectively.

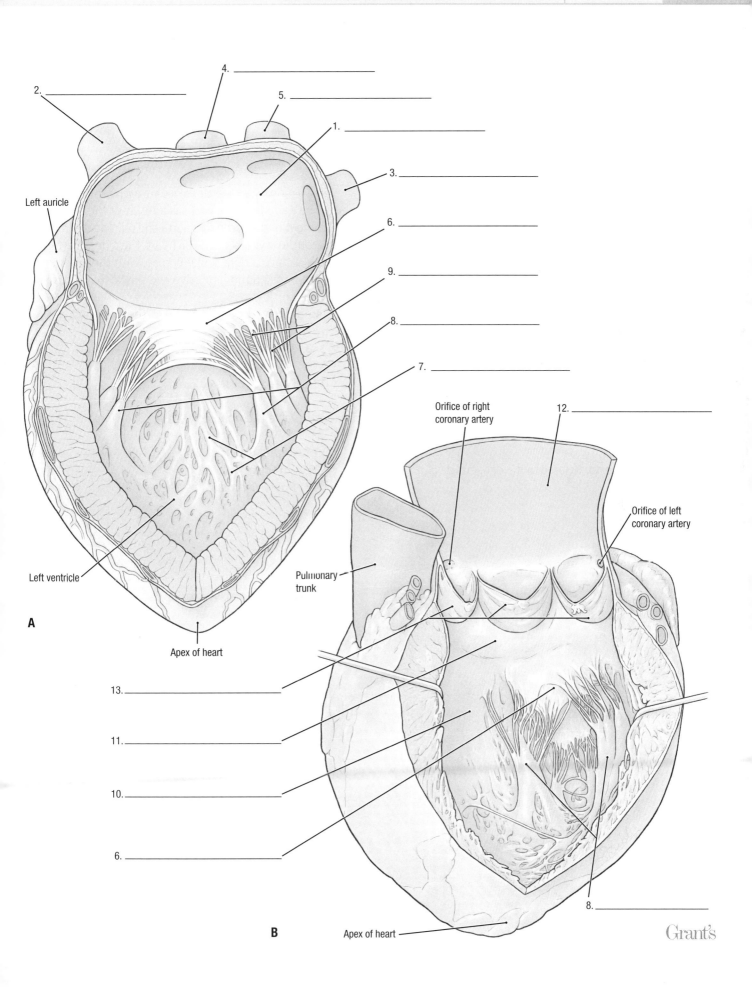

2. _____

4. _____

5. _____

1. _____

3. _____

6. _____

9. _____

8. _____

7. _____

Left auricle

Left ventricle

Apex of heart

A

Orifice of right
coronary artery

12. _____

Orifice of left
coronary artery

Pulmonary
trunk

13. _____

11. _____

10. _____

6. _____

8. _____

B

Apex of heart

Grant's

3.15 AORTIC AND PULMONARY VALVES

From a superior view, the ventricles are positioned anteriorly and to the left, whereas the atria are positioned posteriorly and to the right. The outflow vessels from the ventricles, the ascending aorta and pulmonary trunk, are positioned anterior to the atria.

COLOR each of the following using a different color for each structure:

○ 1. **Right ventricle:** Comprises a majority of the anterior (sternocostal) surface with a smaller portion composed of the left ventricle

○ 2. **Left ventricle:** Comprises only a minor aspect of the anterior (sternocostal) surface and the apex of the heart from the superior view

○ 3. **Left atrium:** Lies primarily in a posterior position with the **_left auricle_** extending anteriorly. Three of the four **_pulmonary veins_** can be visualized entering the left atrium.

○ 4. **Right atrium:** Lies primarily to the right, with the **_right auricle_** extending anteriorly

○ 5. **Superior vena cava:** Lies posterolaterally to the ascending aorta entering the right atrium

○ 6. **Pulmonary trunk:** Related to the left auricle as it curves anteriorly

○ 7. **Ascending aorta:** Related to the right auricle as it curves anteriorly

The pulmonary and aortic valves are each composed of three cusps. The naming of the cusps is a result of the embryologic development of the ascending aorta and pulmonary trunk from a single outflow vessel from the heart, the truncus arteriosus. Both valves have a right and left cusp, with the anterior cusp lying within the pulmonary valve and the posterior cusp lying within the aortic valve.

The pulmonary valve is composed of the following:

○ 8. **Right cusp**
○ 9. **Left cusp**
○ 10. **Anterior cusp**

The aortic valve is composed of the following:

○ 11. **Right cusp**
○ 12. **Left cusp**
○ 13. **Posterior cusp**

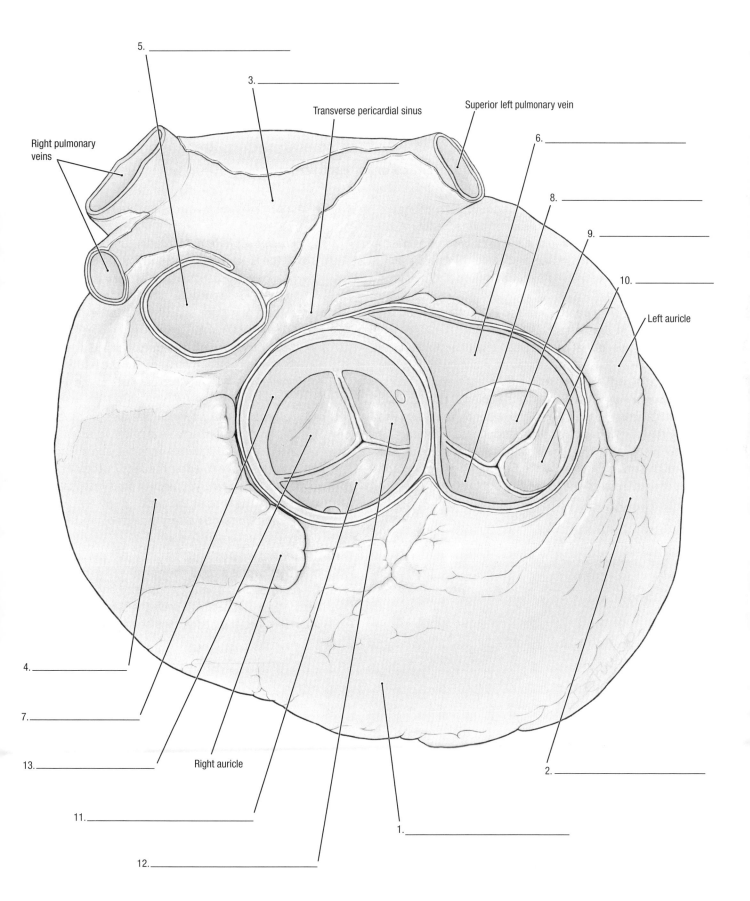

5. _____

3. _____

Transverse pericardial sinus

Superior left pulmonary vein

Right pulmonary veins

6. _____

8. _____

9. _____

10. _____

Left auricle

4. _____

7. _____

13. _____

Right auricle

11. _____

12. _____

1. _____

2. _____

Grant's

| 3.16 | **SUPERFICIAL DISSECTION OF SUPERIOR MEDIASTINUM** |

The sternum, ribs, and pleurae have been removed, to view the contents of the superior mediastinum. The superior mediastinum is superior to the transverse thoracic plane. The transverse thoracic plane passes through the sternal angle and the T4/T5 IV disk.

From anterior to posterior, the contents of the superior mediastinum are as follows: thymus, veins, arteries, trachea, esophagus, and thoracic duct.

COLOR each of the following using a different color for each structure:

○ 1. **Thymus:** Lies immediately posterior to the manubrium and extends inferiorly to the anterior mediastinum before puberty. In the adult, it is rare to observe as much remaining thymus tissue as depicted in this image. The thymus is replaced by fat and fibrous tissue with increasing age.

○ 2. **Right brachiocephalic vein:** Vertically oriented and lies to the right of the trachea

○ 3. **Left brachiocephalic vein:** Obliquely oriented and lies immediately posterior to the thymus and anterior to the proximal portions of the three branches of the arch of aorta

○ 4. **Superior vena cava:** Forms by the union of the right and left brachiocephalic veins. The superior vena cava lies within the right side of the superior mediastinum. The terminal half of the superior vena cava lies in the middle mediastinum inferior to the **fibrous pericardium** and posterolateral to the **ascending aorta**.

The arch of the aorta gives rise to three branches:

○ 5. **Brachiocephalic artery** (trunk): Initially lies anterior to the trachea and posterior to the left brachiocephalic vein. Ascends superolaterally to the right side of the trachea and bifurcates into the right common carotid and right subclavian arteries posterior to the right SC joint.

○ 6. **Left common carotid artery:** Initially lies anterior to the trachea and posterior to the left brachiocephalic vein. Ascends into the neck to the left of the trachea.

○ 7. **Left subclavian artery:** Initially lies posterior to the left brachiocephalic vein and left common carotid artery. Ascends lateral to trachea and left common carotid artery to enter the root of the neck.

○ 8. **Right subclavian artery:** Branch of brachiocephalic artery that enters the root of the neck

○ 9. **Right common carotid artery:** Branch of brachiocephalic artery that enters the neck

○10. **Trachea:** Lies posterior to proximal portions of the branches of the arch of the aorta

○11. **Esophagus:** Lies primarily posterior and to the left of the trachea. Unlike the trachea, the esophagus continues inferiorly into the posterior mediastinum.

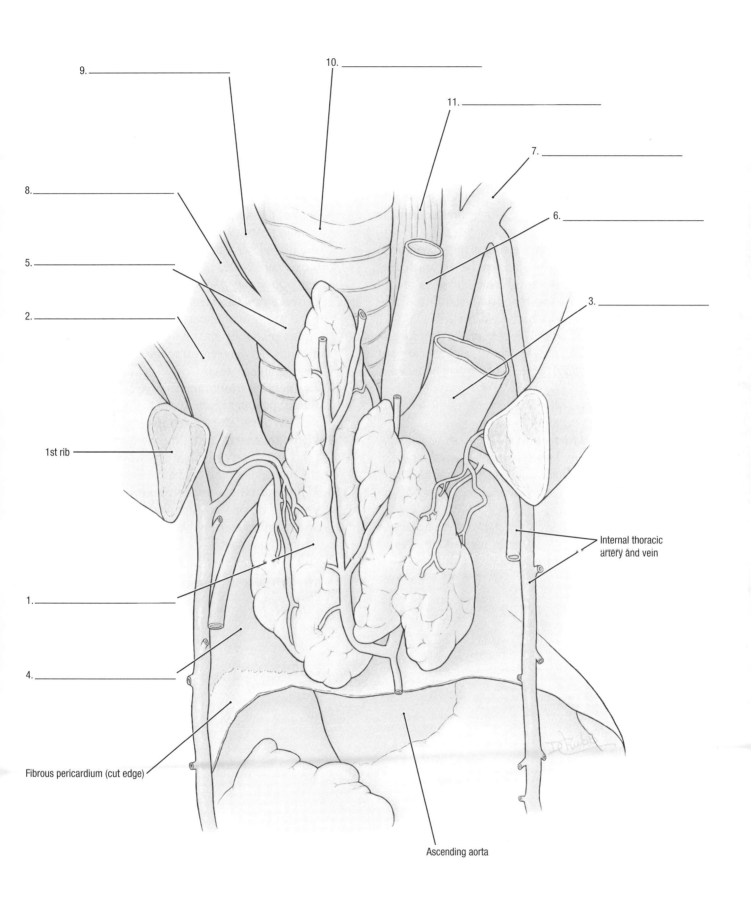

9.

10.

11.

7.

8.

6.

5.

2.

3.

1st rib

Internal thoracic
artery and vein

1.

4.

Fibrous pericardium (cut edge)

Ascending aorta

Grant's

3.17 SUPERIOR MEDIASTINUM WITH THYMUS RESECTED

The thymus has been resected to better visualize the deeper structures of the superior mediastinum. The nerves of the superior mediastinum have been added in this image.

COLOR each of the following using a different color for each structure:

1. **Superior vena cava:** Forms by the union of the left and right brachiocephalic veins

2. **Left brachiocephalic vein:** Less vertically oriented and more than twice as long as the right brachiocephalic vein

3. **Right brachiocephalic vein:** Superior to the superior vena cava on the right side. The union of the left brachiocephalic vein separates it from the superior vena cava.

4. **Arch of the aorta:** Lies posterior to the left brachiocephalic vein and gives rise to three branches:

   5. **Brachiocephalic artery:** Divides into the *right subclavian artery* to supply the right upper limb and *right common carotid artery* to supply the right neck and head

   6. **Left common carotid artery:** Supplies the left neck and head

   7. **Left subclavian artery:** Supplies the left upper limb

8. **Right phrenic nerve:** Travels along the lateral aspect of the right brachiocephalic vein, superior vena cava, and fibrous pericardium. Passes anterior to the root of the right lung.

9. **Left phrenic nerve:** Travels along the lateral surface of the arch of the aorta and fibrous pericardium. Passes anterior to the root of the left lung.

10. **Left vagus nerve:** Enters the superior mediastinum between the left common carotid artery and left subclavian artery and then passes along the lateral aspect of the arch of the aorta. Here, the left vagus nerve passes in a more posterior direction than the left phrenic nerve. Along the lateral aspect of the arch of the aorta, the left vagus nerve gives off branches to the *cardiac plexus* and *pulmonary plexus.*

11. **Left recurrent laryngeal nerve:** Arises from the left vagus nerve at the inferior border of the arch of the aorta, lies within proximity to the ligamentum arteriosum, and ascends between the *trachea* and *esophagus* along their lateral aspects.

12. **Ligamentum arteriosum:** Embryologic remnant between the left pulmonary artery and the arch of the aorta. Lies medial to the left recurrent laryngeal nerve.

13. **Right vagus nerve:** Enters the thorax anterior to the right subclavian artery and then courses posteroinferiorly on the right side of the trachea

14. **Right recurrent laryngeal nerve:** Arises from the right vagus nerve and loops around the right subclavian artery and ascends between the trachea and esophagus along their lateral aspects

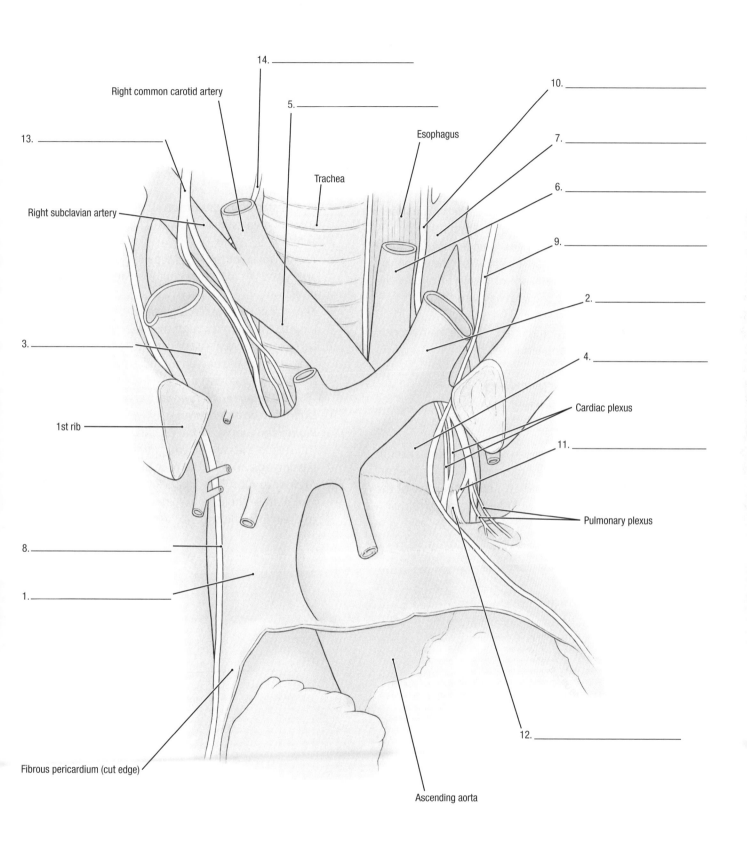

14. _____

Right common carotid artery

5. _____

Esophagus

10. _____

Trachea

13. _____

7. _____

Right subclavian artery

6. _____

9. _____

2. _____

3. _____

4. _____

1st rib

Cardiac plexus

11. _____

Pulmonary plexus

8. _____

1. _____

12. _____

Fibrous pericardium (cut edge)

Ascending aorta

Grant's

3.18 DEEP DISSECTION OF SUPERIOR MEDIASTINUM AND PULMONARY VESSELS

The brachiocephalic veins, superior vena cava, and the arch of aorta and its branches have been cut and mostly removed from this image to demonstrate the deepest structures of the superior mediastinum. The heart has been removed from the middle mediastinum to demonstrate the pulmonary vessels in relation to the **_lungs_** and **_main bronchi_**.

COLOR each of the following using a different color for each structure:

Pulmonary Vessels in the Middle Mediastinum

1. *Right pulmonary artery:* Longer branch from the **_pulmonary trunk_** extending to the hilum of the right lung. At the hilum, lies anterior to the right main bronchus.
2. *Left pulmonary artery:* Shorter branch from the pulmonary trunk extending to the hilum of the left lung. At the hilum, lies superior to the left main bronchus.

   The pulmonary veins lie anteroinferior to the main bronchi of the hilum and the right and left lungs.

3. *Left and right superior pulmonary veins*
4. *Left and right inferior pulmonary veins*

Superior Mediastinum

The **_trachea_** descends into the superior mediastinum anterior to the esophagus slightly right of the median plane. The trachea ends within the superior mediastinum at the level of the sternal angle by dividing into the right and left main (primary) bronchi.

5. *Esophagus:* Extends from the pharynx in the neck to the stomach in the abdomen, passing through the superior and posterior mediastinum. The esophagus enters the superior mediastinum between the trachea and vertebral column.
6. *Arch of aorta (cut):* Passes superiorly over left pulmonary artery and left main bronchus in an anterior-to-posterior direction
7. *Thoracic aorta:* Descends posterior to the root of the left lung to traveling through the posterior mediastinum
8. *Left vagus nerve:* Passes posterior to the root of the left lung entering the posterior mediastinum. Before exiting the superior mediastinum, the left vagus nerve gives off:
    9. *Left recurrent laryngeal nerve*
10. *Ligamentum arteriosum*
11. *Right vagus nerve:* Along with the left vagus nerve contributes to the cardiac and pulmonary plexuses before passing posterior to the root of the right lung
12. *Arch of azygos vein (cut):* Passes superiorly over the root of the right lung in a posterior-to-anterior direction to drain into the superior vena cava

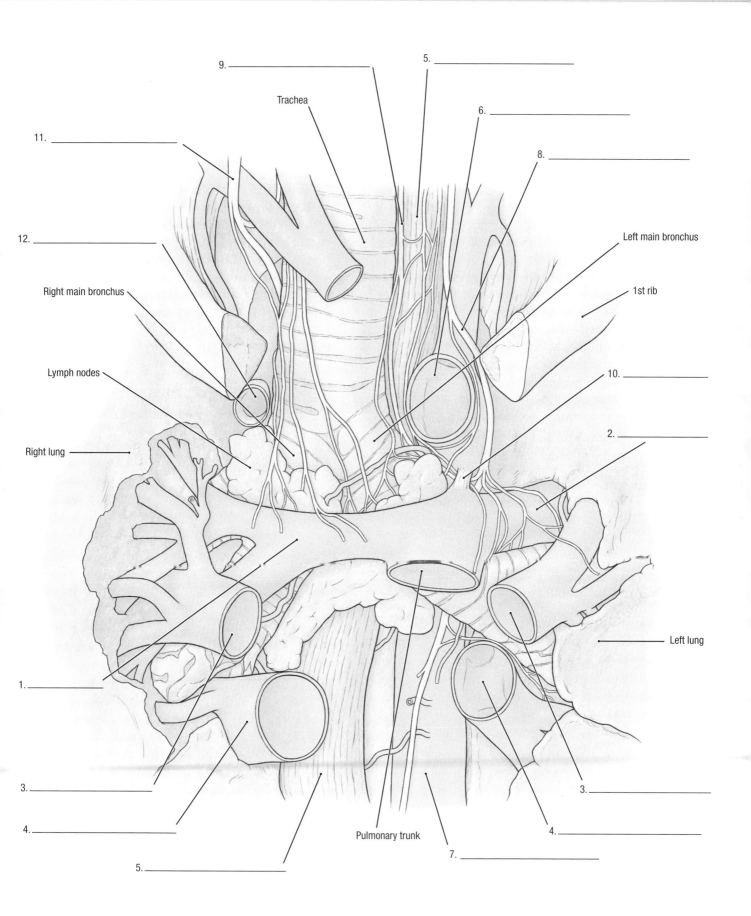

9. _____

5. _____

Trachea

6. _____

11. _____

8. _____

Left main bronchus

12. _____

1st rib

Right main bronchus

Lymph nodes

10. _____

Right lung

2. _____

Left lung

1. _____

3. _____

3. _____

4. _____

4. _____

5. _____

Pulmonary trunk

7. _____

Grant's

3.19   AZYGOS SYSTEM OF VEINS

The azygos system of veins is an asymmetrical network of veins on either side of the vertebral column that drains the back and thoracoabdominal walls and mediastinal viscera. Commonly, there is significant variation in the course and anastomotic connections of the azygos system.

COLOR each of the following using a different color for each structure:

○ 1. *Azygos vein:* Arises on the right side only as a direct connection between the **superior** and **inferior venae cavae**. The azygos vein ascends in the posterior mediastinum along the lateral or anterolateral aspect of the vertebral bodies.

○ 2. *Arch of the azygos vein:* Forms as it passes from a posterior-to-anterior direction over the right root of the lung to join the superior vena cava

○ 3. *Right posterior intercostal veins:* Drain the right posterior thoracic wall primarily to the azygos vein

○ 4. *Hemiazygos vein:* Arises on the left side by the junction of the left subcostal and ascending lumbar veins in the upper posterior abdominal wall. Ascends along the left side of the vertebral column posterior to the thoracic aorta to the level of the T9 vertebra. At this level, it crosses to the right side passing posterior to the thoracic **aorta**, thoracic duct, and esophagus to join the azygos vein.

○ 5. *Accessory hemiazygos vein:* Begins at the medial end of the 4th or 5th intercostal space and descends along the left side of the vertebral column from T5 through T8. Like the hemiazygos vein, it crosses to the right side to join the azygos vein. It may cross independently or may join the hemiazygos vein before joining the azygos vein. It may also have a connection to the left superior intercostal vein.

○ 6. *Left posterior intercostal veins:* Are split in their drainage patterns. The inferior left three posterior intercostal veins along with the inferior esophageal and several mediastinal veins drain into the hemiazygos vein. The 4th to 8th left posterior intercostal veins and left bronchial veins typically drain into the accessory hemiazygos vein.

○ 7. *Left superior intercostal vein:* Typically formed from the 2nd to 4th posterior intercostal veins and typically drains into the **left brachiocephalic vein**. A superior intercostal vein also exists on the right side which typically drains into the arch of the azygos (not shown).

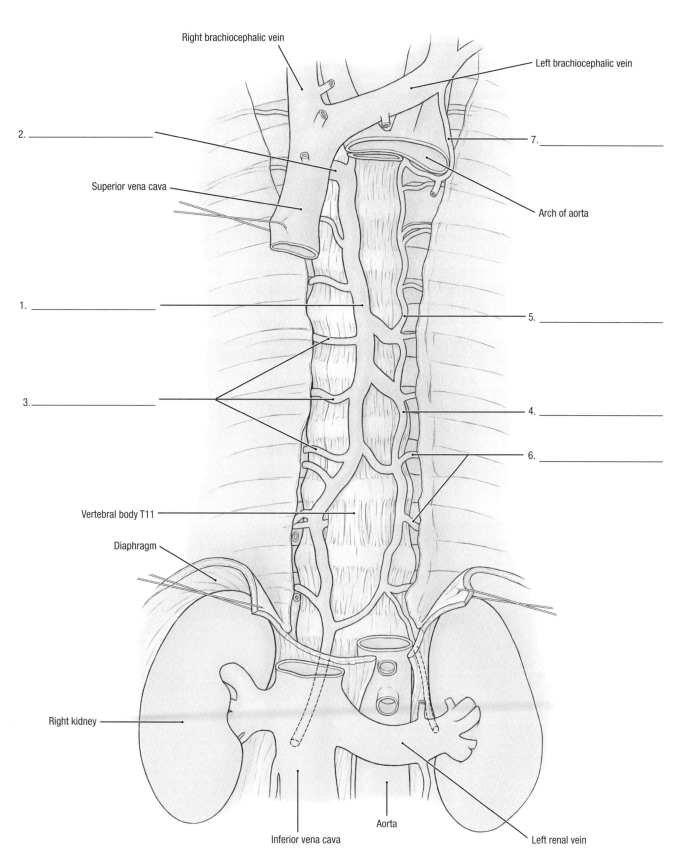

Right brachiocephalic vein

Left brachiocephalic vein

2. _____

7. _____

Superior vena cava

Arch of aorta

1. _____

5. _____

3. _____

4. _____

6. _____

Vertebral body T11

Diaphragm

Right kidney

Inferior vena cava

Aorta

Left renal vein

Grant's

3.20 RIGHT SIDE OF THE MEDIASTINUM

The right lateral thoracic wall and the right lung have been removed. The **_costal_** and **_mediastinal parts of the parietal pleura_** have been removed, except for a portion overlying the anterior thoracic wall and the majority of the lateral aspect of the pericardial sac, respectively. The right side of the mediastinum is dominated by venous structures.

COLOR each of the following using a different color for each structure:

○ 1. **_Azygos vein:_** Receives a majority of the right posterior intercostal veins

○ 2. **_Arch of the azygos vein:_** Courses superiorly over the root of the right lung to drain into the **_superior vena cava_**

○ 3. **_Right superior intercostal vein:_** Formed by the union of the 2nd to 4th right posterior intercostal veins and drains into the arch of the azygos vein

○ 4. **_Trachea:_** Only located in the superior mediastinum between the vascular structures and the esophagus

○ 5. **_Esophagus:_** Located in both the superior and posterior mediastinum anterior to the vertebral bodies

○ 6. **_Right phrenic nerve:_** Travels along the lateral aspect of the **_right brachiocephalic vein_**, superior vena cava, and the fibrous pericardium passing anterior to the root of lung structures en route to the **_diaphragm_**

○ 7. **_Right vagus nerve:_** Travels lateral to the trachea giving off branches to the cardiac and pulmonary plexus, passes medial to the arch of the azygos vein and then posterior to the root of the right lung.

The right vagus nerve, along with the left vagus nerve, forms the **_esophageal plexus_** along the surface of the esophagus.

○ 8. **_Sympathetic trunk:_** Travels along the lateral aspect of the vertebral bodies composed of **_sympathetic ganglia_** and the ascending and descending fibers between them.

○ 9. **_Intercostal nerves_**: Connected to the sympathetic trunk by **_rami communicantes_**

○ 10. **_Greater thoracic splanchnic nerve:_** Forms from branches that arise medially from the T5-T9 levels of the sympathetic trunk

○ 11. **_Posterior intercostal artery:_** Travels through the intercostal space with **_posterior intercostal vein_** superior to it and the intercostal nerve inferior to it forming a neurovascular bundle (vein-artery-nerve; VAN).

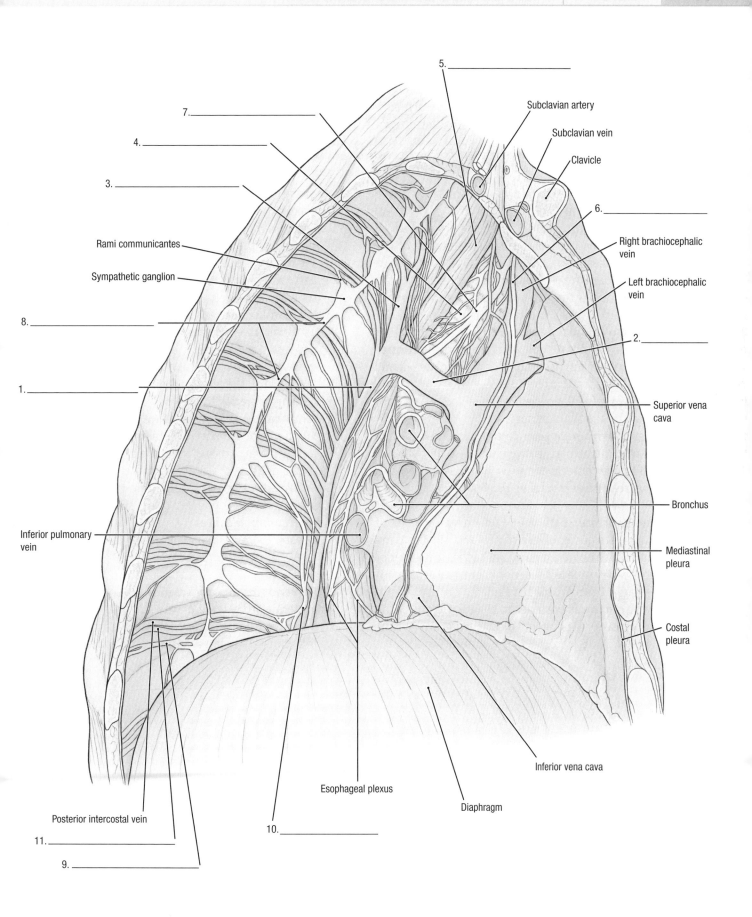

5.

Subclavian artery

Subclavian vein

Clavicle

7.

4.

3.

6.

Rami communicantes

Right brachiocephalic vein

Sympathetic ganglion

Left brachiocephalic vein

8.

2.

1.

Superior vena cava

Bronchus

Inferior pulmonary vein

Mediastinal pleura

Costal pleura

Inferior vena cava

Posterior intercostal vein

Esophageal plexus

11.

Diaphragm

9.

10.

Grant's

3.21 LEFT SIDE OF THE MEDIASTINUM

The left lateral thoracic wall and the left lung have been removed. The **_costal_** and **_mediastinal parts of the parietal pleura_** have been removed except for a portion overlying the anterior thoracic wall and the majority of the lateral aspect of the pericardial sac, respectively. The left side of the mediastinum is dominated by the arterial system.

COLOR each of the following using a different color for each structure:

○ 1. **_Arch of the aorta:_** Courses over the structures of the root of the left lung

○ 2. **_Left common carotid artery:_** Branches from the arch of the aorta and courses through the left side of the superior mediastinum

○ 3. **_Left subclavian artery:_** Branches from the arch of the aorta and courses through the left side of the superior mediastinum

○ 4. **_Descending (thoracic) aorta:_** Descends along the left side of the vertebral bodies posterior to the root of the left lung, giving rise to bronchial, esophageal, and posterior intercostal arteries

○ 5. **_Hemiazygos vein:_** Inferior, vertically oriented vein partially obscured by the thoracic aorta

○ 6. **_Accessory hemiazygos vein:_** Vertically oriented, located superior to the hemiazygos vein, and also partially obscured by the thoracic aorta

○ 7. **_Left posterior intercostal veins:_** Primarily drain into either the accessory hemiazygos or hemiazygos veins

○ 8. **_Left superior intercostal vein:_** Formed by the union of the 2nd to 4th posterior intercostal veins, similar to the right side of the mediastinum. Unlike the right superior intercostal vein, the left superior intercostal vein drains into the **_left brachiocephalic vein._**

○ 9. **_Thoracic duct:_** Lies posterior to the **_esophagus_** in the inferior aspect of the posterior mediastinum. However, at the level of T4-T6 it crosses to the posterolateral aspect of the esophagus and continues to ascend through the superior mediastinum.

○ 10. **_Left phrenic nerve:_** Passes along the lateral aspect of the arch of the aorta and fibrous pericardium anterior to the root of the left lung before piercing the **_diaphragm_**

○ 11. **_Left vagus nerve:_** Passes between the left common carotid and left subclavian arteries to then travel along the lateral aspect of the arch of the aorta posterior to the left phrenic nerve. Inferior to the arch of the aorta, the left vagus nerve gives rise to the **_left recurrent laryngeal nerve,_** which passes posterior to the **_ligamentum arteriosum_**. The left vagus nerve continues to descend passing posterior to the root of the left lung to then form the esophageal plexus with the right vagus nerve.

○ 12. **_Sympathetic trunk:_** Travels along the lateral aspect of the vertebral bodies in the same organizational pattern as the right sympathetic trunk

○ 13. **_Intercostal nerves:_** Course through the intercostal spaces and are connected to the sympathetic trunk by **_rami communicantes_**

○ 14. **_Greater thoracic splanchnic nerve:_** Forms from medially directed fibers from the T5-T9 levels of the sympathetic trunk

○ 15. **_Posterior intercostal arteries:_** Arranged in the same pattern as they were on the left side, with the posterior intercostal vein superior and the intercostal nerve inferior to them in each intercostal space (VAN).

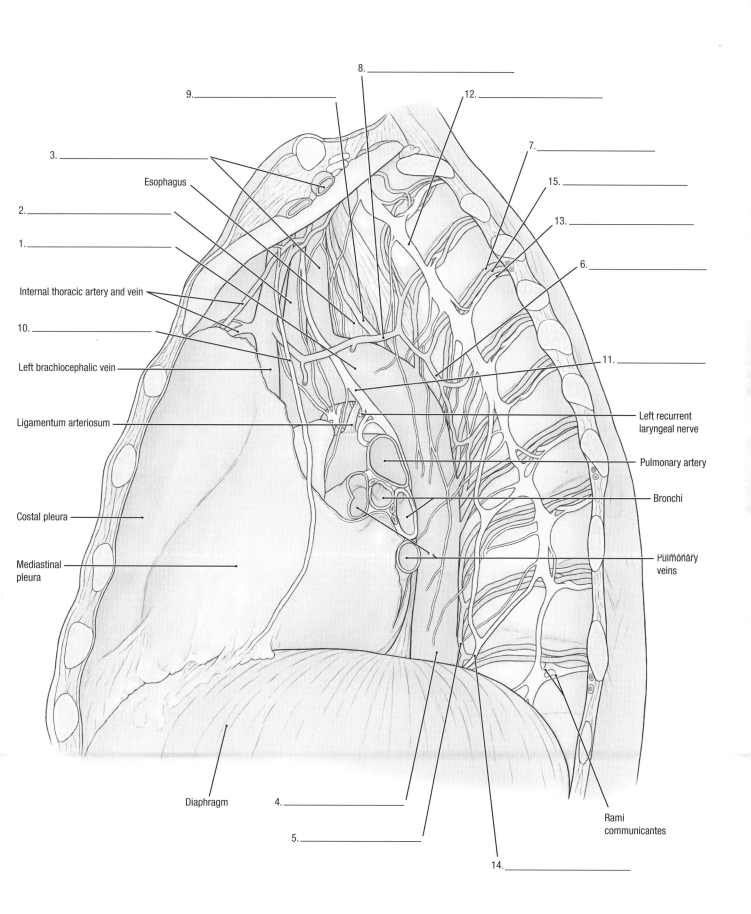

8. _____

9. _____

12. _____

3. _____

Esophagus

7. _____

2. _____

15. _____

1. _____

13. _____

6. _____

Internal thoracic artery and vein

10. _____

11. _____

Left brachiocephalic vein

Ligamentum arteriosum

Left recurrent
laryngeal nerve

Pulmonary artery

Bronchi

Costal pleura

Mediastinal
pleura

Pulmonary
veins

Diaphragm

4. _____

Rami
communicantes

5. _____

14. _____

3.22   DIAPHRAGM AND PERICARDIAL SAC

Superior view of the diaphragm and inferior aspect of the pericardial sac. The diaphragm separates the thoracic and abdominal cavities and is the primary muscle of inspiration. The diaphragmatic pleura has been mostly removed from the diaphragm, except near the reflections to the costal pleura along the thoracic walls and to the mediastinal pleura along the lateral aspects of the mediastinum.

COLOR each of the following using a different color for each structure:

○ 1. *Pericardial sac:* Located on the anteromedial aspect of the diaphragm with two-thirds projecting to the left

○ 2. *Central tendon of the diaphragm:* Located centrally and is shaped like a boomerang extending to the right and left sides

○ 3. *Muscular part of the diaphragm:* Located peripherally as it originates from the superior lumbar vertebrae and costal margin

○ 4. *Inferior vena cava:* Passes through the caval opening in the central tendon just to the right of midline at the level of T8

○ 5. *Costal pleura:* Portion of the parietal pleura that lines the internal aspect of the ribs and sternum

○ 6. *Diaphragmatic pleura:* Portion of the parietal pleura that lines the superior aspect of the diaphragm

The paired *costodiaphragmatic recesses* are potential spaces located between the reflections of the parietal pleura from the costal pleura to the diaphragmatic pleura.

○ 7. *Mediastinal pleura:* Portion of the parietal pleura that lines the lateral aspects of the contents of the mediastinum

The paired *costomediastinal recesses* are potential spaces located posterior to the lateral *sternum* and costal cartilages between the costal pleura and the mediastinal pleura.

○ 8. *Esophagus:* Located posterior to the pericardial sac and passes through the esophageal hiatus of the diaphragm at the level of T10

○ 9. *Thoracic* (descending) *aorta:* Located posterior and to the left of the esophagus and passes through the aortic hiatus, an opening posterior to the diaphragm

○10. *Azygos vein:* Originates in the abdomen via the union of the right subcostal and ascending lumbar veins and typically enters the thoracic cavity via the aortic hiatus

○11. *Thoracic duct:* Medial to the thoracic aorta, posterior to the esophagus, anterior the vertebral bodies, and medial to the azygos vein. The thoracic duct passes through the aortic hiatus into the thoracic cavity from its origin of the cisterna chyli in the abdomen.

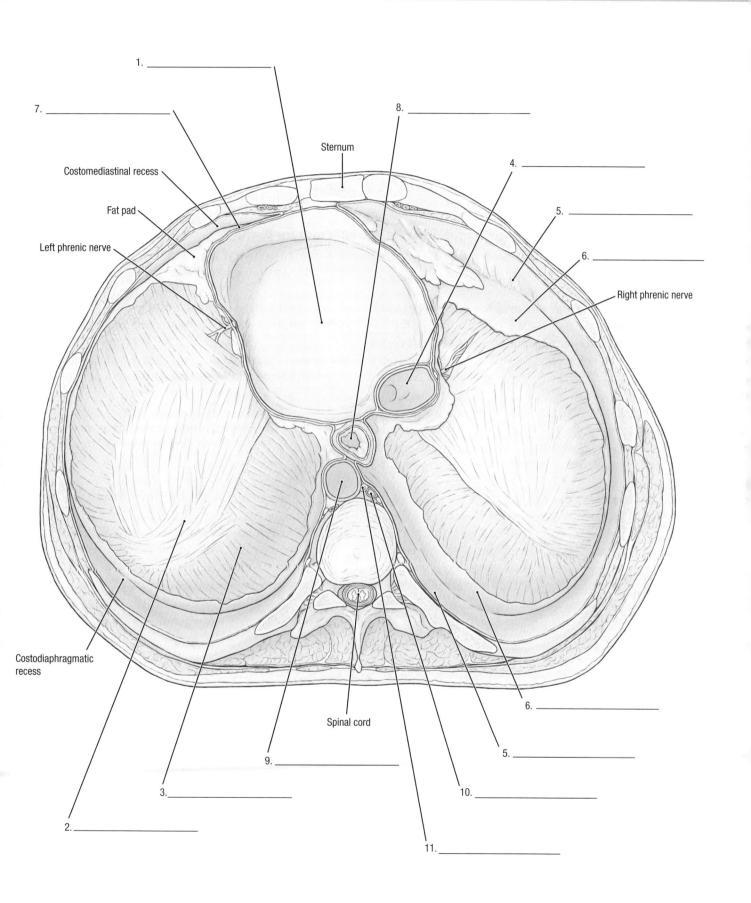

1. _____

7. _____

Sternum

8. _____

4. _____

Costomediastinal recess

5. _____

Fat pad

6. _____

Left phrenic nerve

Right phrenic nerve

Costodiaphragmatic recess

6. _____

Spinal cord

5. _____

9. _____

3. _____

10. _____

2. _____

11. _____

Grant's

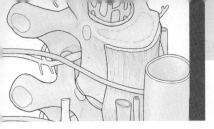

CHAPTER 4

Abdomen

The anterolateral abdominal wall is bounded by the 7th to 10th ribs and xiphoid process of the sternum along with inguinal ligament, iliac crests, pubic crests, and pubic symphysis. From superficial to deep, the wall is composed of skin, subcutaneous tissue, muscle and aponeurosis, deep fascia, and parietal peritoneum.

In this image, the skin and most of the subcutaneous tissue have been removed, except for two small areas along the inferior aspect of the right abdominal wall. The subcutaneous layer is shown reflected on the inferior aspect of the left abdominal wall. The anterior layer of the rectus sheath has been reflected on the left side.

COLOR each of the following structures using a different color for each:

Inferior to the umbilicus, the subcutaneous tissue is arranged in two layers:

○ 1. *Fatty layer of subcutaneous tissue (Camper fascia)*: Variable amount of fatty tissue immediately deep to the skin

○ 2. *Membranous layer of subcutaneous tissue (Scarpa fascia)*: Thin membranous layer deep to superficial fatty layer and superficial to musculoaponeurotic layers

The muscles of the anterolateral wall are arranged similarly to the muscles of the thoracic wall. Three muscles compose the anterolateral wall, with their fibers coursing in varying orientation to each other.

○ 3. *External oblique muscle:* The most superficial of the three anterolateral muscles on each side, primarily courses in an inferomedial direction (like "hands in a pocket"). Superolaterally, fibers interdigitate with the **serratus anterior**. The muscle fibers become the **aponeurosis of the external oblique** at the midclavicular line and

continue to run superficial (anterior) to the rectus abdominis muscle to the **linea alba**.

Unlike the thoracic region, there is no anterior midline vertical bone equivalent to the sternum. Instead, one primary vertical muscle reinforced with the aponeurotic layers of the anterolateral muscles exists in its place to allow for mobility of the intestines and for greater expansion of the abdomen after a large meal or during pregnancy.

○ 4. *Rectus abdominis muscle:* Paired, principal vertical muscle of the anterior abdominal wall. Wider superiorly than inferiorly and separated by the linea alba from each other.

○ 5. *Anterior rectus sheath:* Covers the anterior aspect of the rectus abdominis muscle

○ 6. *Tendinous intersections:* Attachment of the rectus abdominis muscle to the anterior rectus sheath at three or more transverse rows, creating bulging muscles between when tensed ("six pack")

External oblique and Rectus abdominis

Muscle	Proximal Attachment	Distal Attachment	Innervation	Action
External oblique	External surfaces of 5th-12th ribs	Linea alba, pubic tubercle, and anterior half of iliac crest	Thoracoabdominal nerves (T7-T11 spinal nerves) and subcostal nerve	Compresses abdominal viscera and rotates trunk
Rectus abdominis	Pubic symphysis and pubic crest	Xiphoid process and 5th-7th costal cartilages	Thoracoabdominal nerves (anterior rami T6-T11) and subcostal nerve	Flexes trunk and compresses abdominal viscera

Neurovasculature of Anterolateral Abdominal Wall

○ 7. *Superficial epigastric artery and vein:* Branch of the femoral artery/tributary of great saphenous vein running in subcutaneous tissue to/from the umbilicus

○ 8. *Superficial circumflex iliac artery and vein:* Branch of femoral artery/tributary of great saphenous vein running in subcutaneous tissue along inguinal ligament

○ 9. *External pudendal artery and vein:* Branch of femoral artery/tributary of great saphenous vein running in subcutaneous tissue to/from the pubic bone

○ 10. *Lateral abdominal cutaneous branches:* Sensory branches from T7 to T11 that emerge from the musculature of the anterolateral wall to run through the subcutaneous tissue

○ 11. *Anterior abdominal cutaneous branches:* Sensory branches from T7 to T11 that pierce the rectus sheath to enter the subcutaneous tissue. T7-T9 supply the skin superior to the umbilicus; T10 supplies the skin around the **umbilicus** and T11 supplies the skin immediately inferior to the umbilicus.

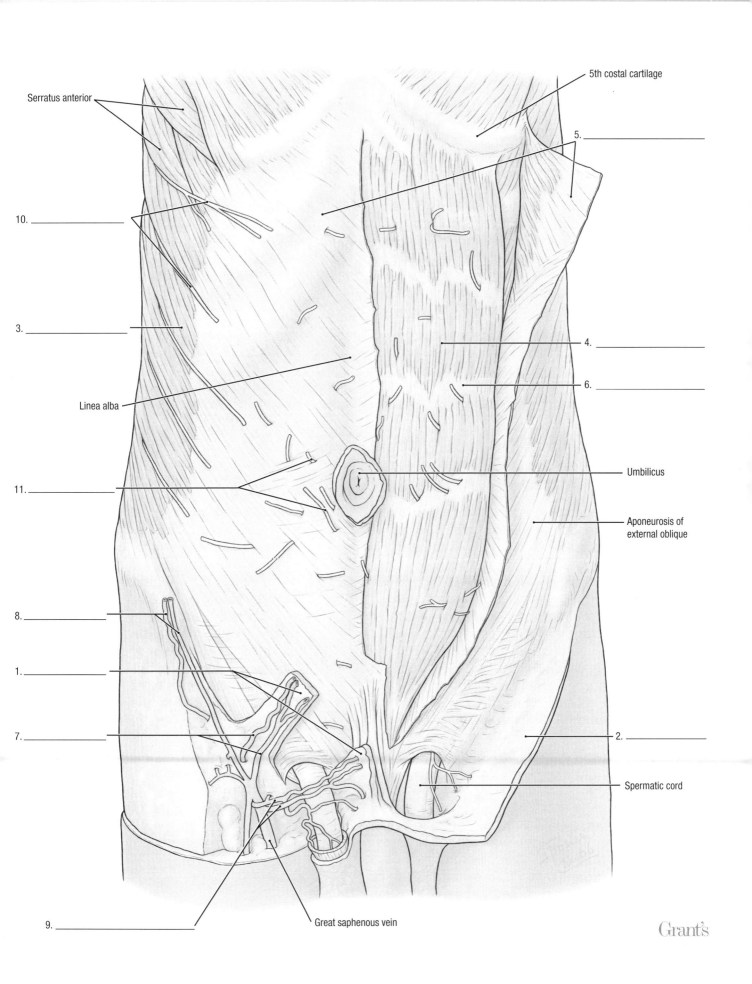

Serratus anterior

5th costal cartilage

5. _____

10. _____

3. _____

4. _____

Linea alba

6. _____

11. _____

Umbilicus

Aponeurosis of
external oblique

8. _____

1. _____

7. _____

2. _____

Spermatic cord

9. _____

Great saphenous vein

Grant's

4.2 DEEP ANTEROLATERAL ABDOMINAL WALL

On the right side, the muscular portion of the ***external oblique*** has been removed, with its aponeurosis and contribution to the anterior rectus sheath left intact. On the left side, the anterior rectus sheath and ***rectus abdominis muscle*** have been removed to demonstrate the posterior layer of the rectus sheath. In addition, the muscular portion of the internal oblique muscle has been cut vertically to reveal the deeper structures of the anterolateral abdominal wall.

COLOR each of the following structures using a different color for each:

◯ 1. *Internal oblique muscle:* Intermediate muscle of the anterolateral abdominal wall. The muscle fibers spread out superomedially perpendicular to the external oblique fibers. Inferior to the level of the **anterior superior iliac spine (ASIS)**, the muscle fibers course in a more horizontal direction. The fibers become aponeurotic at the midclavicular line and continue medially to the **linea alba**.

◯ 2. *Transversus abdominis muscle*: Innermost muscle of the anterolateral abdominal wall. The muscle fibers run transversely. The fibers, like the external and internal oblique, become aponeurotic at the midclavicular line and continue medially to the linea alba.

Internal oblique and Transversus abdominis

Muscle	Proximal Attachment	Distal Attachment	Innervation	Action
Internal oblique	Thoracolumbar fascia, anterior two-thirds iliac crest	Inferior borders of the 10th-12th ribs, linea alba, pecten pubis	Thoracoabdominal nerves (T6-T12) and L1	Compresses and supports abdominal viscera
Transversus abdominis	Internal surfaces of **7**th-12th **costal cartilages**, iliac crest, thoracolumbar fascia	Linea alba, pubic crest, pecten pubis		

Rectus Sheath

◯ 3. *Anterior rectus sheath*: Runs the vertical distance between the costal margin and the pubic bone. The superior two-thirds of the anterior rectus sheath is composed of the interdigitating fibers of the external oblique aponeurosis and half of the internal oblique aponeurotic fibers. The inferior one-third of the anterior rectus sheath is composed of the aponeurotic fibers of all three anterolateral muscles.

◯ 4. *Posterior rectus sheath:* Lies posterior to the rectus abdominis muscle; and unlike the anterior layer of the rectus sheath, only extends the superior two-thirds of the distance between the costal margin and pubic bone. The posterior rectus sheath is composed of half of the internal oblique and the transversus abdominis aponeurotic fibers.

◯5. *Arcuate line*: Demarcates the inferior edge of the posterior rectus sheath. Below the arcuate line, there are no aponeurotic fibers from the anterolateral muscles posterior to the rectus abdominis.

◯ 6. *Transversalis fascia:* Named portion of endoabdominal fascia, a serous membrane lining the internal aspect of the muscles of the abdominal wall. Inferior to the arcuate line, the transversalis fascia lies immediately posterior to the rectus abdominis. Superior to the arcuate line, the transversalis fascia lies immediately posterior to the posterior rectus sheath.

Neurovasculature

◯ 7. *Inferior epigastric artery:* Arises from the external iliac artery superior to the inguinal ligament and courses superiorly in the transversalis fascia to run between the posterior rectus sheath and rectus abdominis muscle to anastomose with the superior epigastric artery

◯ 8. *Superior epigastric artery:* Direct continuation of the internal thoracic artery coursing between the posterior rectus sheath and the rectus abdominis muscle to anastomose with the inferior epigastric artery

◯ 9. *Iliohypogastric nerve:* Terminal superior branch of L1 anterior ramus. Pierces transversus abdominis to course between transversus abdominis and internal oblique muscles and then pierces external oblique aponeuroses of the inferior anterior abdominal wall

◯10. *Ilioinguinal nerve (cut):* Terminal inferior branch of the L1 anterior ramus. Courses between transversus abdominis and internal oblique muscles and then traverses the inguinal canal to emerge via the superficial inguinal ring.

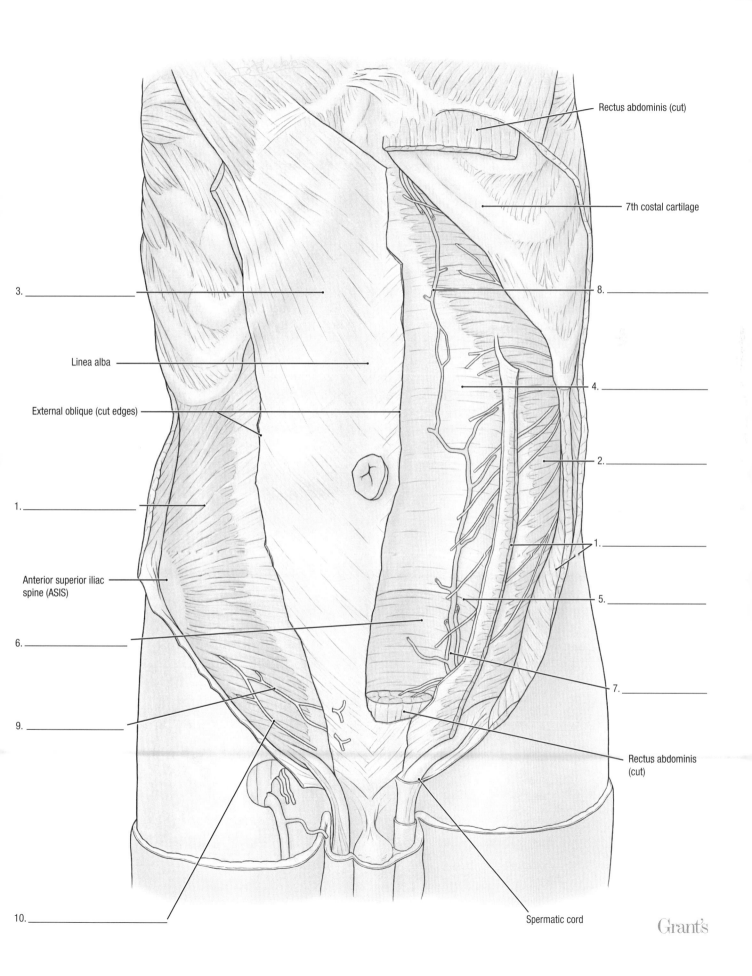

Rectus abdominis (cut)

7th costal cartilage

3. _____

Linea alba _____

External oblique (cut edges) _____

1. _____

Anterior superior iliac
spine (ASIS)

6. _____

9. _____

8. _____

4. _____

2. _____

1. _____

5. _____

7. _____

Rectus abdominis
(cut)

10. _____

Spermatic cord

Grant's

4.3A SUPERFICIAL INGUINAL REGION (MALE) I

The inguinal region extends from the **_Anterior superior iliac spine (ASIS)_** to the **_pubic tubercle_**.

Structures, such as the testis and spermatic cord in the male and the round ligament of the uterus in the female, enter and exit the abdominal cavity via the inguinal canal. The inguinal canal is the oblique passageway connecting the abdominal cavity and perineum through the inferior portion of the anterolateral musculoaponeurotic layers.

---

*COLOR **each of the following structures using a different color for each:***

The **_external oblique aponeurosis_** is expansive in the inferior aspect of the anterior abdominal wall and forms many of the structures of the inguinal region:

○ 1. **_Inguinal ligament_**: Inferiormost fibers of the external oblique aponeurosis running from the ASIS to the pubic tubercle. The inguinal canal lies parallel and superior to the medial half of the inguinal ligament.

○ 2. **_Lacunar ligament:_** Composed of fibers from the inguinal ligament that pass posteriorly to the superior pubic ramus instead of attaching to the pubic tubercle. Lacunar ligament forms the medial boundary of the subinguinal space. Some fibers will continue laterally along the pecten pubis, forming the pectineal ligament (of Cooper).

○ 3. **_Reflected inguinal ligament:_** Composed of fibers from the inguinal ligament that pass superiorly, fanning upward and bypassing the pubic tubercle. This ligament crosses the **_linea alba_** and blends with fibers of the contralateral external oblique aponeurosis.

The superficial inguinal ring is the exit point for the spermatic cord/round ligament of uterus from the inguinal canal located superolateral to the pubic tubercle. The ring appears as a split in the external oblique aponeurosis and not as a prominent "ring" structure.

○ 4. **_Lateral crus:_** Forms the lateral margin of the superficial inguinal ring attaching to the pubic tubercle

○ 5. **_Medial crus:_** Forms the medial margin of the superficial inguinal ring attaching to the pubic crest

○ 6. **_Intercrural fibers:_** Fibers that pass between each crus across the superolateral part of the superficial inguinal ring to help prevent the crura from spreading apart

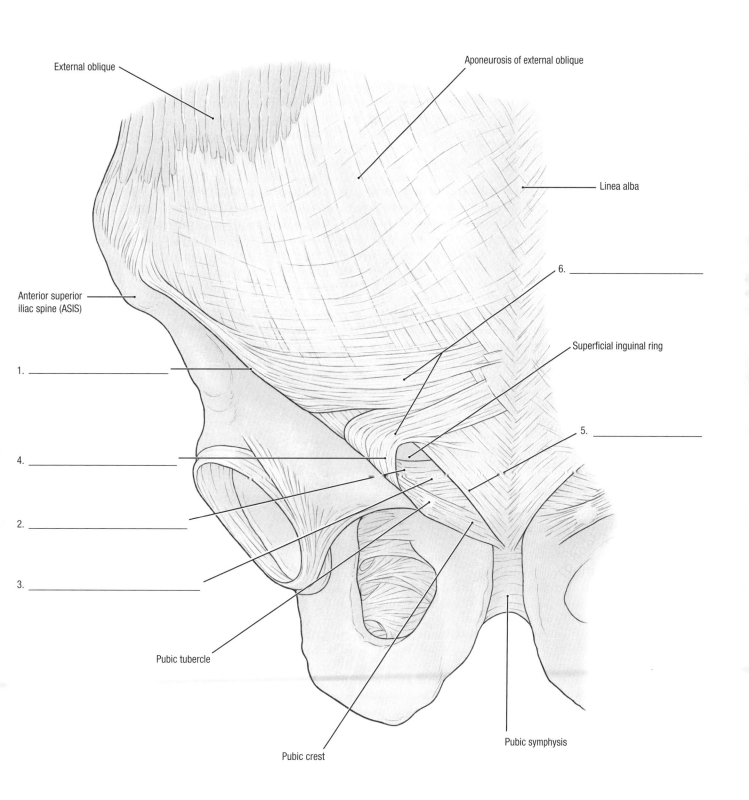

External oblique

Aponeurosis of external oblique

Linea alba

6. _____

Anterior superior
iliac spine (ASIS)

Superficial inguinal ring

1. _____

5. _____

4. _____

2. _____

3. _____

Pubic tubercle

Pubic crest

Pubic symphysis

Grant's

4.3B SUPERFICIAL INGUINAL REGION (MALE) II

On the right side, a large rectangular window has been cut into the ***external oblique muscle and aponeurosis*** with the edges pinned into place. The medial and lateral crura along with the superficial inguinal ring have been removed. The ***superficial inguinal ring*** and crura remain intact on the left side. The ***spermatic cord*** has been cut and portions removed on both sides.

COLOR *each of the following structures using a different color for each:*

1. ***Inguinal ligament:*** Acts as a retinaculum over the subinguinal space and its contents including the hip flexors, ***inguinal lymph nodes***, and ***femoral artery***, ***vein***, and nerve

2. ***Reflected inguinal ligament:*** Superior fibers of the inguinal ligament that do not attach at the pubic tubercle and instead pass upward to the linea alba and blend with the contralateral external oblique aponeurosis

3. ***Lateral crus:*** External oblique aponeurosis fibers that form the lateral margin of the superficial inguinal ring

4. ***Medial crus:*** External oblique aponeurosis fibers that form the medial margin of the superficial inguinal ring

5. ***Intercrural fibers***: Fibers from the external oblique aponeurosis that connect the medial and lateral crura and prevent them from splitting apart

6. ***Internal oblique muscle***: Remains muscular in the inferior anterolateral abdominal wall (unlike the external oblique)

7. ***Cremaster muscle***: Composed of slips of internal oblique muscle fibers and is carried with the testis and spermatic cord as they descend through the internal oblique muscle. Forms the intermediate layer of the spermatic cord coverings

8. ***Conjoint tendon:*** Merged inferiormost aponeurotic fibers of the internal oblique and transversus abdominis superoposterior to the reflected inguinal ligament. Fibers from the internal oblique forming the conjoint tendon attach to the pubic crest.

9. ***Iliohypogastric nerve:*** Pierces through the internal oblique muscle and courses in an inferomedial direction

10. ***Ilioinguinal nerve:*** Pierces through the internal oblique muscle and courses through the inguinal canal, emerging via the superficial inguinal ring

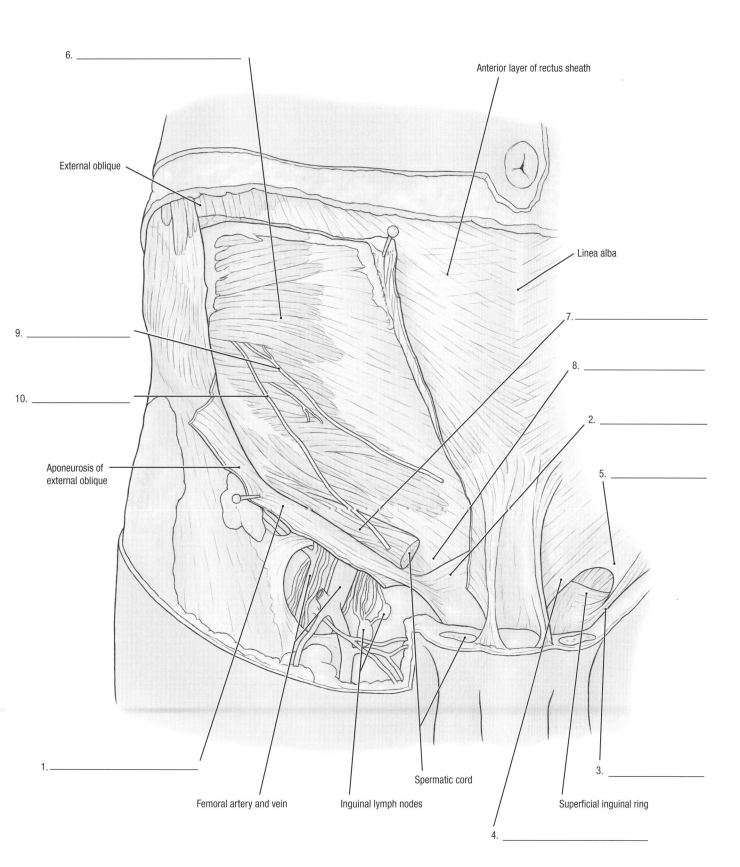

6. _____

Anterior layer of rectus sheath

External oblique

Linea alba

9. _____

7. _____

8. _____

10. _____

2. _____

Aponeurosis of external oblique

5. _____

1. _____

3. _____

Femoral artery and vein

Inguinal lymph nodes

Spermatic cord

Superficial inguinal ring

4. _____

Grant's

4.4A   DEEP INGUINAL REGION (MALE) I

The *external oblique aponeurosis* has been cut and the superficial inguinal ring and crura disrupted. The *internal oblique muscle* has been cut and reflected to reveal the underlying transversus abdominis. The *iliohypogastric* and *ilioinguinal nerves* have been cut as they traveled in the neurovascular plane between the internal oblique and transversus abdominis. The spermatic cord has been retracted inferolaterally with string.

COLOR *each of the following structures using a different color for each:*

◯ 1. *Transversus abdominis muscle:* Fibers pass superior to the *deep inguinal ring* and do not participate in the formation of the inguinal canal or the layers of the spermatic cord

◯ 2. *Transversus abdominis aponeurosis*: Courses inferomedially to the inguinal canal, participating in the formation of the conjoint tendon

◯ 3. *Conjoint tendon:* Inferiormost fibers of the transversus abdominis merge with the *internal oblique aponeurosis*. Fibers from the transversus abdominis attach to the pectineal line.

◯ 4. *Transversalis fascia*: Named portion of endoabdominal fascia that lines the abdominal cavity. First layer penetrated by the descending testes and spermatic cord (or round ligament of uterus in the female) during embryonic development and becomes evaginated. Forms the deep inguinal ring internally at the opening of the evagination.

◯ 5. *Internal spermatic fascia:* Continuation of the transversalis fascia covering the testis and spermatic cord

◯ 6. *Inferior epigastric vessels*: Course medial to the deep inguinal ring from/to external iliac artery/vein, respectively

◯ 7. *Deep circumflex iliac vessels*: Course parallel to the inguinal ligament on the deep aspect of the anterior abdominal wall from/to external iliac artery/vein, respectively

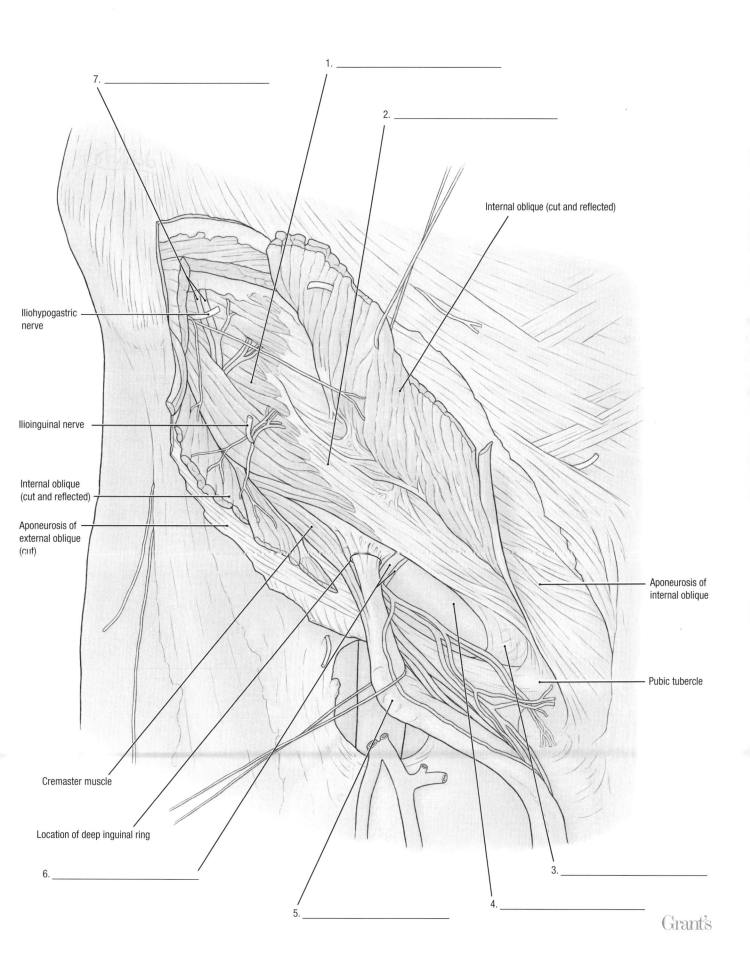

1. _____

2. _____

7. _____

Internal oblique (cut and reflected)

Iliohypogastric nerve

Ilioinguinal nerve

Internal oblique (cut and reflected)

Aponeurosis of external oblique (cut)

Aponeurosis of internal oblique

Pubic tubercle

Cremaster muscle

Location of deep inguinal ring

6. _____

3. _____

5. _____

4. _____

Grant's

4.4B   DEEP INGUINAL REGION (MALE) II

Similar to Section 4.4A, the ***external oblique aponeurosis*** has been cut and the superficial inguinal ring and crura disrupted. The ***internal oblique muscle*** has been cut and reflected to reveal the underlying transversus abdominis. The transversus abdominis and transversalis fascia have been partially cut away, revealing ***extraperitoneal fat*** and the ***external iliac artery and vein***. The spermatic cord has been cut and its components tied together with string.

▌ *COLOR each of the following structures using a different color for each:*

○ 1. ***Transversus abdominis muscle:*** Fibers pass superior to the ***deep inguinal ring*** and do not participate in the formation of the inguinal canal or the layers of the spermatic cord

○ 2. ***Transversus abdominis aponeurosis***: Courses inferomedially to the inguinal canal, participating in the formation of the conjoint tendon

○ 3. ***Conjoint tendon:*** Inferiormost fibers of transversus abdominis merge with the internal oblique aponeurosis. Fibers from the transversus abdominis attach to the pectineal line.

○ 4. ***Transversalis fascia***: Named portion of the endoabdominal fascia that lines the abdominal cavity and comprises the deep inguinal ring

○ 5. ***Spermatic cord***: Composed of the ***testicular vessels*** and the ***ductus deferens***

○ 6. ***Inferior epigastric vessels***: Course medial to the deep inguinal ring from/to external iliac artery/vein, respectively

○ 7. ***Deep circumflex iliac vessels***: Course parallel to the inguinal ligament on the deep aspect of the anterior abdominal wall from/to external iliac artery/vein, respectively

The external iliac artery and vein change names to the ***femoral artery and vein*** as they pass deep to the inguinal ligament.

CLINICAL NOTE: INGUINAL HERNIAS

Abdominal wall hernias are one of the most common surgical problems, with almost 75% occurring in the inguinal region. Of all inguinal hernia repairs, 90% are performed in men. Two types of inguinal hernias exist: indirect and direct. Indirect hernias account for two-thirds of inguinal hernias and are common in younger persons, especially in men. An indirect hernia travels through the ***deep inguinal ring*** (lateral to the ***inferior epigastric vessels***) and then to the inguinal canal, where it is covered by the spermatic cord coverings, and exits via the superficial inguinal ring inside the spermatic cord. Direct hernias are less common and typically occur in adult men because of a weakness in the anterior abdominal wall in the inguinal region. A direct hernia travels medial to inferior epigastric vessels through the parietal peritoneum and transversalis fascia to enter through or near the distal inguinal canal, and exits via the superficial inguinal ring lateral to the spermatic cord.

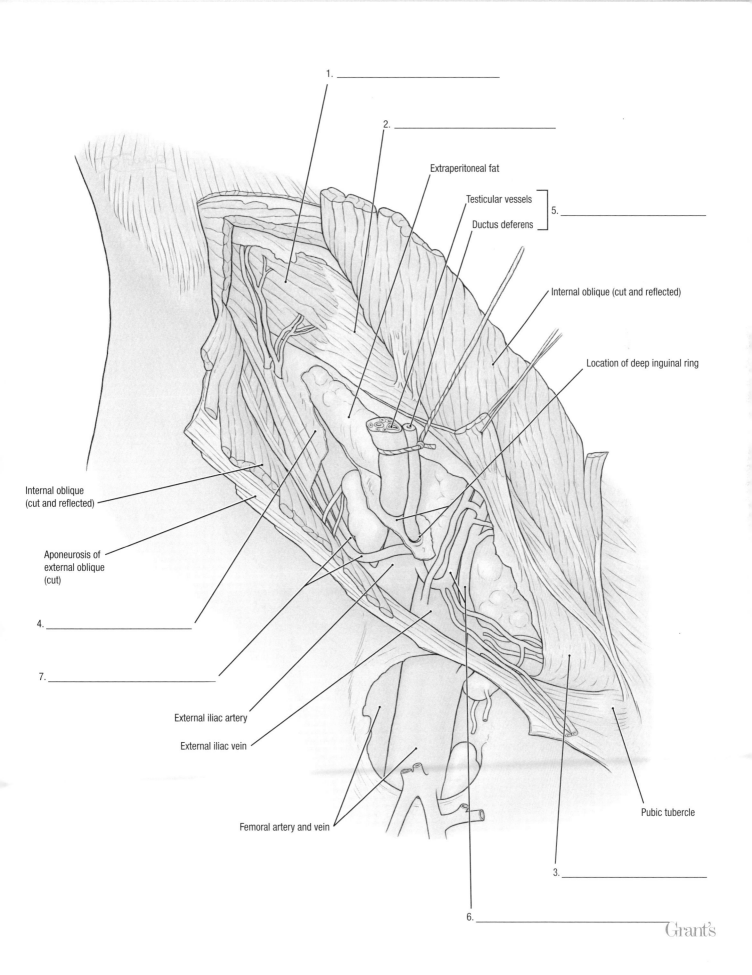

1. _____

2. _____

Extraperitoneal fat

Testicular vessels

Ductus deferens

5. _____

Internal oblique (cut and reflected)

Location of deep inguinal ring

Internal oblique
(cut and reflected)

Aponeurosis of
external oblique
(cut)

4. _____

7. _____

External iliac artery

External iliac vein

Pubic tubercle

3. _____

Femoral artery and vein

6. _____

Grant's

4.5 FEMALE INGUINAL REGION

Similar to the male, the female inguinal region extends from the **ASIS** to the **pubic tubercle**. The structures and relationship of the female anterolateral abdominal wall and inguinal region are similar to those of the male, with the exception that the inguinal structures are less pronounced than those in the male. In addition, the round ligament of the uterus traverses the inguinal canal instead of the testis and spermatic cord.

COLOR each of the following structures using a different color for each:

○ 1. *Fatty layer of subcutaneous tissue:* Immediately deep to skin

○ 2. *Membranous layer of subcutaneous tissue:* Deep to fatty layer and superficial to external oblique aponeurosis in the inguinal region

○ 3. *Lateral crus:* External oblique aponeurosis fibers forming lateral boundary of **superficial inguinal ring**

○ 4. *Medial crus:* External oblique aponeurosis fibers forming medial boundary of superficial inguinal ring

○ 5. *Intercrural fibers:* External oblique aponeurosis fibers crossing from one crus to the other

○ 6. *Round ligament of uterus:* Traverses the inguinal canal from the deep inguinal ring to the superficial inguinal ring; fans out to insert into the **labium majus**

CLINICAL NOTE: FEMORAL HERNIA

Femoral hernias are rare, comprising only about 1 in every 20 groin hernias, and are more common in women because of their wider pelves. The hernia courses deep to the inguinal ligament and emerges inferolateral to the pubic tubercle, medial to the femoral vein, and lateral to the lacunar ligament. Strangulation (loss of blood supply) to the herniated intestine may occur because the space of the femoral herniation is narrow and the boundaries rigid.

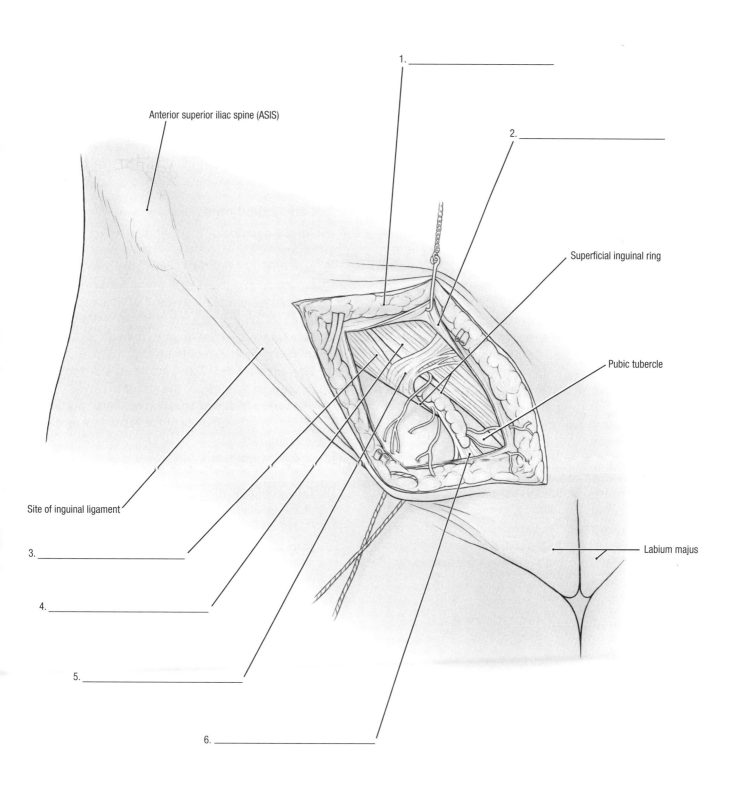

1. _____

2. _____

Anterior superior iliac spine (ASIS)

Superficial inguinal ring

Pubic tubercle

Site of inguinal ligament

Labium majus

3. _____

4. _____

5. _____

6. _____

4.6A and B   SPERMATIC CORD AND TESTES

Figure A depicts the inguinal region, spermatic cord, and testes. On the right, the *aponeurosis of the external oblique* has been cut to reveal the *internal oblique* and *conjoint tendon*. On the left, the external oblique and internal oblique have been cut to expose the *transversus abdominis* and *transversalis fascia* along with the layers of the spermatic cord.

Figure B depicts the internal structures of the testis with the epididymis and ductus deferens.

COLOR each of the following structures using a different color for each:

Coverings of the Testes and Spermatic Cord

○ 1. *Internal spermatic fascia*: Forms as the testis and spermatic cord descended through the transversalis fascia of the anterolateral abdominal wall. Covers the extent of the testis, epididymis, and spermatic cord.

○ 2. *Cremasteric muscle and fascia*: Forms as the testis and spermatic cord descended through the internal oblique muscle and muscle. Covers the extent of the testis, epididymis, and spermatic cord superficial to the internal spermatic fascia.

○ 3. *External spermatic fascia*: Forms as the testis and spermatic cord descended through the superficial ring of the external oblique aponeurosis. Covers the extent of the testis, epididymis, and spermatic cord superficial to the cremaster muscle and fascia.

During the descent of the testis, a portion of the peritoneal cavity is pulled inferiorly with the testis. The connection to the peritoneal cavity regresses and a separate, closed sac is left surrounding the testis.

○ 4. *Parietal layer of tunica vaginalis*: Deep to the internal spermatic fascia at the level of the testis and inferior spermatic cord

○ 5. *Visceral layer of tunica vaginalis:* Covers the surface of the testis, except where the testis attaches to the epididymis and spermatic cord and a portion of the epididymis

○ 6. *Cavity of tunica vaginalis:* Potential space between the parietal and visceral layers of tunica vaginalis typically filled with a small amount of fluid to allow the testis to move freely in the scrotum

Testes and Epididymis

○ 7. *Tunica albuginea:* Tough, fibrous outer surface of the testes

○ 8. *Seminiferous tubules:* Long, highly coiled small tubes arranged into lobules comprising a majority of the internal structure of the testes. Developing sperm travel along the seminiferous tubules to the straight tubules.

○ 9. *Rete testis:* Collection of canals from the straight tubules in the mediastinum of the testis

○ 10. *Efferent ductules:* Transport newly developed sperm to the epididymis from the rete testis

○ 11. *Head of epididymis:* Superior expanded portion resting on the superior pole of the testis that receives the efferent ductules

○ 12. *Body of epididymis:* Main component of the tightly coiled duct of the epididymis

○ 13. *Tail of epididymis:* Tapering continuation of the duct of the epididymis leading to ductus deferens

○ 14. *Ductus deferens:* Duct of the spermatic cord that transports sperm from the epididymis to the ejaculatory duct

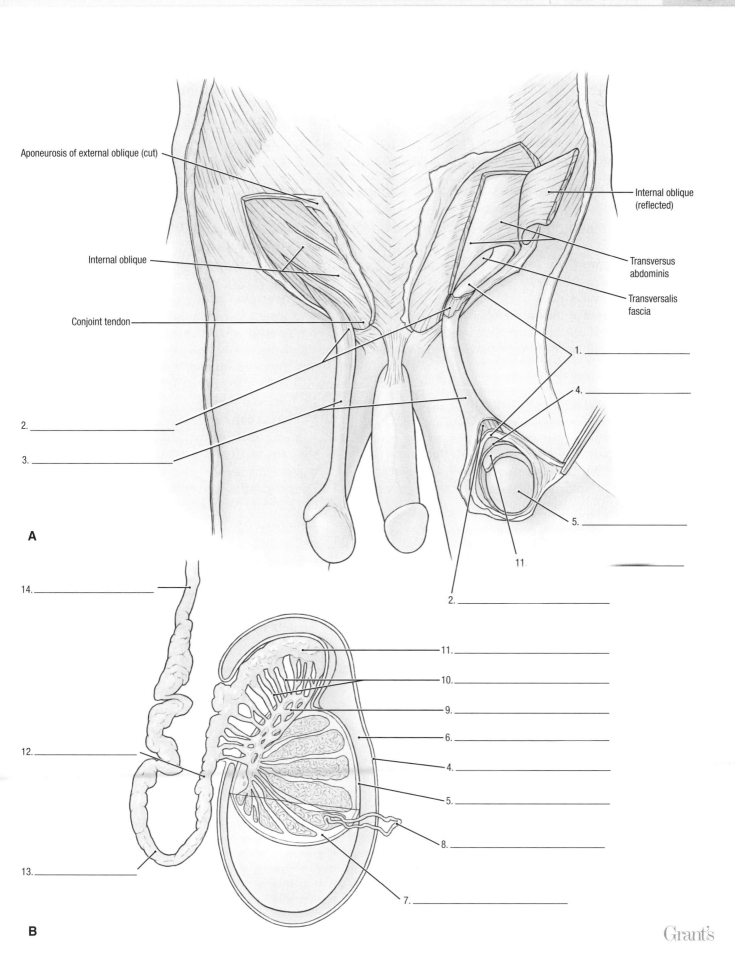

Aponeurosis of external oblique (cut)

Internal oblique (reflected)

Internal oblique

Transversus abdominis

Transversalis fascia

Conjoint tendon

1. _____

4. _____

2. _____

3. _____

5. _____

11. _____

A

14. _____

2. _____

11. _____

10. _____

9. _____

12. _____

6. _____

4. _____

5. _____

8. _____

13. _____

7. _____

B

4.7 INTERNAL ASPECT OF ANTEROLATERAL ABDOMINAL WALL

The anterolateral abdominal wall has been removed and the internal aspect displayed. On the left side of the specimen, the layers of the anterolateral abdominal wall from superficial to deep are visible in the cut edges: ***external oblique***, ***internal oblique***, ***transversus abdominis***, ***transversalis fascia***, and parietal peritoneum. On the right side of the specimen, the parietal peritoneum has been removed and a vertical cut made in the ***transversalis fascia*** deep to the rectus abdominis to reveal the arcuate line.

▌ *COLOR each of the following structures using a different color for each:*

○ 1. *Parietal peritoneum*: Lies deep (internal) to the transversalis fascia

○ 2. *Falciform ligament:* Double layer of peritoneum coursing from the liver to the parietal peritoneum, covering the anterior abdominal wall

○ 3. *Round ligament of the liver:* Embryological remnant of the umbilical vein coursing in the inferior free edge of the falciform ligament from the ***umbilicus*** to the liver

Along the internal aspect, three structures course from the inferior anterolateral abdominal wall toward the umbilicus:

○ 4. *Inferior epigastric vessels:* Most lateral structures

○ 5. *Umbilical artery*: Lies medial to the inferior epigastric vessels and is typically obliterated as it travels along the anterior abdominal wall

The urachus is an embryological remnant that lies in the midline, traveling superiorly from the ***urinary bladder***.

As the parietal peritoneum falls over structures on the deep aspect of the anterolateral abdominal wall, three ridges and three depressions form:

○ 6. *Lateral umbilical fold:* Forms as the parietal peritoneum lies over the inferior epigastric vessels on each side
Lateral inguinal fossa lies lateral to the lateral umbilical ligament.

○ 7. *Medial umbilical fold:* Forms as the parietal peritoneum lies over the umbilical artery on each side
Medial inguinal fossa lies between the lateral and medial umbilical ligaments.

○ 8. *Median umbilical fold:* Forms as parietal peritoneum lies over the urachus
Supravesical fossa lies between the medial and median umbilical ligaments.

○ 9. *Transversalis fascia:* Lies superficial to the parietal peritoneum and immediately deep to the muscles of the anterolateral abdominal wall.

Forms the ***deep inguinal ring*** as the structures of the spermatic cord descend through the inguinal region:

○ 10. *Testicular vessels*

○ 11. *Ductus deferens*

○ 12. *Iliopubic tract:* Inferiormost thickening of the fibers of the transversalis fascia running parallel and deep to the inguinal ligament

○ 13. *Deep circumflex iliac vessels:* Parallel the course of the iliopubic tract on the deep aspect of the anterolateral abdominal wall

○ 14. *Rectus abdominis muscle:* Inferior one-third is directly covered by transversalis fascia posteriorly

○ 15. *Posterior rectus sheath:* Directly related to the posterior aspect of the superior two-thirds of the rectus abdominis muscle

○ 16. *Arcuate line:* Inferior margin of the posterior rectus sheath

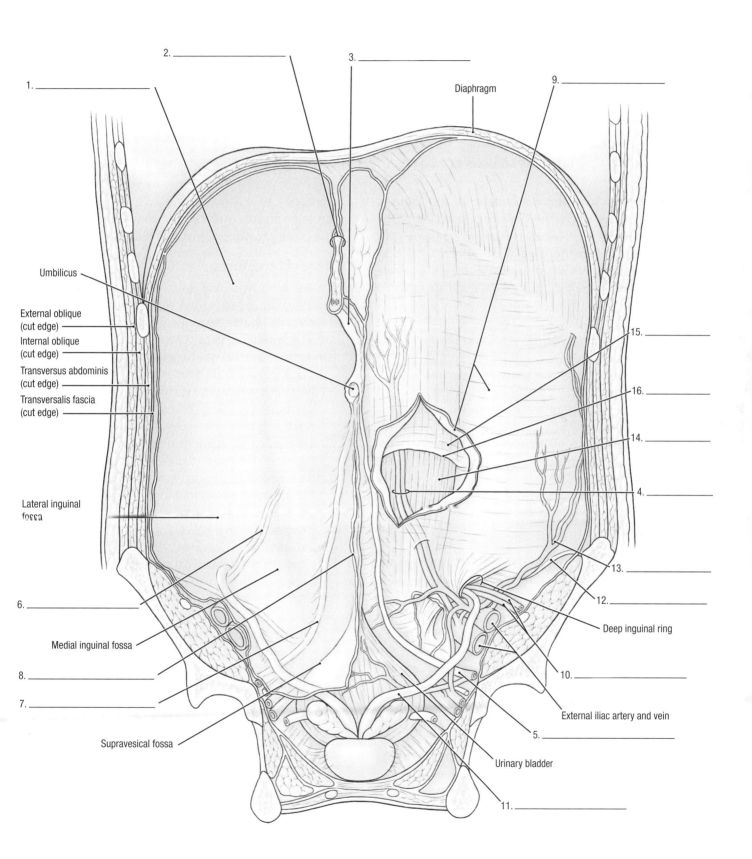

2. _____

3. _____

Diaphragm

9. _____

1. _____

Umbilicus

External oblique
(cut edge) _____

Internal oblique
(cut edge) _____

Transversus abdominis
(cut edge) _____

Transversalis fascia
(cut edge) _____

Lateral inguinal
fossa

15. _____

16. _____

14. _____

4. _____

13. _____

12. _____

Deep inguinal ring

6. _____

Medial inguinal fossa

8. _____

7. _____

10. _____

Supravesical fossa

External iliac artery and vein

5. _____

Urinary bladder

11. _____

Grant's

4.8   PERITONEAL CAVITY

The ***anterolateral abdominal*** and anterior thoracic walls have been removed to reveal the contents of the abdominal cavity. ***External oblique***, ***internal oblique***, ***transversus abdominis***, and ***rectus abdominis*** muscles are visible along the cut edges.

The peritoneum is a continuous serous membrane that consists of two layers: parietal peritoneum lining the internal aspect of the abdominopelvic cavity and visceral peritoneum investing certain abdominal viscera. Parietal peritoneum not only lines the internal aspect of the anterolateral abdominal wall (deep to the endoabdominal fascia) but also lines the inferior surface of the diaphragm and the anterior or superior surfaces of the abdominopelvic structures not located within the peritoneal cavity (retroperitoneal and subperitoneal structures).

COLOR each of the following structures using a different color for each:

○ 1. ***Diaphragm***: Separates the abdominal and thoracic cavities. Superiorly covered by diaphragmatic pleura except where it is pierced by the ***inferior vena cava*** and related to the ***pericardial sac***. Inferiorly lined by peritoneum except at the bare area of the liver where the peritoneum reflects away from the diaphragm.

Peritoneal Organs

- Intraperitoneal organs invaginated into the peritoneal cavity during embryonic development and are almost completely covered with visceral peritoneum in the adult. The first layer pierced by a pin on an intraperitoneal organ is the visceral peritoneum. Intraperitoneal organs include the liver, spleen, very proximal and distal duodenum, tail of the pancreas, jejunum, ileum, cecum, appendix, transverse colon, and sigmoid colon. Two other intraperitoneal organs are the:

○ 2. ***Stomach***

○ 3. ***Gallbladder***

- Retroperitoneal organs are located posterior to the peritoneal cavity and have the parietal peritoneum covering their anterior surfaces. Retroperitoneal organs include the kidneys, suprarenal glands, ureters, and the continuation of the ***descending aorta*** and inferior vena cava inferior to the diaphragm.
- Secondarily retroperitoneal organs invaginated into the peritoneal cavity in the developing embryo, but were then pushed back to the posterior wall because of the developing gut and the peritoneal layers fused. Secondarily retroperitoneal organs include most of the duodenum, most of the pancreas (except the tail), ascending colon, and descending colon. Subperitoneal organs are located inferior to the peritoneal cavity and are covered by parietal peritoneum on their superior surfaces. Subperitoneal organs include the urinary bladder, uterus, and rectum.

Peritoneal Structures

With multiple organs in one peritoneal cavity, multiple peritoneal connections and structures are created within the cavity:

- Mesentery: Double layer of peritoneum that connects an intraperitoneal organ to the body wall
- Omentum: Double layer of peritoneum that connects the stomach and proximal duodenum to an adjacent organ
  - The greater omentum runs from the greater curvature of the stomach and proximal duodenum to the diaphragm, spleen, and transverse colon.
  - ○4. ***Gastrocolic ligament***: Primary component of the greater omentum that descends like an apron over the small intestine, and then folds back to attach to the transverse colon and its mesentery creating a four-layered peritoneal structure. Fat is typically deposited within the layers of the gastrocolic ligament.
  - ○5. ***Gastrosplenic ligament***: Connects the greater curvature of the stomach to the hilum of the spleen; smaller component of greater omentum
- Ligament: Double layer of peritoneum that connects an organ to another organ or body wall
  - ○ 6. ***Falciform ligament***: Courses from the anterior abdominal wall to the liver dividing the liver into the following:
    - ○ 7. ***Right lobe***
    - ○ 8. ***Left lobe***
  - ○ 9. ***Round ligament of liver (ligamentum teres):*** Embryological remnant of the umbilical vein (not composed of parietal peritoneum) located in the free edge of the falciform ligament

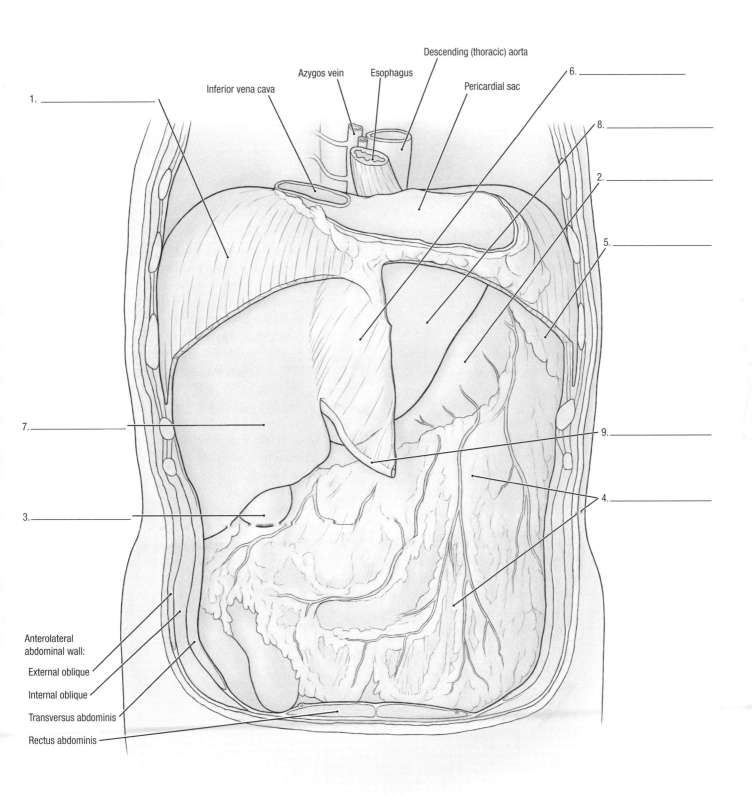

Descending (thoracic) aorta

Azygos vein   Esophagus

Inferior vena cava   Pericardial sac

6. _____

1. _____

8. _____

2. _____

5. _____

7. _____

9. _____

4. _____

3. _____

Anterolateral
abdominal wall:

External oblique

Internal oblique

Transversus abdominis

Rectus abdominis

4.9 STOMACH AND OMENTA

Most of the diaphragm, left lobe and a portion of the right lobe of the liver, and the falciform ligament have been removed to demonstrate the relationships of the omentum with the stomach (***bold black line outlines the missing components of the liver***).

COLOR each of the following structures using a different color for each:

Parts of the Stomach

○ 1. *Fundus:* Dilated superior portion related to the left dome of the ***diaphragm***

○ 2. *Body*: Main portion between fundus and pyloric region

○ 3. *Pyloric region:* Outflow portion shaped like a funnel with an antrum area associated with the body of the stomach that leads into the canal just distal to the first part of the duodenum

Relationships to the Stomach

The fourth part of the stomach, the cardia, is the inlet portion of the stomach related to the esophagus (not visible in this image).

○ 4. *Duodenum:* Receives contents from the pyloric region of the stomach

○ 5. *Liver:* Connected to the stomach and first part of duodenum via the lesser omentum, to the diaphragm via the coronary ligaments, and to the anterior abdominal wall via the falciform ligament

The peritoneal cavity is divided into the greater and lesser peritoneal sacs because of the development and rotation of the stomach. The greater sac comprises most of the peritoneal cavity. The lesser peritoneal sac (omental bursa) is positioned posterior to the stomach and lesser omentum. At the ***free edge of the lesser omentum***, the greater peritoneal sac communicates with the lesser peritoneal sac (omental bursa) via the ***omental (epiploic) foramen***.

○ 6. *Lesser omentum:* Double layer of peritoneum attaching the liver to the ***lesser curvature of the stomach*** (hepatogastric ligament) and to the first part of the duodenum (hepatoduodenal ligament)
   • Contained within the hepatoduodenal ligament of the lesser omentum is the portal triad: common bile duct, proper hepatic artery, and hepatic portal vein.
   • Parallel to the lesser curvature of the stomach, the left and right gastric arteries anastomose within the hepatogastric ligament. ***Tributaries of the right and left gastric arteries*** spread out from the lesser curvature along the stomach.

○ 7. *Gastrocolic ligament:* Main component of the greater omentum descending from the ***greater curvature of the stomach*** to fold upon itself and attach onto the transverse colon.

○ 8. *Transverse colon*: Obscured by the attachment of the gastrocolic ligament from the anterior view

○ 9. *Left and right gastro-omental (epiploic) arteries:* Anastomose within the gastrocolic ligament parallel to the greater curvature of the stomach. Tributaries from these arteries supply the stomach along the greater curvature.

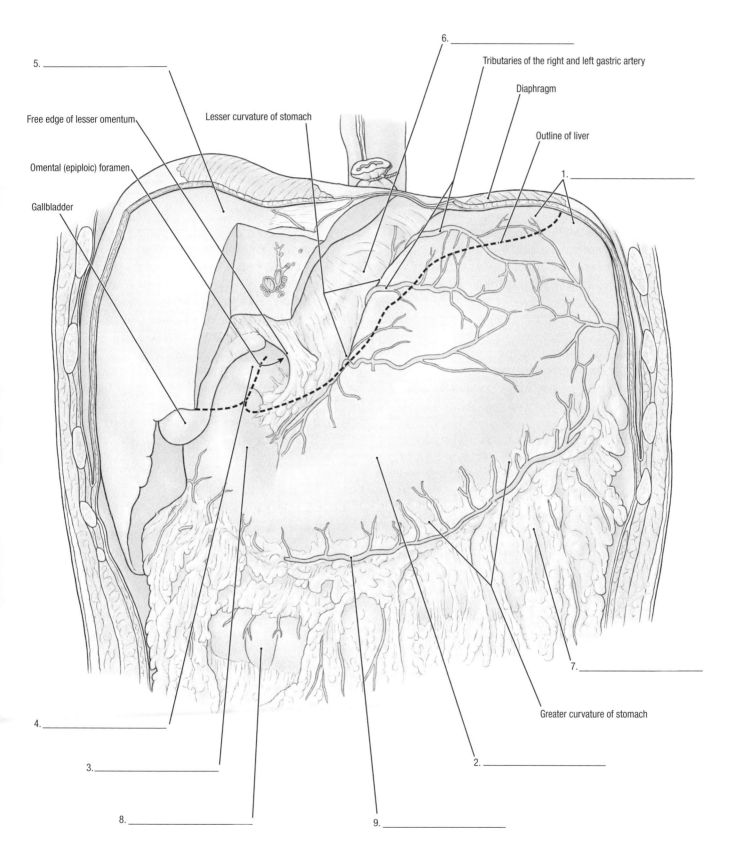

6. _____

Tributaries of the right and left gastric artery

Diaphragm

Outline of liver

5. _____

Free edge of lesser omentum

Lesser curvature of stomach

Omental (epiploic) foramen

1. _____

Gallbladder

4. _____

3. _____

7. _____

Greater curvature of stomach

2. _____

8. _____

9. _____

Grant's

4.10   POSTERIOR RELATIONSHIPS TO THE STOMACH

The *stomach*, *lesser omentum*, and *gastrocolic ligament* form the anterior wall of the lesser peritoneal sac (omental bursa). All three structures have been cut in a sagittal plane and reflected to the left and right to reveal the space of the omental bursa.

Small windows have been cut into the parietal peritoneum of the posterior wall to reveal structures that lie posterior to the lesser peritoneal sac. The lesser peritoneal sac (omental bursa) is a saclike peritoneal cavity between the parietal peritoneum overlying the retroperitoneal organs at this level, such as the *pancreas*, and the visceral peritoneum covering the posterior aspect of the stomach, the lesser omentum, and the gastrocolic ligament. A *superior recess* extends to the diaphragm and coronary ligaments of liver. The omental bursa permits free movement of the stomach on the structures posterior to it.

The omental bursa freely communicates with the greater sac via the omental foramen located posterior to the free edge of the lesser omentum (*rod passing from greater sac to omental bursa*).

COLOR each of the following structures using a different color for each:

○ 1. ***Transverse mesocolon***: Connects the ***transverse colon*** to the posterior abdominal wall. Also forms the posterior wall of the inferior aspect of the omental bursa. The transverse mesocolon adheres to the parietal peritoneum, forming the remainder of the posterior border of the omental bursa at the inferior border of the pancreas.

A window has been cut into the parietal peritoneum superior to the pancreas to reveal the three branches of the celiac trunk. The celiac trunk provides blood supply to foregut structures and the spleen.

○ 2. ***Left gastric artery:*** Immediately passes into the lesser omentum and parallels the lesser curvature of the stomach. Gives rise to an esophageal artery and will anastomose with the right gastric artery.

○ 3. ***Splenic artery:*** Courses tortuously to the left along the superior aspect of the pancreas
○ 4. ***Common hepatic artery:*** Courses to the right toward the liver
○ 5. ***Hepatic portal vein***: Travels through the hepatoduodenal ligament of the lesser omentum with the proper hepatic artery and common bile duct

Additional windows cut into the transverse mesocolon reveal the vessels supplying the midgut:

○ 6. ***Superior mesenteric artery***
○ 7. ***Superior mesenteric vein***

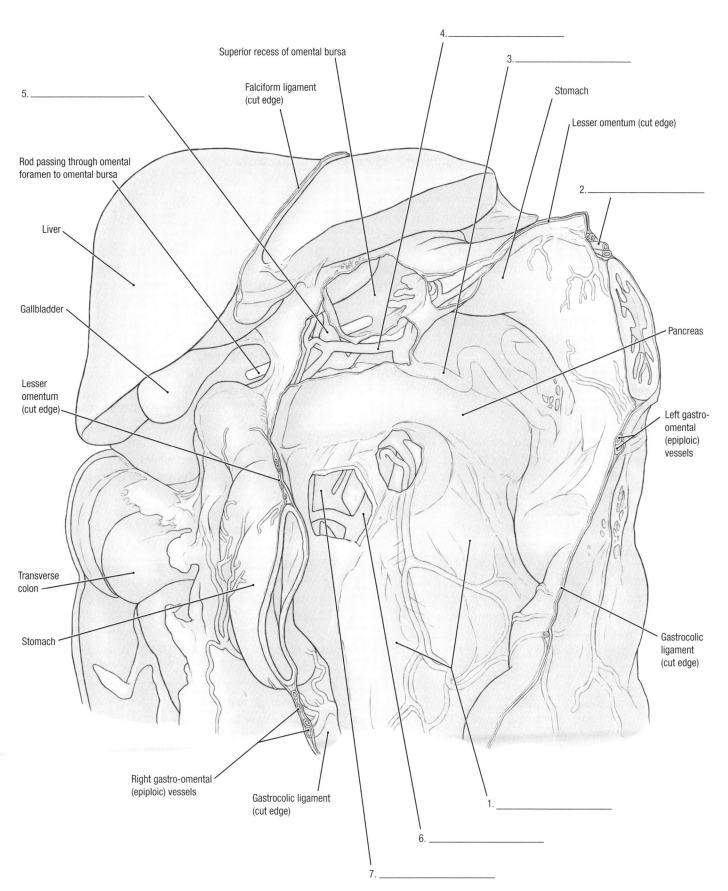

4. _____

3. _____

Superior recess of omental bursa

Stomach

Falciform ligament (cut edge)

Lesser omentum (cut edge)

5. _____

2. _____

Rod passing through omental foramen to omental bursa

Liver

Pancreas

Gallbladder

Lesser omentum (cut edge)

Left gastro-omental (epiploic) vessels

Transverse colon

Gastrocolic ligament (cut edge)

Stomach

Right gastro-omental (epiploic) vessels

Gastrocolic ligament (cut edge)

1. _____

6. _____

7. _____

4.11 CELIAC TRUNK AND FORMATION OF HEPATIC PORTAL VEIN

The parietal peritoneum of the posterior wall of the lesser peritoneal sac has been mostly removed. In addition, most of the left lobe of the *liver* and a section of the body of the *pancreas* have been removed. The *stomach* has been cut in a sagittal plane and reflected to the right and left sides.

A *rod* passes through the location of the omental foramen. The description that follows provides the typical branching pattern of the celiac trunk; however, variation is common. The branches of the celiac trunk are named for the structures that they pass to and supply.

COLOR each of the following structures using a different color for each:

○ 1. **Celiac trunk:** Arises from the abdominal aorta inferior to the aortic hiatus and gives rise to branches that supply the stomach, esophagus, proximal duodenum, liver and biliary apparatus, pancreas, and spleen.

○ 2. **Left gastric artery:** Arises from the celiac trunk and passes within the lesser omentum, paralleling the lesser curvature of the stomach while giving off several small branches. Anastomoses with the right gastric artery.

○ 3. **Esophageal branch:** Arises from the left gastric artery to supply the distal esophagus

○ 4. **Splenic artery:** Arises from the celiac trunk and meanderingly courses to the left along the superior border of the pancreas, sending off numerous branches to the body of the pancreas

○ 5. **Left gastro-omental (epiploic) artery:** Arises from the splenic artery at the hilum of the *spleen* to pass within the greater omentum along the greater curvature of the stomach to anastomose with the right gastro-omental artery

○ 6. **Short gastric artery:** Usually four to five small arteries that arise from the splenic artery at the hilum of the spleen and then course through the gastrosplenic ligament to supply the fundus of the stomach

○ 7. **Common hepatic artery:** Arises from the celiac trunk and courses to the right, passing anterior to the hepatic portal vein

○ 8. **Gastroduodenal artery:** Arises from the common hepatic artery and descends posterior to the first part of the duodenum. Gives rise to branches that supply the distal stomach, proximal duodenum, and pancreas.

○ 9. **Right gastro-omental (epiploic) artery:** Arises from the gastroduodenal artery and passes within the gastrocolic ligament parallel to the greater curvature of the stomach to anastomose with the left gastro-omental artery

○ 10. **Anterior superior pancreaticoduodenal artery:** Arises from the gastroduodenal artery and travels along the anterior surface of the head of the pancreas supplying it and proximal portions of the duodenum

○ 11. **Proper hepatic artery:** Continuation of the common hepatic artery after the origin of the gastroduodenal artery, courses through the hepatoduodenal ligament for a variable length with hepatic portal vein and *common bile duct* before bifurcating into the following:

○ 12. **Right hepatic artery:** Courses to the right lobe of the liver, giving rise to the cystic artery to the *gallbladder*

○ 13. **Left hepatic artery:** Courses to the left lobe of the liver

○ 14. **Right gastric artery:** Arises variably from the common hepatic, proper hepatic, or gastroduodenal artery and courses within the lesser omentum to parallel the lesser curvature of the stomach to anastomose with the left gastric artery

○ 15. **Superior mesenteric artery (SMA):** Arises from the abdominal aorta immediately inferior to the celiac trunk to supply midgut structures

○ 16. **Superior mesenteric vein (SMV):** Drains midgut structures to the hepatic portal vein

○ 17. **Splenic vein:** Courses along the posterior aspect of the pancreas to the hepatic portal vein

○ 18. **Inferior mesenteric vein (IMV):** Drains hindgut structures to the splenic vein, the superior mesenteric vein, or the confluence (joining) of the splenic and superior mesenteric veins

○ 19. **Hepatic portal vein:** Forms posterior to the *neck of the pancreas* as the splenic and superior mesenteric veins merge and course through the hepatoduodenal ligament with the proper hepatic artery and common bile duct

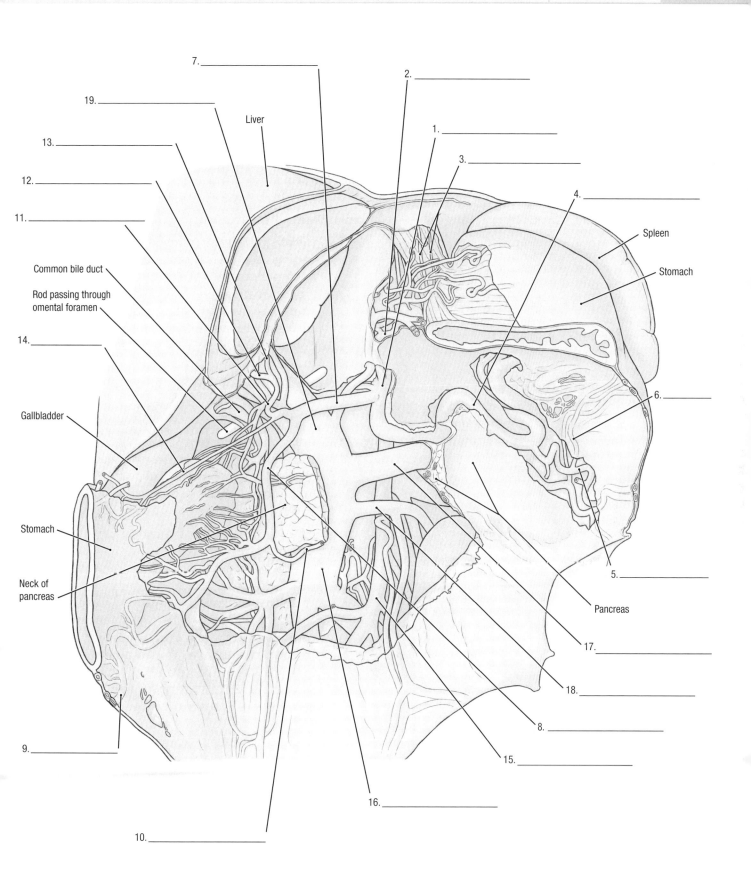

7.
2.
19.
1.
13.
3.
12.
4.
11.
Spleen
Common bile duct
Stomach
Rod passing through
omental foramen
14.
6.
Gallbladder
Stomach
5.
Neck of
pancreas
Pancreas
17.
18.
8.
9.
15.
16.
10.

Liver

4.12 PANCREAS AND DUODENUM

The pancreas and duodenum have been isolated from the liver and from most of the stomach. The *spleen* has been pulled superolaterally away from the tail of the pancreas. The superior mesenteric vessels have been cut because they extended into the *mesentery of the small intestine.*

COLOR each of the following structures using a different color for each:

Pancreas

The pancreas is secondarily retroperitoneal (except the tail) in the adult at the level of L1 and L2 vertebral bodies.

1. *Head of the pancreas*: Sits in the C-shape of the duodenum to the right of the superior mesenteric vessels. The uncinate process projects medially from the inferior aspect of the head posterior to the superior mesenteric artery (SMA).
2. *Neck of the pancreas:* Lies anterior to the superior mesenteric vessels and the formation of the hepatic portal vein
3. *Body of the pancreas:* Continues from the neck lying to the left of the superior mesenteric vessels. The posterior aspect of the body is in direct contact with the abdominal aorta, SMA, *splenic vessels*, *left suprarenal gland*, and renal vessels to the *left kidney*
4. *Tail of the pancreas:* Lies anterior to the left kidney and is closely related to the splenic hilum ("the tail of the pancreas tickles the spleen")

Duodenum

The duodenum is mostly secondarily retroperitoneal, except at the very beginning and end as it transitions from and to intraperitoneal organs of the stomach and *jejunum*. The duodenum is the first, shortest, and most fixed part of the small intestine. It begins at the *pylorus* on the right side, takes a C-shaped course, and ends at the duodenojejunal junction on the left side. The duodenum is divided into four parts:

5. *First (superior) part:* Continues from the *pylorus*, is overlapped by the gallbladder and liver, and is attached to the liver by the hepatoduodenal ligament
6. *Second (descending) part:* Runs inferiorly to the right and parallel to the *inferior vena cava* and is pierced posteriorly by the hepatopancreatic ampulla (union of the main pancreatic duct and common bile duct)
7. *Third (horizontal/inferior) part:* Runs transversely to the left anterior to the inferior vena cava, aorta, and psoas major muscle. The SMA and vein pass anterior to the distal portion of the third part.

Fourth (ascending) part is hidden by the mesentery of the small intestine and branches of the superior mesenteric vessels. The fourth part runs superiorly to the inferior border of the pancreas along the left side of the *abdominal aorta*. The distal aspect turns anteriorly to join the jejunum at the duodenojejunal flexure (junction).

Portal Triad

The *portal triad* is located within the hepatoduodenal ligament and consists of the following:

8. *Hepatic portal vein:* Forms posterior to the neck of the pancreas and courses posterior to the proper hepatic artery and common bile duct
9. *Proper hepatic artery*: Arises from the common hepatic artery after the origin of the gastroduodenal artery and courses to the liver anterior to the hepatic portal vein
10. *Common bile duct:* Courses posterior to the head of the pancreas

Vasculature of the Pancreas and Duodenum

11. *Supraduodenal artery:* Typically arises from the proper hepatic artery to supply the first part of the duodenum
12. *Gastroduodenal artery*: Supplies the posterior aspect of the head of the pancreas and proximal duodenum (proximal to entry of hepatopancreatic ampulla in the second part) by the posterior superior pancreaticoduodenal artery

The gastroduodenal artery then bifurcates after coursing posterior to the first part of the duodenum into the *right gastro-omental artery* and the:

13. *Anterior superior pancreaticoduodenal artery:* Supplies the anterior aspect of the head and proximal duodenum before the entry of the hepatopancreatic ampulla
14. *Superior mesenteric vein:* Passes anterior to the distal portion of the third part of the duodenum to unite with the splenic vein to form the hepatic portal vein posterior to the neck of the pancreas
15. *Superior mesenteric artery*: Branches from the abdominal aorta, passes posterior to the body of the pancreas, and then passes anterior to the distal portion of the third part of the duodenum and uncinate process of the pancreas. The SMA supplies the duodenum distal to the entry of hepatopancreatic ampulla in the second part of the duodenum and the head of the pancreas via the inferior pancreaticoduodenal arteries.
16. *Anterior inferior pancreaticoduodenal artery*: Branches from the SMA and courses along the anterior aspect of the head of the pancreas to anastomose with the anterior superior pancreaticoduodenal artery

The posterior inferior pancreaticoduodenal artery anastomoses with the posterior superior pancreaticoduodenal artery along the posterior aspect of the head of the pancreas.

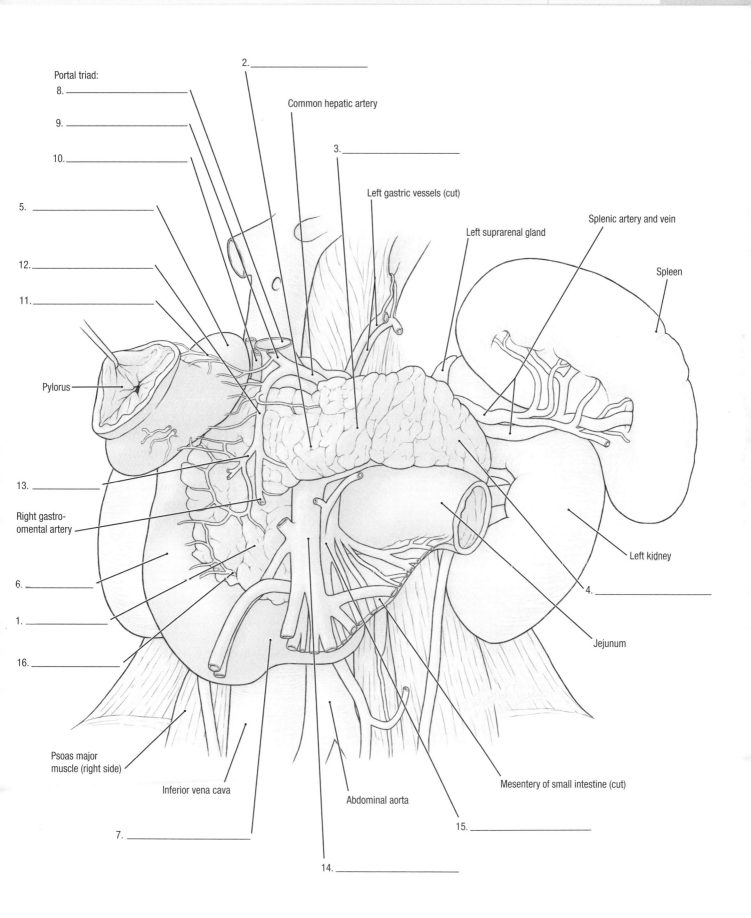

Portal triad:

8. _____

9. _____

10. _____

5. _____

12. _____

11. _____

Pylorus

13. _____

Right gastro-
omental artery

6. _____

1. _____

16. _____

Psoas major
muscle (right side)

Inferior vena cava

7. _____

2. _____

Common hepatic artery

3. _____

Left gastric vessels (cut)

Left suprarenal gland

Splenic artery and vein

Spleen

Left kidney

4. _____

Jejunum

Mesentery of small intestine (cut)

Abdominal aorta

15. _____

14. _____

4.13A INTESTINES IN SITU

The anterior abdominal wall has been cut, with the **_rectus abdominis_** muscles reflected inferiorly. The **_gastrocolic ligament_** has been reflected superiorly to reveal the small intestine, with the terminal portion of the ileum reflected to reveal the appendix.

COLOR each of the following structures using a different color for each:

Small Intestine

Most of the small intestine is composed of the jejunum and ileum. No clear line demarcates the jejunum from the ileum grossly.

○ 1. *Jejunum*: Mostly lies in the left upper quadrant
○ 2. *Ileum*: Mostly lies in the right lower quadrant
○ 3. *Mesentery of the small intestine (mesentery, true mesentery):* Fan-shaped double layer of peritoneum that attaches the jejunum and ileum to the posterior abdominal wall

Large Intestine

The large intestine includes the cecum, appendix, ascending colon, transverse colon, descending colon, sigmoid colon, rectum, and anal canal. The large intestine frames the right, superior, left, and inferior sides of the centrally located jejunum and ileum. Several distinct features of the large intestine distinguish it from the small intestine.

○ 4. *Omental appendices*: Fatty projections hanging from the four parts of the colon
Teniae coli: Three bands of longitudinal smooth muscle that run from the beginning of the ascending colon to the beginning of the rectum

Haustra: Bubble-like sacs of the intestinal wall between the tenia coli
○ 5. *Cecum*: First part of the large intestine and is continuous with the ascending colon. It is a blind pouch inferior to the ileocecal junction. Typically lies in the right iliac fossa.
○ 6. *Appendix:* Blind diverticulum of the cecum usually located posterior to the cecum, but is variable in its position
○ 7. *Ascending colon:* Passes superiorly on the right side from the cecum to the right lobe of the liver, where it turns to the left at the **_right colic (hepatic) flexure_** to become the transverse colon.
○ 8. *Transverse colon:* Longest and most mobile portion of the large intestine, crossing the abdomen from the right colic to **_left colic (splenic) flexure_**. The transverse mesocolon fuses with parietal peritoneum at the inferior border of the pancreas.
○ 9. *Descending colon*: Passes inferiorly on the left side from the left colic flexure to the left iliac fossa, where it is continuous with the sigmoid colon.
○ 10. *Sigmoid colon:* Characterized by an S-shaped loop connecting the descending colon to the rectum.

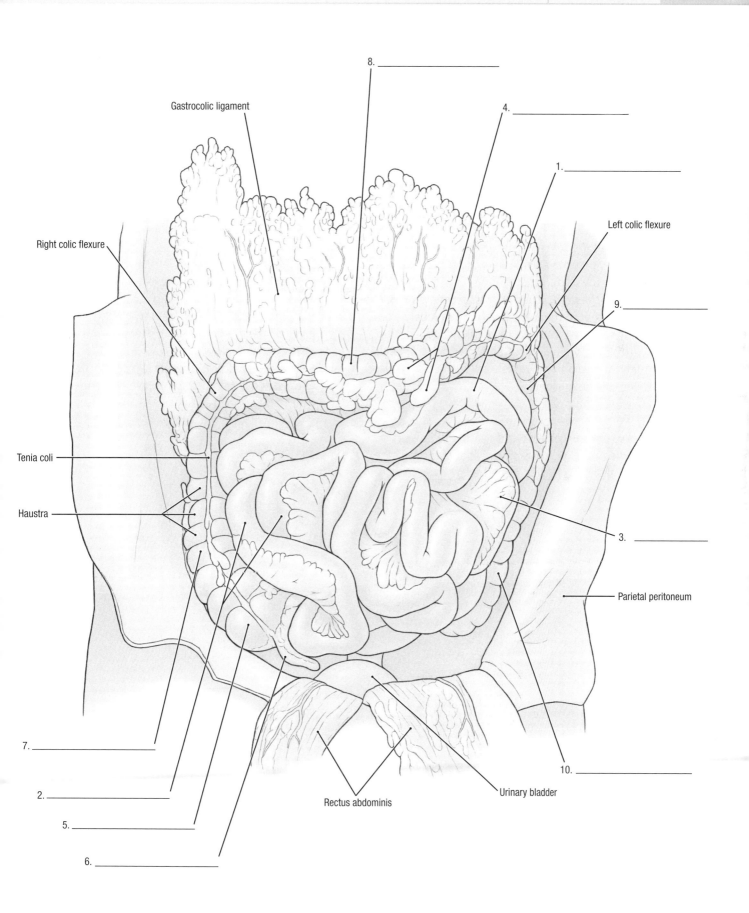

8. _____

4. _____

1. _____

Gastrocolic ligament

Left colic flexure

Right colic flexure

9. _____

Tenia coli

Haustra

3. _____

Parietal peritoneum

7. _____

10. _____

2. _____

Urinary bladder

5. _____

Rectus abdominis

6. _____

4.13B MESENTERY OF THE SMALL INTESTINE AND SIGMOID MESOCOLON

Similar to Section 4.13A, the anterior abdominal wall has been cut and reflected with the **_rectus abdominis_** muscles reflected inferiorly. The **_gastrocolic ligament_** has again been reflected superiorly to reveal the small intestine. In addition, the small intestines have been elevated superiorly to reveal their mesentery and the sigmoid colon elevated to reveal the sigmoid mesocolon.

COLOR each of the following structures using a different color for each:

Small Intestine

○ 1. *Jejunum*: Mostly lies in the left upper quadrant beginning at the **_duodenojejunal junction (flexure)_**

○ 2. *Ileum*: Mostly lies in the right lower quadrant ending at the ileocolic junction

○ 3. *Mesentery of the small intestine (mesentery, true mesentery):* The root of the mesentery runs obliquely from the duodenojejunal junction to the ileocolic junction, crossing the abdominal **_aorta_** and inferior vena cava. The superior mesenteric vessels course between the two layers of the mesentery.

Large Intestine

○ 4. *Transverse colon:* Longest and most mobile portion of the large intestine, crossing the abdomen from the right colic to left colic flexures. The **_left colic flexure_** is typically located more superior than the right colic flexure.

○ 5. *Descending colon*: Passes inferiorly on the left side from the left colic flexure to the left iliac fossa, where it is continuous with the sigmoid colon

○ 6. *Sigmoid colon:* Extends from the left iliac fossa to the level of the S3 vertebra connecting the descending colon to the rectum

○ 7. *Sigmoid mesocolon:* Double layer of peritoneum connecting the sigmoid colon to the posterior abdominal wall

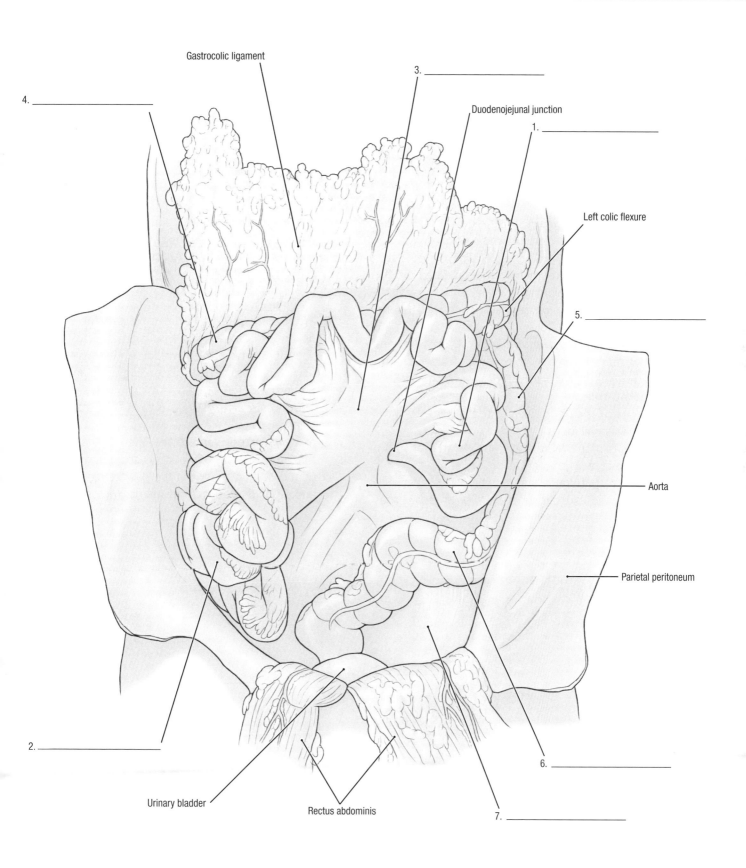

Gastrocolic ligament

3. _____

Duodenojejunal junction

4. _____

1. _____

Left colic flexure

5. _____

Aorta

Parietal peritoneum

2. _____

Urinary bladder

Rectus abdominis

6. _____

7. _____

Grant's

4.14   SUPERIOR MESENTERIC ARTERY (SMA)

The jejunum, ileum, and proximal large intestine along with their arterial supply, the SMA, have been isolated from the remainder of the abdominal cavity. A portion of the peritoneum of the mesentery of the small intestine and transverse mesocolon has been stripped off to demonstrate the branching pattern of the SMA. Branches arising from the left side of the SMA supply the *jejunum* and *ileum*, whereas branches arising from the right side supply the large intestine from the cecum to the middle of the *transverse colon*.

COLOR each of the following structures using a different color for each:

○ 1. *Superior mesenteric artery*: Arises from the abdominal aorta at the level of L1 vertebra and supplies derivatives of the midgut

○ 2. *Jejunal artery*: Numerous jejunal arteries arise from the SMA to supply the jejunum

  ○ 3. *Arcades of the jejunum*: Jejunal arteries unite to form simple, large loops

  ○ 4. *Vasa recta of the jejunum*: Long, straight arteries arising from the arcades to the wall of the jejunum

○ 5. *Ileal artery:* Numerous ileal arteries arise from the SMA to supply the ileum

  ○ 6. *Arcades of the ileum*: Ileal arteries unite to form complex, small loops

  ○ 7. *Vasa recta of the ileum*: Short, straight arteries arising from the arcades to the wall of the ileum

○ 8. *Ileocolic artery:* Terminal branch of the SMA that courses directly to the ileocolic junction with branches that supply the terminal ileum and proximal colon including the *cecum* and *ascending colon*

○ 9. *Appendicular artery*: Arises from the ileocolic artery, passes posterior to the terminal portion of the ileum to travel through the mesoappendix to reach the *appendix*

○ 10. *Right colic artery:* Courses toward the right colic flexure. This artery may arise independently or from a common trunk with the middle colic artery off of the SMA. Supplies the distal ascending colon and proximal transverse colon.

○ 11. *Middle colic artery*: Courses toward the middle of the transverse colon

○ 12. *Marginal artery:* Parallels the length of the colon and is formed by the anastomotic connections from the ileocolic, right colic, middle colic of the SMA, along with left colic and sigmoid arteries of the inferior mesenteric artery

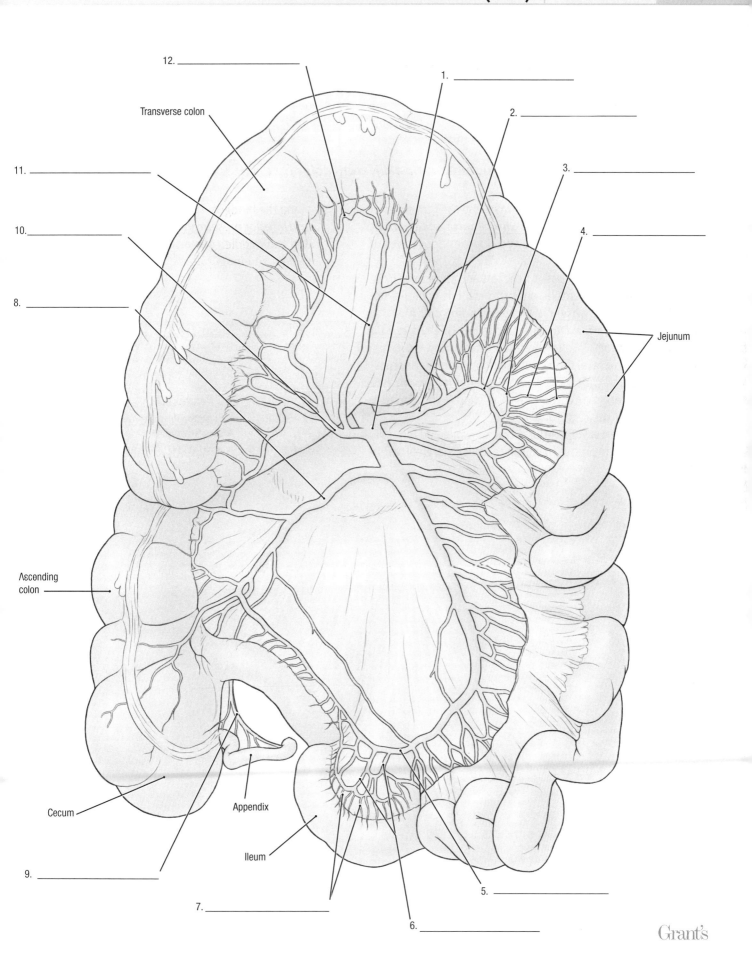

12. _____

Transverse colon

11. _____

10. _____

8. _____

Ascending
colon _____

Cecum _____

9. _____

1. _____

2. _____

3. _____

4. _____

Jejunum

Appendix

Ileum

7. _____

6. _____

5. _____

4.15   INFERIOR MESENTERIC ARTERY (IMA)

The root of the mesentery of the small intestine has been cut from the duodenojejunal junction to the ileocolic junction. Portions of the 2nd to 4th portions of the **duodenum** are visible through the portion of the remaining root of the mesentery and parietal peritoneum of the posterior abdominal wall. The **SMA** and many of its branches have been cut except for the **middle colic artery**.

COLOR each of the following structures using a different color for each:

○ 1. **Inferior mesenteric artery (IMA)**: Arises 2-3 cm superior to the bifurcation of the **abdominal aorta** into the **right and left common iliac arteries**. Supplies derivatives of the hindgut.

○ 2. **Left colic artery**: Passes to the left and superiorly from the inferior mesenteric artery to the left colic flexure between the **transverse** and **descending colon**.

○ 3. **Sigmoid arteries:** Descend to the left to the **sigmoid colon** (usually two to three branches)

○ 4. **Superior rectal artery**: Continuation of the inferior mesenteric artery after the sigmoid arteries have branched off; descends into the pelvis to supply the superior portion of the rectum

○ 5. **Marginal artery:** Superior rectal, sigmoid, and left colic arteries anastomose to continue as the marginal artery along the hindgut. The **anastomosis between superior and inferior mesenteric arteries** at the left colic artery and the middle colic artery marks the transition from midgut to hindgut at the left colic flexure.

CLINICAL NOTE: ABDOMINAL AORTIC ANEURYSM

An aneurysm is a focal dilatation in an artery with at least a 50% increase in the vessel's normal diameter; in the abdominal aorta, the enlargement in diameter can be 3 cm or more. As the vessel wall becomes progressively weaker, the aneurysm enlarges, and risk of spontaneous rupture increases. Most abdominal aortic aneurysms (AAAs) occur inferior to the renal arteries and superior to the **common iliac arteries**, often near the inferior mesenteric artery. Most AAAs are asymptomatic (until a rupture) and are detected as incidental findings on diagnostic imaging.

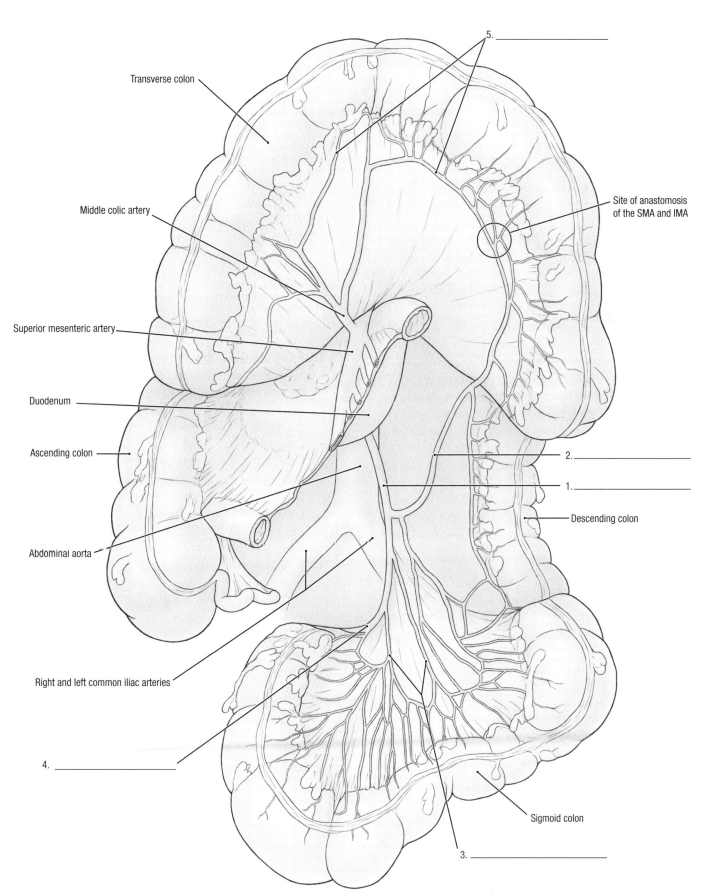

5. _____

Transverse colon

Site of anastomosis
of the SMA and IMA

Middle colic artery

Superior mesenteric artery

Duodenum

Ascending colon

2. _____

1. _____

Descending colon

Abdominal aorta

Right and left common iliac arteries

4. _____

Sigmoid colon

3. _____

4.16A and B LIVER

The liver and gallbladder have been isolated from the abdominal cavity. Figure A depicts the liver from an anterior (diaphragmatic) view, whereas Figure B is from the posteroinferior (visceral surface) view.

COLOR each of the following structures using a different color for each:

Peritoneal Structures

○ 1. *Falciform ligament*: Attaches the liver to the anterior abdominal wall, dividing the liver into right and left lobes

    ○ 2. *Round ligament of the liver (ligamentum teres):* Located in the inferior free edge of the falciform ligament formed by the obliterated umbilical vein

○ 3. *Coronary ligament:* Two-layer peritoneal structure attaching the liver to the diaphragm. The anterior layer is formed by the bifurcation of the falciform ligament at the superior border of the liver into right and left extensions (Figure A). The posterior layer is a continuation laterally from the *lesser omentum* (Figure B).

○ 4. *Bare area of the liver:* Area between the two diverging layers of the coronary ligament on the posterior aspect of the liver, where there is a lack of visceral peritoneum covering the surface of the liver (Figure B)

○ 5. *Right triangular ligament:* Site where the two layers of the coronary ligament meet laterally on the right (Figure B)

○ 6. *Left triangular ligament:* Site where the two layers of the coronary ligament meet laterally on the left

Porta Hepatis

On the visceral surface of the liver, a right and left sagittal fissure are connected centrally to form the *porta hepatis*, a transverse fissure where the portal triad structures enter and leave the liver.

    The portal triad structures are within the lesser omentum and include the following:

○ 7. *Hepatic portal vein*

○ 8. *Common bile duct*

○ 9. *Proper hepatic artery*

The right sagittal fissure contains the following:

○ 10. *Inferior vena cava*: Lies in the superior aspect of the right sagittal fissure and receives blood from the liver via the hepatic veins

○ 11. *Gallbladder*: Lies in the inferior aspect of the right sagittal fissure

Lobes of the Liver

Externally, the liver is divided into two anatomical lobes and two accessory lobes by the peritoneum reflections and fissures.

○ 12. *Right lobe:* Lies to the right of the falciform ligament anteriorly and is separated posteriorly by the right sagittal fissure from the quadrate and caudate lobes

○ 13. *Left lobe:* Lies to the left of the falciform ligament anteriorly and is separated posteriorly by the left sagittal fissure from the quadrate and caudate lobes

○ 14. *Quadrate lobe:* Lies between the gallbladder and the left sagittal fissure anteroinferior to the porta hepatis

○ 15. *Caudate lobe:* Lies between the inferior vena cava and the left sagittal fissure posterosuperior to the porta hepatis. Typically has a process resembling a "tail," earning it the name caudate even though it is not in a caudal anatomical position.

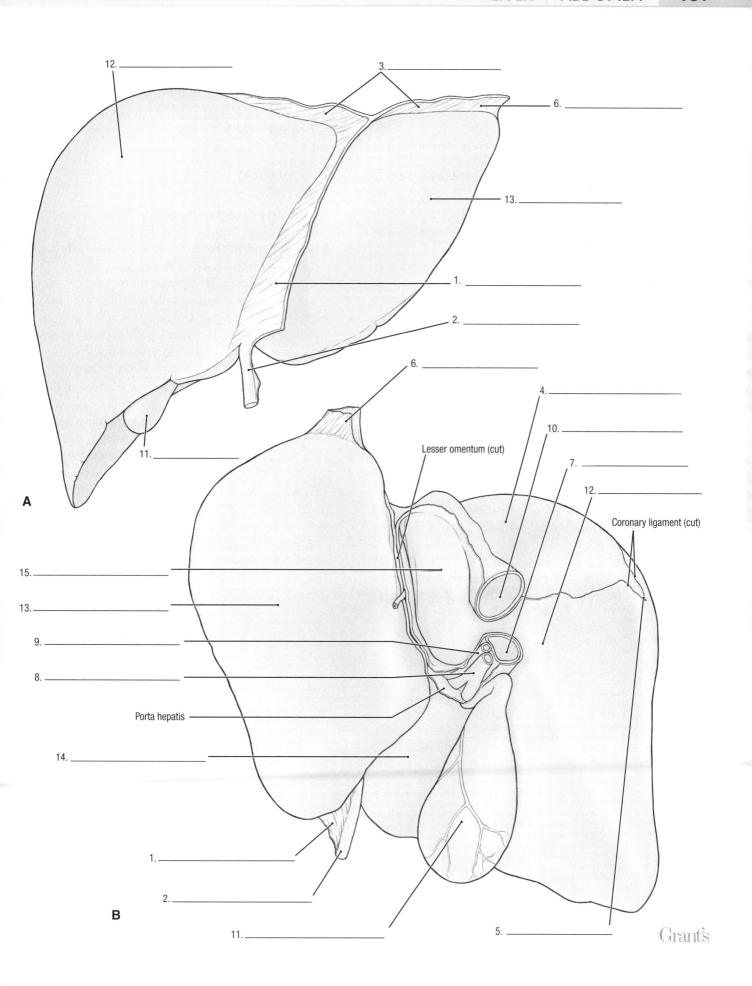

12. _____

3. _____

6. _____

13. _____

1. _____

2. _____

11. _____

A

6. _____

4. _____

10. _____

7. _____

12. _____

Coronary ligament (cut)

Lesser omentum (cut)

15. _____

13. _____

9. _____

8. _____

Porta hepatis _____

14. _____

1. _____

2. _____

11. _____

5. _____

B

4.17A and B   GALLBLADDER AND BILIARY SYSTEM

The visceral surface of the liver has been elevated in Figure A to demonstrate the porta hepatis.

The gallbladder, extrahepatic biliary system, and pancreatic ducts have been isolated with the duodenum. The gallbladder has been elevated in Figure B (in anatomical position, the body of the gallbladder lies anterior to the *superior part of the duodenum*).

COLOR each of the following structures using a different color for each:

○ 1. **Gallbladder:** Lies on the visceral surface of the liver between the right and *quadrate lobes*. The gallbladder has three parts (Figure B):

  ○ 2. **Fundus**: Wide blunt end that usually projects outward from the inferior border of the liver

  ○ 3. **Body**: Main portion that contacts the visceral surface of the liver, transverse colon, and superior part of duodenum

  ○ 4. **Neck**: Narrow, tapering end opposite the fundus

○ 5. **Cystic duct:** Connects the neck of the gallbladder to the common hepatic duct. The mucosa of the neck spirals, assisting to keep the cystic duct open and allowing bile to easily enter the gallbladder.

○ 6. **Right hepatic duct:** Drains bile from the right lobe of the liver

○ 7. **Left hepatic duct:** Drains bile from the left, quadrate, and *caudate lobes* of the liver

○ 8. **Common hepatic duct**: Union of the left and right hepatic ducts almost immediately after leaving the porta hepatis

○ 9. **(Common) bile duct:** Union of the common hepatic duct and the cystic duct. Passes within the lesser omentum (hepatoduodenal ligament) with the *hepatic portal vein* and *proper hepatic artery*. Passes posterior to the superior part of the duodenum.

○ 10. **Main pancreatic duct**: Courses horizontally through the tail, body, and head of the pancreas (Figure B)

○ 11. **Hepatopancreatic ampulla**: Union of the main pancreatic duct and common bile duct to the left of the *descending part of the duodenum* in the head of pancreas (Figure B). The ampulla pierces through the mucosa and opens into the duodenum at the major duodenal papilla (internal duodenal landmark).

○ 12. **Accessory pancreatic duct**: Courses through the head of the pancreas superior to the main pancreatic duct to open independently in the descending part of the duodenum (Figure B). When present, forms a minor duodenal papilla superior to the major duodenal papilla.

The gallbladder receives its blood supply from the following:

○ 13. **Cystic artery**: Typically branches from the *right hepatic artery* in the cystohepatic triangle (of Calot) between the cystic duct, common hepatic duct, and the visceral surface of the liver (Figure A)

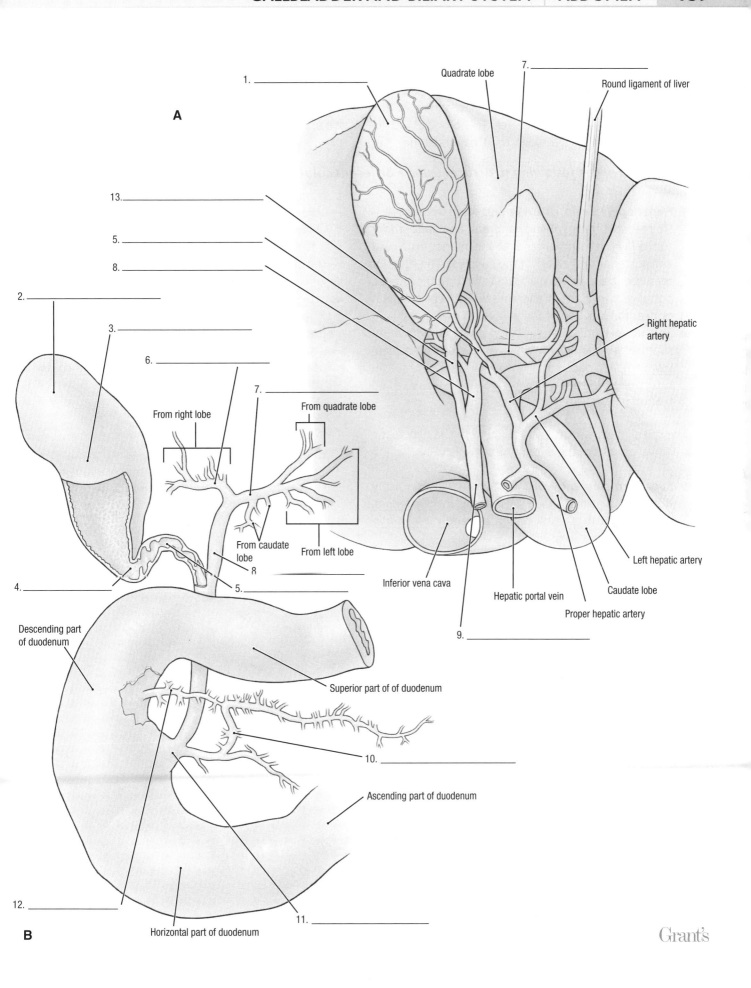

A

1. _____

Quadrate lobe

7. _____

Round ligament of liver

Right hepatic artery

13. _____

5. _____

8. _____

2. _____

3. _____

6. _____

From right lobe

7. _____

From quadrate lobe

From caudate lobe

From left lobe

8

4. _____

5. _____

Inferior vena cava

Hepatic portal vein

Proper hepatic artery

Left hepatic artery

Caudate lobe

9. _____

Descending part of duodenum

Superior part of of duodenum

10. _____

Ascending part of duodenum

12. _____

11. _____

Horizontal part of duodenum

B

Grant's

4.18   PORTAL VENOUS SYSTEM

The hepatic portal vein collects blood from the abdominal gastrointestinal tract as well as the spleen, pancreas, and gallbladder and carries it to the liver. This blood is rich in nutrients from absorption through the small intestines, but reduced in oxygen. The blood is processed through the liver before moving through the hepatic veins to the inferior vena cava and the heart.

COLOR each of the following structures using a different color for each:

○ 1. **Hepatic portal vein**: Drains venous blood from the gastrointestinal tract, **spleen**, **pancreas**, and **gallbladder** to the **liver**. It forms anterior to the inferior vena cava and posterior to the neck of the pancreas. The superior mesenteric and splenic veins unite to form the hepatic portal vein, with the inferior mesenteric vein joining at or near the junction of the two veins.

○ 2. **Splenic vein** drains venous blood primarily from areas supplied by the splenic artery including the spleen, **stomach**, and pancreas:
  ○ 3. **Left gastro-omental vein**
  ○ 4. **Short gastric vein**

The splenic vein also receives blood from the pancreatic veins and variably from the inferior mesenteric vein.

○ 5. **Superior mesenteric vein** drains venous blood primarily from areas supplied by the SMA, including the **duodenum**, pancreas, small intestine, **cecum**, **appendix**, **ascending colon**, and transverse colon:
  ○6. **Right gastro-omental vein**
  ○7. **Jejunal and ileal**
  ○8. **Ileocolic vein**

○9. **Right colic vein**
○10. **Middle colic vein**

The superior mesenteric vein also receives blood from the pancreaticoduodenal veins and variably from the inferior mesenteric vein.

○ 11. **Inferior mesenteric vein** drains venous blood primarily from areas supplied by the inferior mesenteric artery, including the **descending colon**, **sigmoid colon**, and superior **rectum**:
  ○12. **Superior rectal vein**
  ○13. **Sigmoid vein**
  ○14. **Left colic vein**
○ 15. **Right and left gastric veins** typically drain directly into the hepatic portal vein or into the splenic vein because there is not a venous equivalent to the celiac trunk.

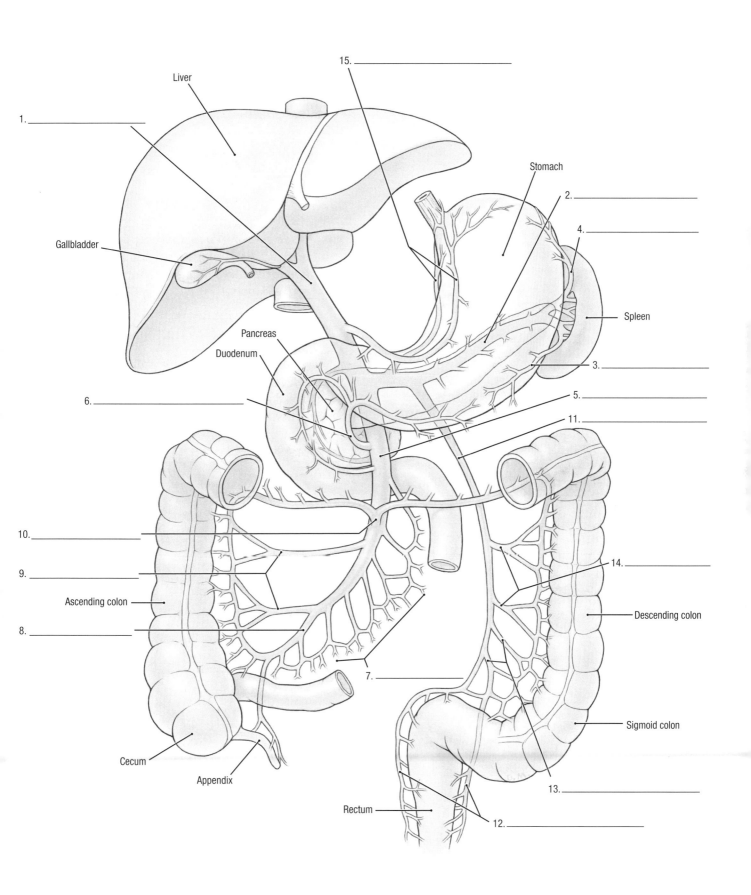

15. _____

Liver

1. _____

Stomach

2. _____

4. _____

Gallbladder

Spleen

Pancreas

Duodenum

3. _____

6. _____

5. _____

11. _____

10. _____

9. _____

Ascending colon

8. _____

14. _____

Descending colon

7. _____

Cecum

Sigmoid colon

Appendix

13. _____

Rectum

12. _____

Grant's

4.19 PORTACAVAL SYSTEM

Portions of the hepatic portal venous system and the caval venous system are shown. Communication between the portal venous system and the caval system occurs at the level of the venules, where structures and organs that drain portally are in close proximity to structures and the body wall that drain through the caval system.

COLOR each of the following structures using a different color for each:

The following areas of the caval system are most likely to communicate with the hepatic portal venous system:

○ 1. **Inferior vena cava**
○ 2. **Common iliac vein**: Right and left unite to form the inferior vena cava
○ 3. **External iliac vein**: Drains lower limb and unites with internal iliac vein to form common iliac vein
○ 4. **Internal iliac vein**: Drains the pelvis and perineum and unites with external iliac vein to form the common iliac vein
○ 5. **Azygos vein**

There are four sites of portocaval (portal-systemic) anastomoses:

I. Esophageal

○ 6. **Esophageal veins**: Drain into azygos vein (caval)
○ 7. **Left gastric vein**: Esophageal branches (portal)

II. Umbilical

○ 8. **Epigastric veins**: Drain umbilicus and anterior abdominal wall to branches of external iliac vein (caval)
○ 9. **Paraumbilical veins**: Course from umbilical area with round ligament of liver to portal vein

III. Rectal

○ 10. **Middle and inferior rectal veins**: Drain anal canal and lower rectum to the internal iliac artery (caval)
○ 11. **Superior rectal vein**: Drains rectum to **inferior mesenteric vein** (portal)

IV. Retroperitoneal

○ 12. **Retroperitoneal veins**: Veins of posterior abdominal wall drain into inferior vena cava
○ 13. **Colic veins**: Veins draining the ascending and descending colon drain into the portal vein and are in close approximation to the veins of the posterior abdominal wall

---

CLINICAL NOTE: PORTAL HYPERTENSION

The hepatic portal vein carries ~1500 mL/min of blood to the liver. Obstruction of portal venous flow, commonly from cirrhosis, results in an increase in portal venous pressure. Normal portal vein pressure is between 5 and 10 mm Hg. Complications such as varices and ascites occur at 12 mm Hg or greater. As the pressure rises in the hepatic portal vein, the pressure also rises in its tributaries. The increased volume of blood in the tributaries may produce varicose veins (enlarged, gnarled veins), especially at the locations of portacaval anastomoses. The veins may become so enlarged that their walls rupture, resulting in hemorrhage that may be fatal in the case of ruptured esophageal varices.

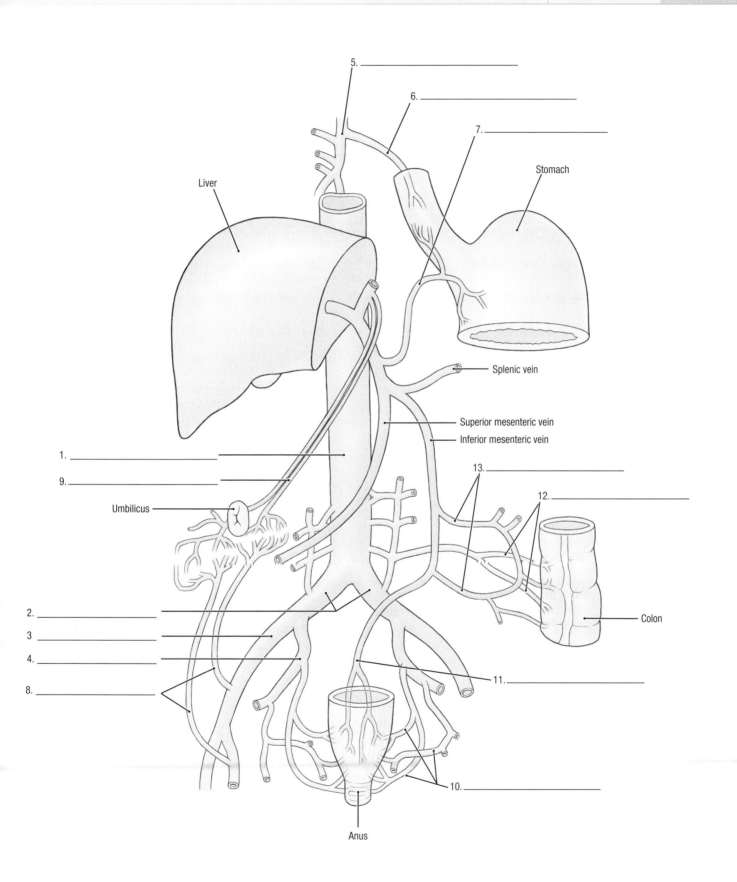

5. _____

6. _____

7. _____

Stomach

Liver

Splenic vein

Superior mesenteric vein

Inferior mesenteric vein

1. _____

9. _____

13. _____

12. _____

Umbilicus

Colon

2. _____

3. _____

4. _____

11. _____

8. _____

10. _____

Anus

4.20 POSTERIOR ABDOMINAL WALL

The abdominal portion of the gastrointestinal tract has been removed, except the ***descending*** and ***sigmoid colon***. The celiac trunk and superior mesenteric arteries have been cut near their origin from the abdominal aorta. The pancreas, gallbladder, and liver have also been removed, with the ***hepatic veins*** cut as they drained to the inferior vena cava.

COLOR each of the following structures using a different color for each:

○ 1. **Abdominal aorta**: Begins at the aortic hiatus of the diaphragm at T12 and ends at the level of L4 vertebra by dividing into the right and left ***common iliac arteries***

The abdominal aorta gives rise to several branches:

○ 2. **Celiac trunk:** Arises immediately below the aortic hiatus of the diaphragm

○ 3. **Celiac ganglion:** Collection of postganglionic sympathetic cell bodies at the base of the celiac trunk involved in sending postganglionic sympathetic fibers along the branches of the celiac trunk to foregut structures and spleen

○ 4. **Superior mesenteric artery:** Arises immediately inferior to the celiac trunk and passes anterior to left renal vein along with the third part of duodenum and uncinate process of pancreas (not shown)

○ 5. **Inferior mesenteric artery:** Arises one vertebral level superior to the bifurcation of the aorta into the common iliac arteries

○ 6. **Renal arteries:** Paired arteries that arise immediately inferior to the SMA and initially course posterior to the renal veins

○ 7. **Gonadal (testicular/ovarian) arteries:** Paired arteries that arise between the renal arteries and the inferior mesenteric artery and course inferiorly

○ 8. **Inferior phrenic arteries:** Paired arteries that arise at the level of the celiac trunk and course along the inferior aspect of diaphragm

○ 9. **Subcostal arteries:** Paired arteries that arise inferior to the SMA and course along the inferior aspect of the 12th rib

○ 10. **Median sacral artery:** Arises from the posterior aspect of the aorta immediately superior to the bifurcation of the aorta and descends along the sacrum into the pelvis

○ 11. **Inferior vena cava:** Begins anterior to the L5 vertebra by the union of the ***common iliac veins***

Most veins of the posterior abdominal wall drain into the inferior vena cava:

○ 12. **Right renal vein**

○ 13. **Right gonadal vein**

○ 14. **Left renal vein:** Courses anterior to the aorta and posterior to the SMA to drain into the inferior vena cava. Receives the venous drainage of the following:

○ 15. **Left gonadal vein**

○ 16. **Left suprarenal vein**

○ 17. **Right kidney:** Related to the liver, duodenum, and ascending colon anteriorly

○ 18. **Left kidney:** Related to the stomach, ***spleen***, pancreas, jejunum, and descending colon anteriorly

○ 19. **Ureter:** Muscular ducts that run inferiorly from the renal hilum to pass over the pelvic brim into the pelvis to the bladder

○ 20. **Right suprarenal gland:** Pyramidal shaped; situated over the superior aspect of the right kidney

○ 21. **Left suprarenal gland**: Crescent shaped; situated medial to the superior aspect of the left kidney

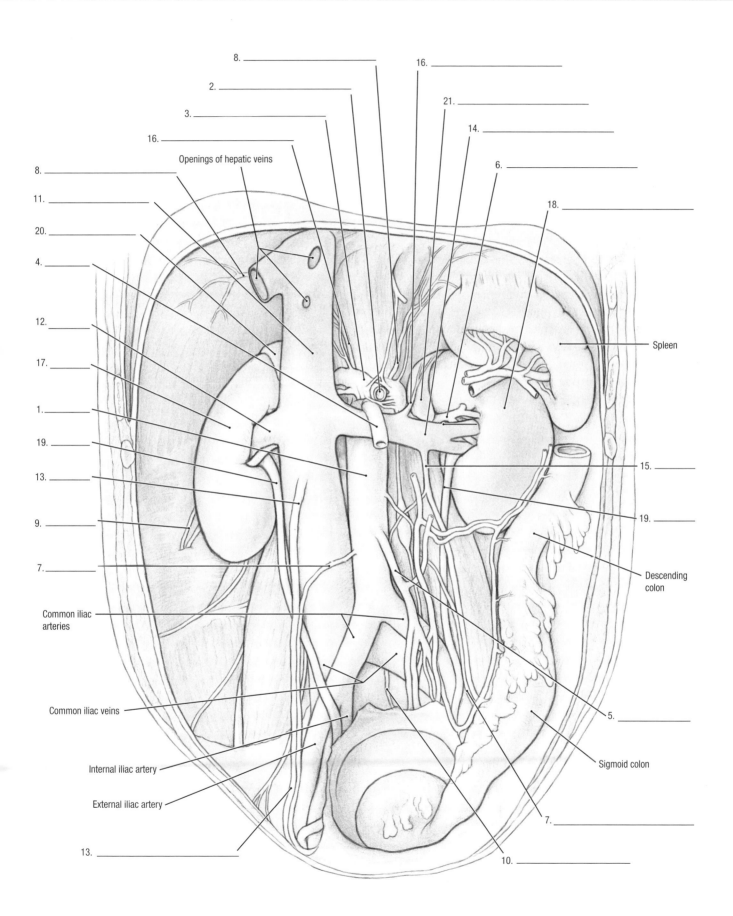

8.

2.

3.

16.

Openings of hepatic veins

8.

11.

20.

4.

12.

17.

1.

19.

13.

9.

7.

Common iliac
arteries

Common iliac veins

Internal iliac artery

External iliac artery

13.

16.

21.

14.

6.

18.

Spleen

15.

19.

Descending
colon

5.

Sigmoid colon

7.

10.

Grant's

4.21A and B KIDNEY

In Figure A, a portion of the anterior aspect of the kidney has been removed to reveal the space of the ***renal sinus*** and the structures within the sinus. Figure B depicts a coronal section of the kidney demonstrating the internal structures of the kidney.

COLOR each of the following structures using a different color for each:

1. *Fibrous capsule*: Adhered to the surface of the kidney
2. *Renal cortex*: Outer portion of the kidney deep to the fibrous capsule
3. *Renal column*: Extension of the renal cortex interiorly between the renal medullary pyramids
4. *Renal medulla*: Innermost portion of the kidney usually segmented
5. *Renal pyramids*: Typical formation of renal medulla in between the renal columns
6. *Renal papilla:* Apex of the renal pyramid that protrudes and excretes urine into a minor calyx
7. *Minor calyx:* First component of the collecting system that forms the ureter
8. *Major calyx:* Merging of two to four minor calyces

9. *Renal pelvis:* Merging of two to three major calyces to form the superior dilated portion of the ureter within the space of the renal sinus
10. *Ureter:* Formed by the narrowing of the renal pelvis
11. *Perinephric fat:* Surrounds the kidneys, renal vessels, and collecting system filling the renal sinus

CLINICAL NOTE: KIDNEY STONES (RENAL CALCULI)

Kidney stones (renal calculi) can form and become lodged within the calyces of the kidney, ureters, or urinary bladder. If the stone is larger than the renal pelvis or the ureter, it will cause distension of the muscular tube resulting in renal colic. Common patient presentation includes sudden onset of severe flank pain that radiates inferiorly and anteriorly with or without nausea and vomiting. Approximately 80% to 85% of kidney stones pass spontaneously, with only 20% of patients requiring hospitalization.

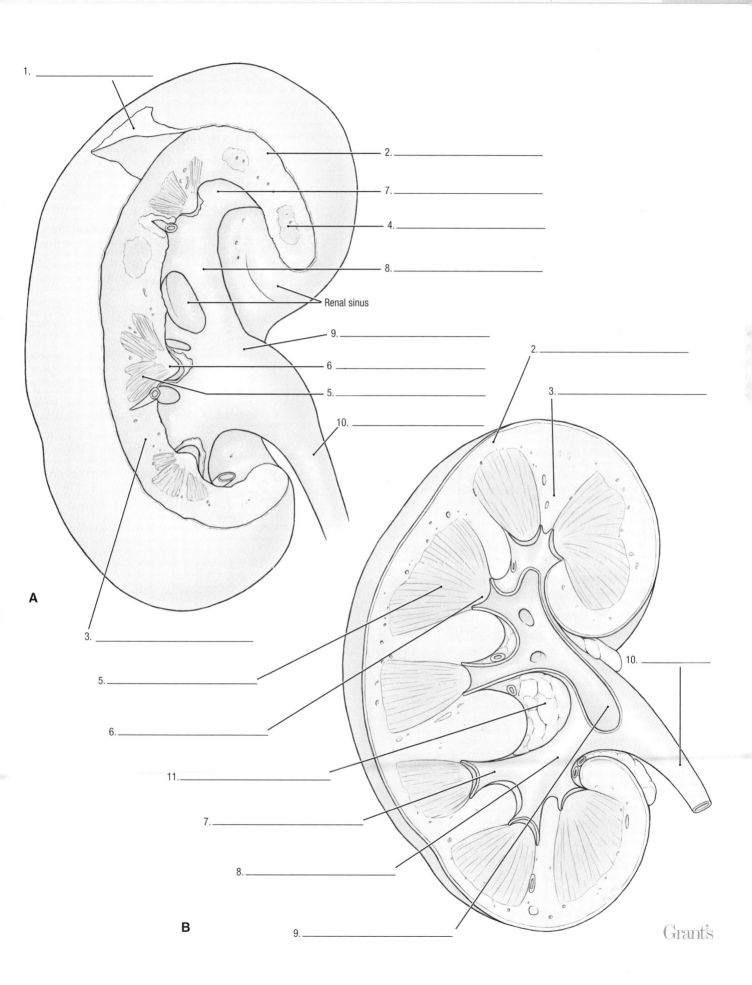

1. _____

2. _____

7. _____

4. _____

8. _____

Renal sinus

9. _____

6. _____

5. _____

10. _____

A

3. _____

5. _____

6. _____

11. _____

7. _____

8. _____

B

2. _____

3. _____

10. _____

9. _____

Grant's

4.22 NERVES AND MUSCLES OF POSTERIOR ABDOMINAL WALL

Abdominopelvic cavity contents have been removed to reveal the muscles and nerves of the posterior abdominal wall. On the left, the psoas major muscle has also been removed to reveal the formation of the lumbar plexus.

COLOR each of the following structures using a different color for each:

Muscles of the Posterior Abdominal Wall

○ 1. *Psoas major muscle*: Lies lateral to the lumbar vertebrae and passes inferolaterally deep to inguinal ligament to the lesser trochanter of the femur

○ 2. *Psoas minor muscle*: Lies superficial to the psoas major, if present

○ 3. *Iliacus muscle*: Lies lateral to the inferior part of the psoas major muscle, with most of its fibers joining the psoas major to form the iliopsoas muscle

○ 4. *Quadratus lumborum*: Lies lateral to the superior part of the psoas major muscle and medial to the *transversus abdominis muscle*

Muscle	Proximal Attachment	Distal Attachment	Innervation	Action
Psoas major	Transverse processes of lumbar vertebrae and vertebral bodies T12-L5	Lesser trochanter of femur	Anterior rami of L1-L3	1. Acting with iliacus, flexes thigh 2. Acting superiorly, flexes vertebral column laterally
Psoas minor	Vertebral bodies of T12-L1	Pectineal line and iliopectineal eminence	Anterior rami of L1-L2	Balances the trunk with psoas major
Iliacus	Superior two-thirds of iliac fossa and ala of sacrum	Lesser trochanter of femur	Femoral nerve (L2-L4)	Acting with psoas major, flexes thigh
Quadratus lumborum	Medial half of 12th ribs and lumbar transverse processes	Iliac crest	Anterior rami of T12 and L1-L4	Extends and laterally flexes vertebral column

Nerves of Posterior Abdominal Wall

○ 5. *Subcostal nerve*: Anterior ramus of T12 that arises in the thorax, passes posterior to the *lateral arcuate ligament* of the diaphragm, and courses inferolaterally on the anterior surface of quadratus lumborum

Lumbar plexus is composed of the anterior rami of L1-L4 and forms several named branches:

○ 6. *Iliohypogastric nerve:* Branch of the anterior ramus of L1; enters abdomen posterior to *medial arcuate ligament* and courses inferolaterally on the anterior surface of the quadratus lumborum inferior to the subcostal nerve

○ 7. *Ilioinguinal nerve:* Branch of anterior ramus of L1; enters abdomen posterior to medial arcuate ligament and courses inferolaterally on the anterior surface of quadratus lumborum inferior to the iliohypogastric nerve

○ 8. *Genitofemoral nerve:* Forms from L1 to L2, pierces the psoas major, courses along its anterior surface, and divides into *genital and femoral branches*

○ 9. *Lateral cutaneous nerve of the thigh:* Arises from L2 to L3, runs lateral to the psoas major and along the anterior surface of the iliacus muscle to enter the thigh deep to the inguinal ligament

○10. *Femoral nerve:* Forms from L2 to L4, runs deep to the psoas major, and then emerges from the lateral border of the psoas major to pass deep to the inguinal ligament to the anterior thigh

○11. *Obturator nerve:* Arises from L2 to L4, emerges medial to the psoas major, and passes into the lesser pelvis

○12. *Lumbosacral trunk:* Forms from L4 to L5 passing over the ala of the sacrum, descends into the lesser pelvis, and participates in the sacral plexus

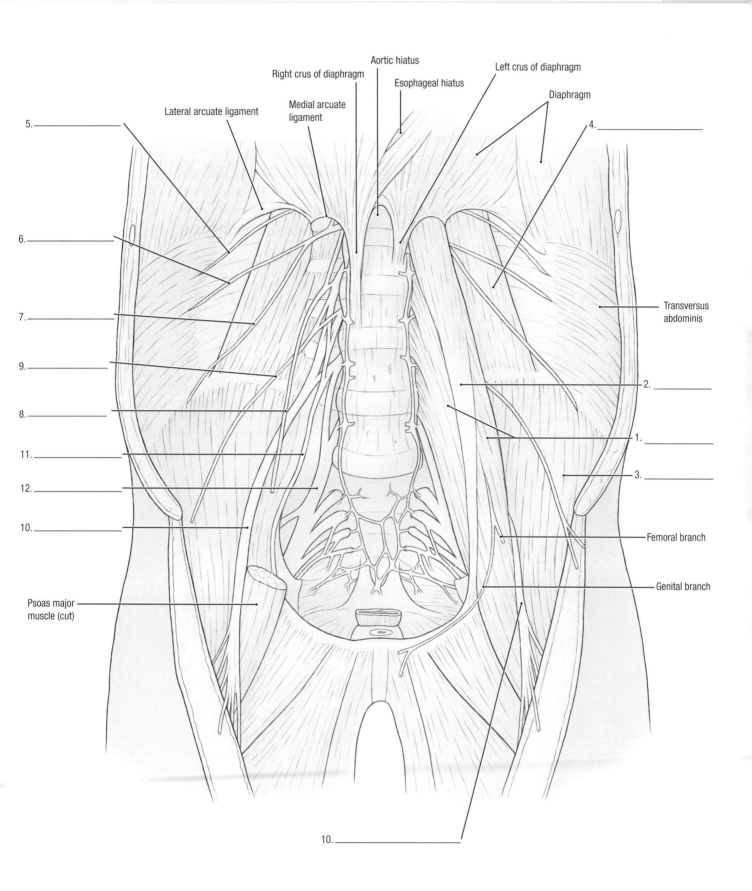

Lateral arcuate ligament

Right crus of diaphragm

Medial arcuate ligament

Aortic hiatus

Esophageal hiatus

Left crus of diaphragm

Diaphragm

5.

6.

7.

9.

8.

11.

12.

10.

Psoas major muscle (cut)

4.

Transversus abdominis

2.

1.

3.

Femoral branch

Genital branch

10.

Grant's

4.23 INFERIOR VIEW OF DIAPHRAGM

The inferior view of the diaphragm demonstrates the structures formed as the diaphragm attaches to inferior thoracic cage and superior lumbar vertebra. The ***psoas major*** muscle has been removed.

COLOR each of the following structures using a different color for each:

○ 1. **Central tendon:** Central aponeurotic portion surrounded by the muscular portion of the diaphragm peripherally

○ 2. **Caval opening**: Aperture located in the central tendon primarily for the inferior vena cava located at the level of the T8/9 IV disk

○ 3. **Esophageal hiatus**: Aperture in the muscular portion of the right crus at the level of T10 vertebra

○ 4. **Aortic hiatus**: Aperture posterior to the median arcuate ligament of the diaphragm at the T12 vertebra level

○ 5. **Left crus**: Musculotendinous band arising from L1 to L2 vertebrae, forming a portion of the aortic hiatus

○ 6. **Right crus**: Musculotendinous band arising from L1 to L4 vertebrae forming a portion of the aortic hiatus and forms the esophageal hiatus

○ 7. **Median arcuate ligament**: Arches over the anterior aspect of the aorta uniting the right and left crura

○ 8. **Medial arcuate ligament**: Thickening of fascia over the psoas major muscle

○ 9. **Lateral arcuate ligament**: Thickening of fascia over the ***quadratus lumborum*** muscle

CLINICAL NOTE: DIAPHRAGMATIC RUPTURE

Rupture of the diaphragm is most likely to occur from blunt or penetrating trauma. Most blunt trauma injuries to the diaphragm are from motor vehicle crashes. The impact either distorts the chest wall, creating a separation between the diaphragm and its attachments, or creates tears along the posterolateral wall of the diaphragm. The posterolateral wall of the diaphragm is the weakest component of the diaphragm because of its intermittent attachment points to the muscles of the posterior abdominal wall. Most diaphragmatic ruptures occur on the left side (80% to 90%) because of the presence of the liver on the right side in close relationship to the diaphragm. If the rupture is large enough, a traumatic diaphragmatic hernia may occur in which the stomach, small intestine, transverse colon, or spleen may pass through the rupture into the thoracic cavity.

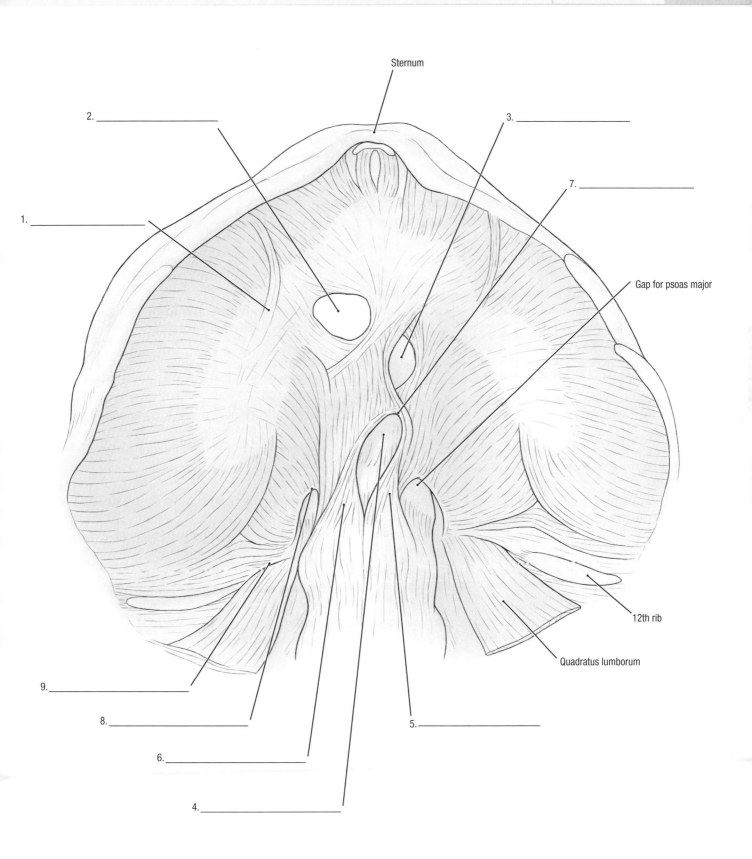

Sternum

2. _____

3. _____

7. _____

1. _____

Gap for psoas major

12th rib

Quadratus lumborum

9. _____

8. _____

5. _____

6. _____

4. _____

Grant's

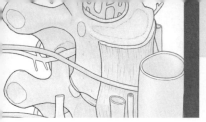

CHAPTER 5

Pelvis and Perineum

5.1A and B PELVIC GIRDLE

The pelvic girdle is a basin-shaped ring of bones that connects the vertebral column to the femurs. The pelvic girdle transfers the weight to the lower limbs during standing and walking and also protects the true pelvic organs and some of the more inferior abdominal viscera. The anatomic position of the pelvic girdle is with the **_anterior superior iliac spine_** (**_ASIS_**) and pubic symphysis located in the same vertical plane, which places the pelvis in an oblique plane to the abdomen.

COLOR each of the following structures using a different color for each:

In the adult, the pelvic girdle is composed of three bones: the sacrum and the right and left hip bones (coxal, os coxae), which are the fusion of the ilium, ischium, and pubis bones.

○ 1. **Sacrum:** Formed by the fusion of five sacral vertebrae and defines the posterior wall of the bony pelvis
  ○ 2. **Sacral promontory:** Anterior midline projection of the body of S1
  ○ 3. **Ala of sacrum:** "Wings" of S1 that sweep laterally from the promontory (right and left) that articulate laterally with the posterior surface of a hip bone at the **_sacroiliac joints_**

Coxal (hip; innominate; os coxae) bones define the anteroinferior and lateral walls of the bony pelvis. Each hip bone contains an **_obturator foramen_** along the anterior aspect.

○ 4. **Acetabulum:** Formed by all three hip bones and articulates with the head of the femur
○ 5. **Pubic symphysis:** Fibrocartilaginous pad that joins the hip bones anteriorly. The **_pubic arch_** is located immediately inferior to the pubic symphysis and the paired **_ischiopubic rami_**

The ilium forms the superior and lateral part of hip bone. The iliac crest forms the superior boundary of the ilium. The ASIS is the anterior projection from the iliac crest. Inferior to the ASIS, a minor projection, the **_anterior inferior iliac spine,_** **_(AIIS)_** is also present.

○ 6. **Iliac fossa:** Anteromedial concave surface of the ala of the ilium
○ 7. **Arcuate line:** Inferior to iliac fossa and contributes to the formation of the pelvic brim

The ischium forms the posteroinferior part of hip bone (in the anatomic position)

○ 8. **Ischial ramus:** Forms part of the obturator foramen and will join with the pubis to form the ischiopubic ramus
○ 9. **Ischial spine:** Small, pointed posteromedial projection for the attachment of the sacrospinous ligament

The pubis forms the anteroinferior part of the hip bone (in the anatomic position).

○10. **Superior pubic ramus:** Contributes to acetabulum
○11. **Inferior pubic ramus:** Contributes to the formation of the obturator foramen and ischiopubic ramus
○12. **Pubic tubercle:** Prominent protuberance of the superior ramus lateral to the pubic symphysis
○13. **Pubic crest:** Thickening of the pubis between the pubic tubercle and the pubic symphysis
○14. **Pectin pubis (pectineal line):** Oblique ridge along the superior ramus lateral to the pubic tubercle

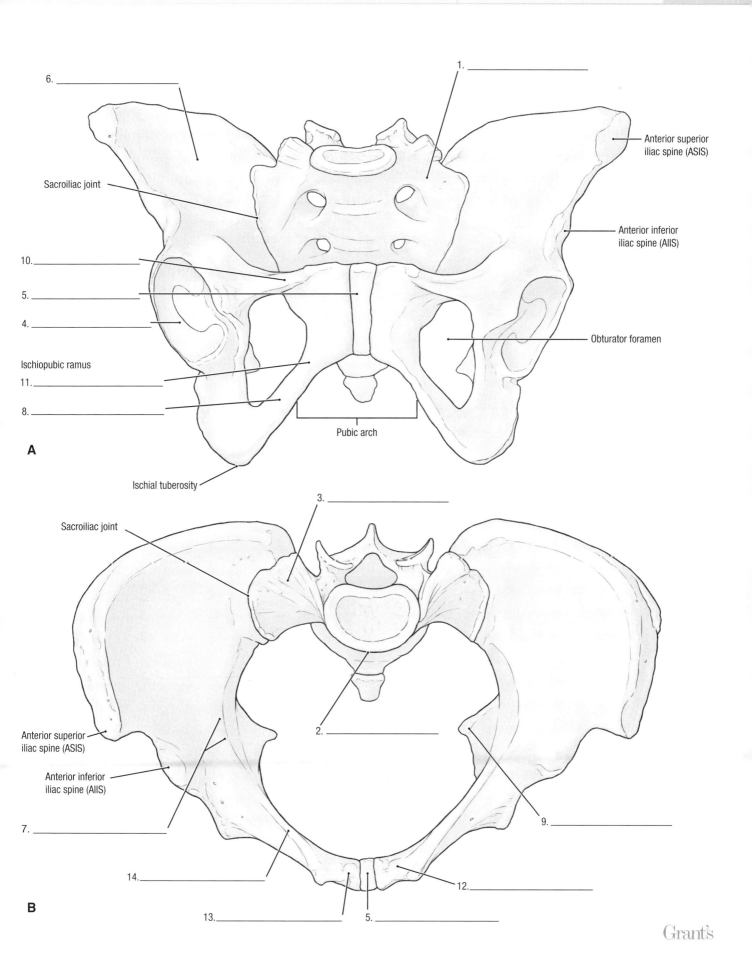

6. _____

1. _____

Anterior superior
iliac spine (ASIS)

Sacroiliac joint

Anterior inferior
iliac spine (AIIS)

10. _____

5. _____

4. _____

Ischiopubic ramus

Obturator foramen

11. _____

8. _____

Pubic arch

A

Ischial tuberosity

3. _____

Sacroiliac joint

Anterior superior
iliac spine (ASIS)

Anterior inferior
iliac spine (AIIS)

2. _____

7. _____

9. _____

14. _____

12. _____

13. _____   5. _____

B

Grant's

5.2A and B   PELVIC COMPARTMENTS AND LIGAMENTS

Pelvic Compartments

The pelvis is divided into a greater (false) pelvis and a lesser (true) pelvis. The two compartments of the pelvis are delineated by the bony **pelvic brim**. The greater pelvis lies superior to the pelvic brim bounded by the ala of the ilium and primarily contains abdominal viscera. The lesser pelvis lies inferior to the pelvic brim and primarily contains pelvis viscera.

The bony components of the pelvic brim are as follows:
- Sacral promontory (S1 vertebra) and sacral ala (wings)
- Right and left linea terminalis formed by the union of the following:
  - Pubic crest
  - Pecten pubis
  - Arcuate line of the ilium

COLOR each of the following structures using a different color for each:

Pelvic Ligaments

The sacroiliac joints are strong, weight-bearing compound joints and are the most immobile synovial joints of the body.

Weight is transferred from the axial skeleton to the ilia via the sacroiliac ligaments:

○ 1. **Anterior sacroiliac ligament:** Thin, anterior portion of the fibrous joint capsule

○ 2. **Posterior sacroiliac ligament:** Fibers run obliquely upward and outward from the sacrum as posterior continuation of the interosseous sacroiliac ligaments

○ 3. **Sacrotuberous ligament:** Passes from posterior ilium and lateral sacrum/coccyx to the **ischial tuberosity**, forming the sciatic foramen

○ 4. **Sacrospinous ligament:** Passes from lateral sacrum/coccyx to the ischial spine, subdividing the sciatic foramen into the greater and lesser sciatic foramina

○ 5. **Greater sciatic foramen:** Point of exit for structures entering/exiting the pelvis posteriorly to/from the lower limb or perineum

○ 6. **Lesser sciatic foramen:** Route for structures destined for the perineum

○ 7. **Obturator membrane:** Spans the obturator foramen except for a small defect to permit the passage of the obturator nerve and vessels

○ 8. **Inguinal ligament:** Spans the distance between the **ASIS** and **pubic tubercle**, acting as a retinaculum for structures entering/exiting the pelvis anteriorly to/from the lower limb

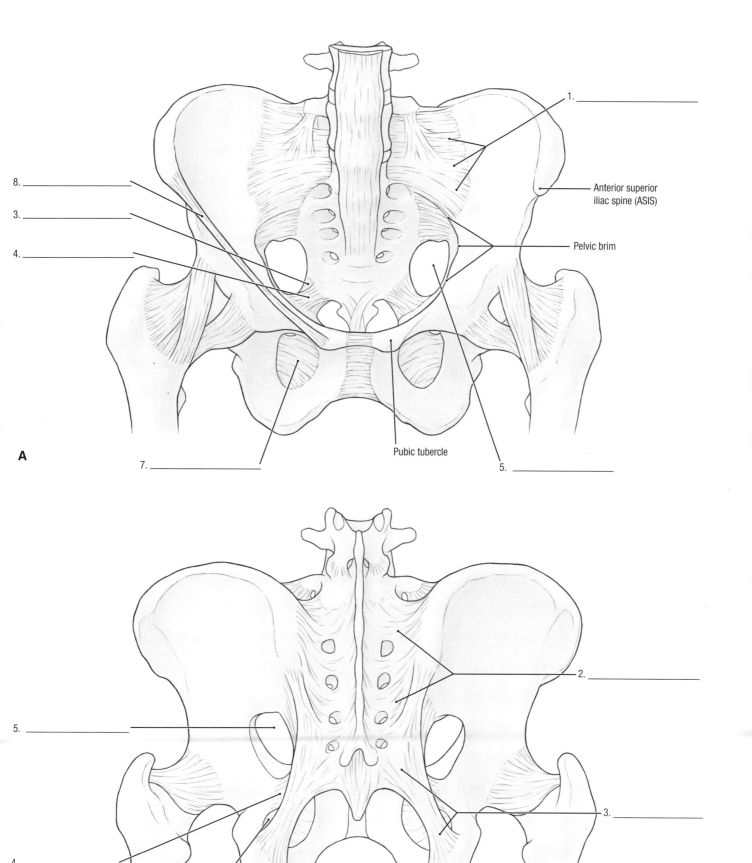

1. _____

Anterior superior
iliac spine (ASIS)

8. _____

3. _____

4. _____

Pelvic brim

Pubic tubercle

7. _____

5. _____

A

2. _____

5. _____

3. _____

4. _____

Ischial tuberosity

6. _____

B

Grant's

5.3A and B   MUSCLES OF THE LESSER PELVIS

In Figure A, the majority of the muscles of the pelvic diaphragm that separate the pelvis from the perineum have been removed along with the obturator internus fascia. In Figure B, all of the muscles of the pelvic diaphragm and the obturator internus fascia are intact. The internal iliac vasculature has been cut, to view the musculature of the pelvic walls. The ***external iliac artery and vein*** remain intact superior to the ***pelvic brim***.

COLOR each of the following structures using a different color for each:

There are no muscles that cross from the greater pelvis into the lesser pelvis. All the muscles of the lesser pelvis have their origins inferior to the pelvic brim.

Obturator Internus

○ 1. *Obturator internus:* Fills the obturator foramen on its inner (deep) surface, forming the muscular wall for the anterolateral walls of both the lesser pelvis and perineum

○ 2. *Obturator fascia:* Fascia covering the deep (inner) aspect of the obturator internus muscle

○ 3. *Tendinous arch of the levator ani:* Central thickening of the obturator internus fascia that provides the origin of the levator ani muscles of the pelvic diaphragm

Pelvic Diaphragm

The pelvic diaphragm is a funnel-shaped muscular sling or hammock composed of two groups of muscles, the ***levator ani*** and the coccygeus, on each side that meet in the midline (except where pelvic viscera exit the pelvis to the perineum). The pelvic diaphragm closes off the inferior pelvic aperture and thereby separates the lesser pelvis from the perineum.

○ 4. *Coccygeus:* Triangular sheet of muscle that lies against the posterior portion of the iliococcygeus muscle

The levator ani forms a majority of the pelvic diaphragm and is composed of three muscles:

○ 5. *Puborectalis:* Thicker, narrower, medial portion

○ 6. *Pubococcygeus:* Wider, but thinner intermediate portion

○ 7. *Iliococcygeus:* Thinnest, posterolateral portion

Piriformis

○ 8. *Piriformis:* Forms the posterolateral wall of the inner (deep) surface of the lesser pelvis superior to the coccygeus to exit via the greater sciatic foramen

Neurovascular Structures

○ 9. *Anterior rami of S1-S3:* Travel along the deep surface of the piriformis, forming components of the sacral plexus

○ 10. *Obturator nerve:* Formed by anterior rami of L2-L4 of the lumbar plexus, courses into the lesser pelvis, and exits the lesser pelvis with the obturator artery and vein to the medial thigh by a small defect in the obturator membrane. Does not innervate the obturator internus muscle.

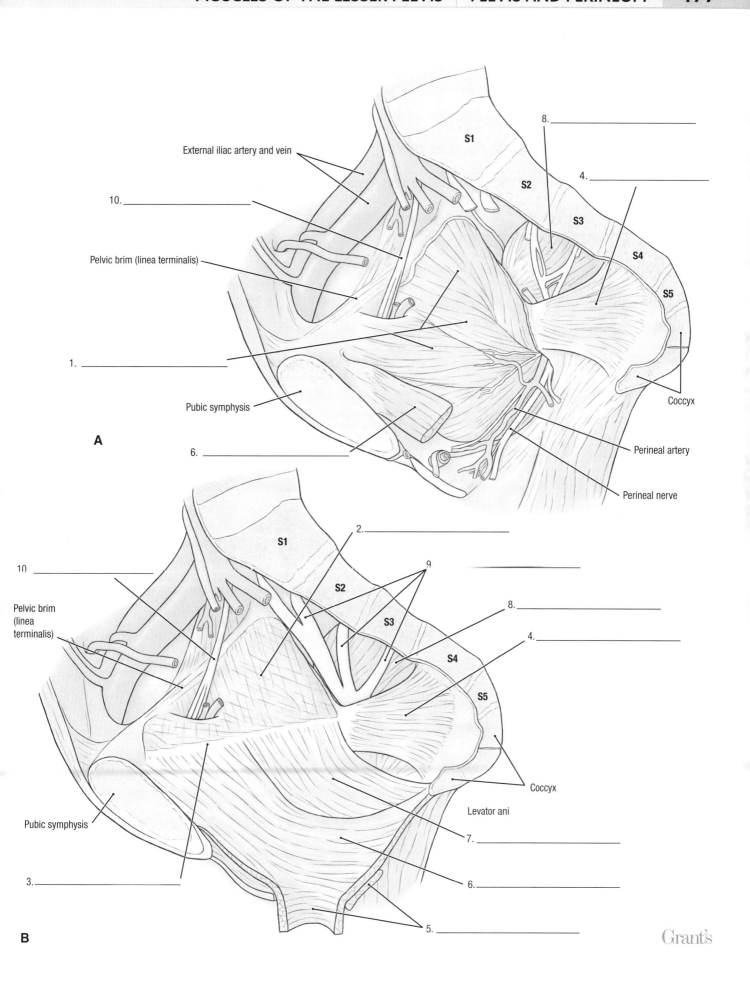

S1

S2

8. _____

4. _____

External iliac artery and vein

10. _____

S3

S4

S5

Pelvic brim (linea terminalis)

1. _____

Pubic symphysis

Coccyx

A

Perineal artery

6. _____

Perineal nerve

S1

2. _____

10 _____

S2

9

Pelvic brim
(linea
terminalis)

S3

8. _____

S4

4. _____

S5

Coccyx

Levator ani

7. _____

Pubic symphysis

3. _____

6. _____

5. _____

B

Grant's

5.4   SUPERIOR VIEW OF THE FLOOR AND WALLS OF THE PELVIS

From the superior view, the muscles of the pelvic diaphragm blend together, forming the bowl or funnel shape of the floor of the pelvis. Centrally, the muscles of the levator ani are hidden by a thickening of the endopelvic fascia, the ***tendinous arch*** ***of pelvic fascia***. On the left side, a window has been cut into the tendinous arch of pelvic fascia to display the puborectalis muscle. In addition, a string retracts the rectum. The muscles of the pelvis are the same in both males and females.

COLOR each of the following structures using a different color for each:

Muscles of the Lesser Pelvis

Muscle	Proximal Attachment	Distal Attachment	Innervation	Action
◯ 1. *Obturator internus*	Obturator membrane, deep surface of ilium and ischium	Greater trochanter of femur	Nerve to obturator internus (L5-S2)	Rotates hip laterally
◯ 2. *Piriformis*	Deep surface of S2-S4, sacrotuberous ligament		Anterior rami of S1-S2	Rotates hip laterally; abducts hip joint
◯ 3. *Levator ani (pubococcygeus, puborectalis, iliococcygeus)*	◯ 4. *Tendinous arch of levator ani*, body of pubis, ischial spine	Median raphe, coccyx, perineal body, walls of pelvic viscera	Nerve to levator ani (S4)	Elevates against increased intra-abdominal pressure
◯ 5. *Coccygeus*	Ischial spine	Coccyx and inferior sacrum	Nerve to coccygeus (S4-S5)	Elevates against increased intra-abdominal pressure

Urogenital Hiatus

◯ 6. *Urogenital hiatus:* Space anteriorly between the two sets of levator ani in the midline for the passage of the **urethra** and the vagina (in females). Inferiorly (in the perineum), the space is reinforced by a second layer, the perineal membrane, to prevent prolapse of organs.

Neurovascular Structures

◯ 7. *Obturator artery:* Branch of the internal iliac artery that travels with the obturator nerve and vein through a defect in the obturator membrane to reach the medial thigh

◯ 8. *Inferior gluteal artery:* Branch of the internal iliac artery that travels through the greater sciatic foramen with the piriformis muscle to reach the gluteal region

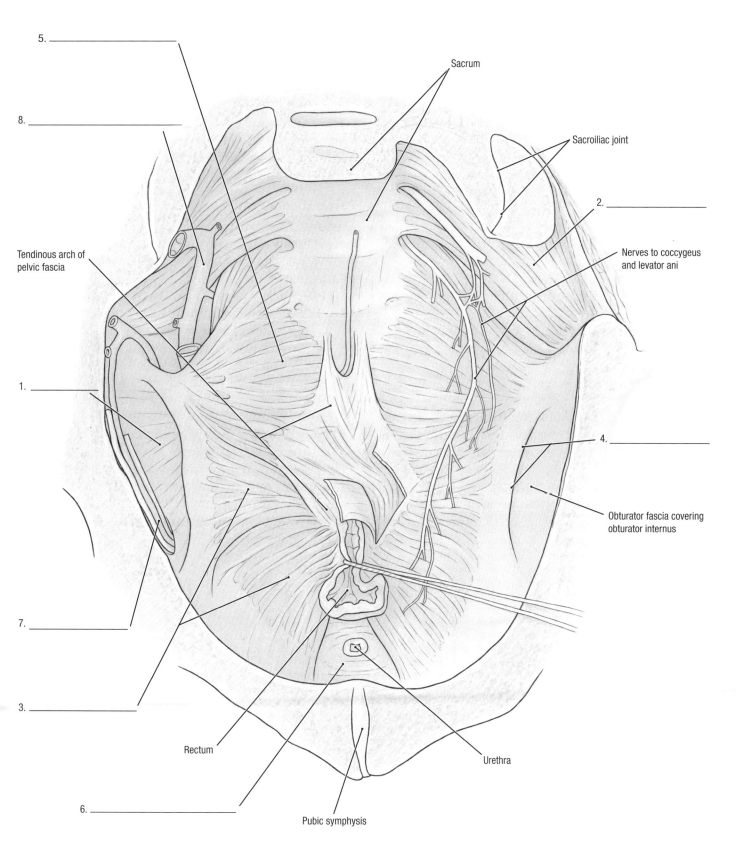

5. _____

8. _____

Sacrum

Sacroiliac joint

2. _____

Nerves to coccygeus
and levator ani

Tendinous arch of
pelvic fascia

1. _____

4. _____

Obturator fascia covering
obturator internus

7. _____

3. _____

Rectum

Urethra

6. _____

Pubic symphysis

Grant's

5.5 BOUNDARIES OF THE PERINEUM

The majority of the contents of the perineum have been removed revealing an inferior view of the pelvic diaphragm. Most of the external anal sphincter has been removed on the right side to reveal the *__internal anal sphincter__*. A string retracts the *__skin around the anus__* to reveal the remaining portion of the external anal sphincter on the right and a hook also retracts the puborectalis on the right side.

COLOR *each of the following structures using a different color for each:*

The perineum is the diamond-shaped shallow compartment between the thighs at the inferior border of the trunk inferior to the pelvic diaphragm. Because of the hammock/sling shape of the pelvic diaphragm, the perineum is the shallowest centrally, with gradually more depth peripherally. The boundaries of the perineum are as follows:

◯ 1. *Pubic symphysis:* Anterior
◯ 2. *Ischiopubic rami:* Anterolateral
◯ 3. *Ischial tuberosities:* Lateral
◯ 4. *Sacrotuberous ligament:* Posterolateral (along with gluteus maximus muscle)
◯ 5. *Coccyx:* Posterior (along with inferior sacrum)
  Inferior aspect of pelvic diaphragm: Superior
  Skin: Inferior

Urogenital and Anal Triangles

The perineum is divided into a urogenital triangle and anal triangle by a line passing through the ischial tuberosities. The urogenital triangle comprises the anterior part of the perineum, lying superficial (inferior) to the urogenital hiatus of the levator ani and spanning the space of the pubic arch (formed by the two ischiopubic rami). The anal triangle comprises the posterior part of the perineum, again lying superficial (inferior) to the pelvic diaphragm.

◯ 6. *Perineal body:* Mass of connective tissue and muscle at the central point of the perineum
◯ 7. *External anal sphincter:* Surrounds the anal canal in the anal triangle

Pelvic Diaphragm

The pelvic diaphragm forms the superior boundary of the perineum because it separates the perineum from the true pelvis. The pelvic diaphragm is composed of the group of levator ani muscles and the coccygeus.

  Levator ani:
  ◯ 8. *Puborectalis:* Most medial pair of the levator ani muscles, forming a sling around the junction of the rectum and anal canal
  ◯ 9. *Pubococcygeus:* Wider portion of the levator ani and lateral to the puborectalis
  ◯ 10. *Iliococcygeus:* Posterolateral and thinnest portion of the levator ani
◯ 11. *Coccygeus:* Lies posterior to the iliococcygeus
◯ 12. *Urogenital hiatus:* Space of the anterior gap of the levator ani muscles, allowing for the passage of the urethra (and vagina in females) from the true pelvis to the perineum. In men, the *__prostate__* and *__prostatic urethra__* can be visualized through the urogenital hiatus from the perineum.

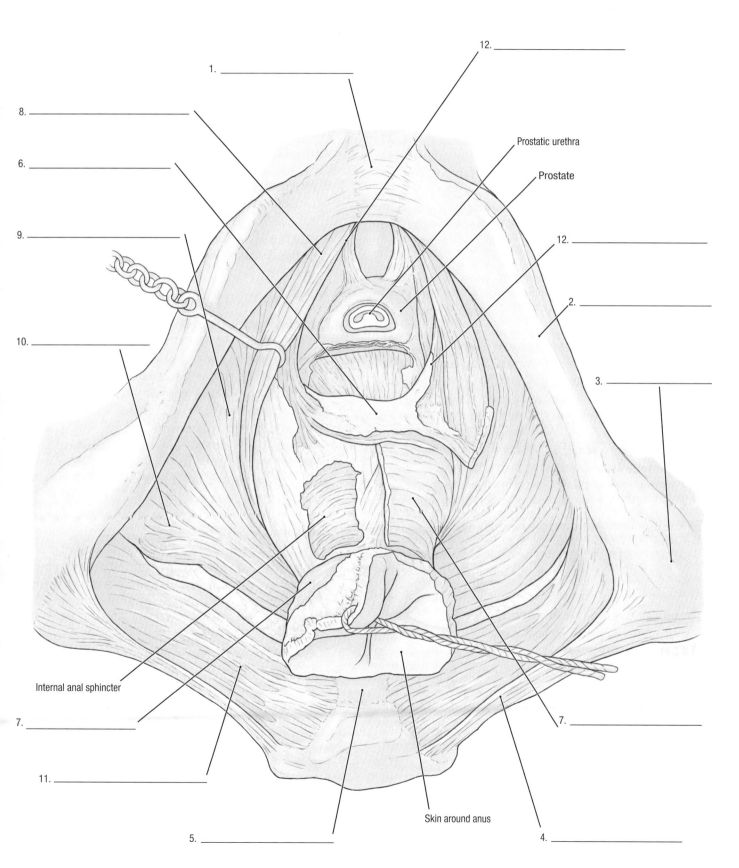

12. _____

1. _____

8. _____

Prostatic urethra

6. _____

Prostate

9. _____

12. _____

2. _____

10. _____

3. _____

Internal anal sphincter

7. _____

7. _____

11. _____

Skin around anus

5. _____

4. _____

Grant's

5.6 SUPERFICIAL DISSECTION—MALE SUPERFICIAL PERINEAL POUCH

The shaft of the penis has been transversely cut. The membranous layer of the subcutaneous tissue has also been cut to open the superficial perineal pouch.

COLOR each of the following structures using a different color for each:

Anal Triangle of the Perineum

Ischioanal (ischiorectal) fossae are primarily fat-filled spaces located on either side of the anal canal. They are wedge shaped, wide inferiorly and narrow superiorly, between the perianal skin and the inferior surface of the pelvic diaphragm. The posterior boundary of each ischioanal fossa is formed by the _**gluteus maximus muscle**_ along with the sacrotuberous ligament.

○ 1. _**External anal sphincter:**_ Forms part of the medial boundary of each ischioanal fossa
○ 2. _**Levator ani:**_ Forms the superomedial wall of each ischioanal fossa
○ 3. _**Obturator fascia forming pudendal canal:**_ Deep surface of the obturator internus muscle is covered by the obturator fascia, forming the lateral wall of the ischioanal fossa. The obturator fascia also forms the pudendal canal as it covers the internal pudendal artery and vein and pudendal nerve.
○ 4. _**Inferior rectal (anal) artery:**_ Branch of internal pudendal artery as it courses through the pudendal canal. Pierces through the obturator fascia and courses through the fat of the ischioanal fossa to supply the external anal sphincter and surrounding perianal skin.
○ 5. _**Inferior rectal (anal) nerve:**_ Branch of the pudendal nerve as it courses through the pudendal canal. Pathway and distribution are similar to the inferior rectal artery.

Urogenital Triangle of Perineum

Unlike the anal triangle, the urogenital triangle is divided into two pouches (spaces), superficial and deep, by the perineal membrane. The layers of the urogenital triangle, from superficial to deep, are as follows: skin (and associated external genitalia), subcutaneous tissue (superficial fatty layer and membranous layer), superficial perineal pouch (lies between membranous layer and perineal membrane), perineal membrane, deep perineal pouch (lies between perineal membrane and pelvic diaphragm), and inferior surface of pelvic diaphragm.

In males, the superficial fatty layer of the subcutaneous fascia is diminished.

○ 6. _**Membranous layer of subcutaneous tissue (Colles fascia):**_ Laterally attaches to the ischiopubic rami, posteriorly adheres to the perineal membrane (does not extend into the anal triangle), continuous with Scarpa's fascia of the abdominal wall, and in males continuous with the dartos fascia of the scrotum and penis

Superficial Perineal Pouch Contents

○ 7. _**Ischiocavernous muscle:**_ Paired muscles covering the crura of penis and attached to the ischiopubic rami and perineal membrane. Maintains erect state by forcing blood from cavernous spaces within the crura into distal parts of _**corpora cavernosa**_ of the penis.
○ 8. _**Bulbospongiosus muscle:**_ Paired muscles covering bulb of penis, acting as a constrictor that are joined at midline raphe. Aids in emptying of ejaculate or urine of spongy urethra in the bulb of the penis.
○ 9. _**Superficial transverse perineal muscle:**_ Paired muscles at the posterior edge of the urogenital triangle that act like cross beams to stabilize the superficial perineal region
○ 10. _**Perineal artery:**_ Branch of the internal pudendal artery supplying contents of the superficial perineal pouch
○ 11. _**Posterior scrotal artery:**_ Terminal branches of perineal artery supplying the posterior skin of scrotum
○ 12. _**Posterior scrotal nerve:**_ Terminal branches of the perineal nerve supplying the posterior skin of the scrotum
○ 13. _**Perineal membrane:**_ Thin sheet of connective tissue forming the boundary between the superficial and deep perineal pouches of the urogenital triangle
○ 14. _**Perineal body:**_ Site of muscle fiber convergence of the superficial transverse perineal, bulbospongiosus, external anal sphincter, along with muscles of the deep perineal pouch and the rectum located posterior to the bulb of the penis and anterior to the anus

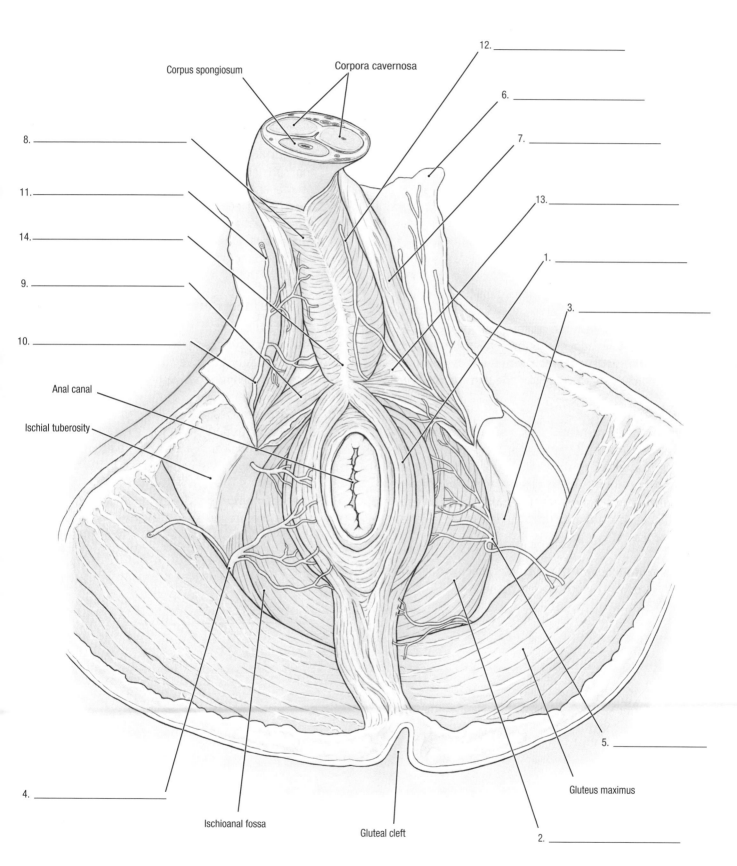

12. _____

6. _____

7. _____

Corpus spongiosum

Corpora cavernosa

13. _____

8. _____

1. _____

11. _____

3. _____

14. _____

9. _____

10. _____

Anal canal

Ischial tuberosity

Gluteus maximus

5. _____

4. _____

Ischioanal fossa

Gluteal cleft

2. _____

Grant's

5.7   INTERMEDIATE DISSECTION—MALE SUPERFICIAL PERINEAL POUCH

The membranous layer of subcutaneous fascia (Colles fascia) and muscles of the superficial perineal pouch have been removed to demonstrate the erectile tissue of the root of the penis and perineal membrane. On the right side, the *external anal* *sphincter* has been cut and reflected to show the internal anal sphincter. A metal probe elevates the muscle fibers from the external anal sphincter contributing to the cut *perineal body*.

COLOR each of the following structures using a different color for each:

○ 1. *Levator ani:* Forms the superior boundary (and a portion of the medial boundary) of both the anal and urogenital triangles. The full extent of the levator ani in the urogenital triangle is not visible because it lies superior to the perineal membrane.

○ 2. *Prostate:* Visible through the urogenital hiatus of the levator ani (does not extend inferiorly into the perineum)

○ 3. *Obturator fascia:* Lines the deep aspect of the obturator internus muscle, forming the lateral boundary of both the anal and urogenital triangles. The full extent of the obturator fascia in the urogenital triangle is not visible because it lies superior to the perineal membrane.

○ 4. *Sacrotuberous ligament:* Forms the posterior boundary of the perineum (along with the *gluteus maximus*)

Anal Triangle

The external anal sphincter forms a broad band around the inferior two-thirds of the anal canal and is under voluntary control. It is attached to the perineal body anteriorly and to the *coccyx* posteriorly via the *anococcygeal body/ligament*. It then blends superiorly with the levator ani. The external anal sphincter is often described as having three indistinct parts or zones:

○ 5. *Subcutaneous part:* Immediately deep to skin and associated with subcutaneous tissue

○ 6. *Superficial part:* Deep to subcutaneous part of external anal sphincter and surrounds lowermost fibers of the internal anal sphincter

○ 7. *Deep part:* Deepest portion of external anal sphincter and surrounds portion of the internal anal sphincter

○ 8. *Internal anal sphincter:* Thickening of the circular muscle layer surrounding upper two-thirds of the anal canal and is controlled by the autonomic nervous system

Superficial Perineal Pouch of Urogenital Triangle

○ 9. *Crus of penis:* Paired structures attached to the inferior and internal surface of ischiopubic rami anterior to ischial tuberosity and covered by ischiocavernous muscle. Each crus is continuous with the corpora cavernosa in the body of the penis.

○ 10. *Bulb of penis:* Enlarged midline structure that is pierced by the bulbous part of the spongy urethra and covered by bulbospongiosus muscle. The bulb of the penis is continuous with the corpus spongiosum of the body of the penis.

○ 11. *Perineal membrane:* Spans the breadth of the pubic arch in the urogenital triangle, separating superficial and deep perineal pouches and providing support for the erectile tissue

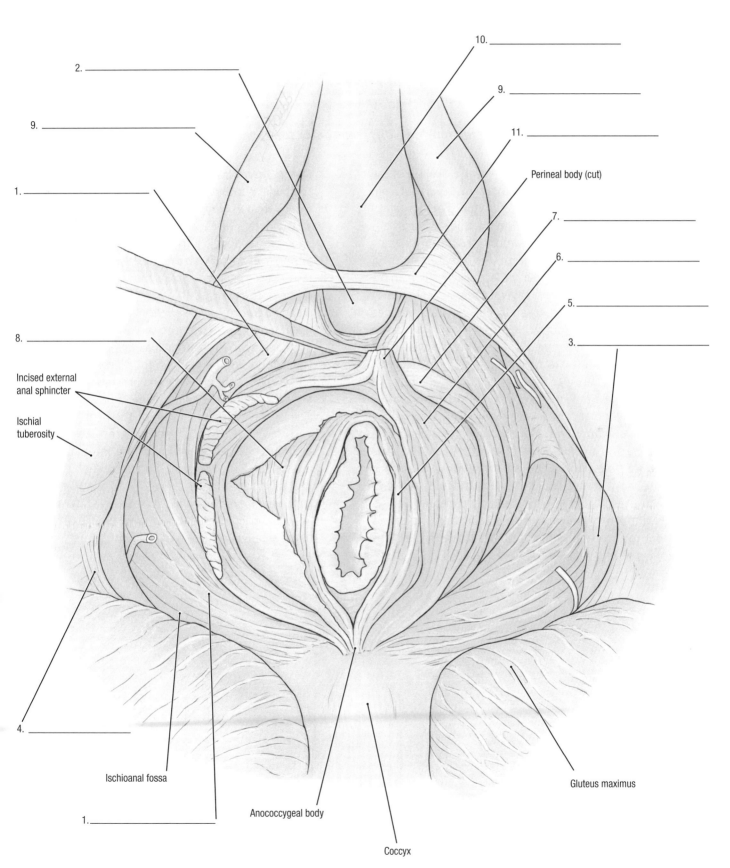

2. _____

9. _____

1. _____

8. _____

Incised external
anal sphincter

Ischial
tuberosity

4. _____

Ischioanal fossa

1. _____

Anococcygeal body

Coccyx

10. _____

9. _____

11. _____

Perineal body (cut)

7. _____

6. _____

5. _____

3. _____

Gluteus maximus

5.8A and B LAYERS OF THE PENIS

The anatomic position of the penis is in the erect state. Thus, structures are described as located on dorsal and ventral surfaces of the penis. The penis is divided into two parts: the root and the body. The root of the penis is located in the superficial perineal pouch and is composed of the two crura and the bulb of the penis. The body of the penis is the free, pendulous portion that is suspended from the pubic symphysis. Figure A depicts the lateral view of the penis with the portions of the skin and fascial layers reflected, whereas Figure B depicts a transverse section through the body of the penis.

COLOR each of the following structures using a different color for each:

1. *Corpus spongiosum:* Lies on the ventral surface of the penis and contains the _spongy urethra_. Separated from the corpora cavernosa by its own _tunica albuginea_ to prevent the corpus spongiosum from becoming as engorged with blood as the corpora cavernosa, allowing the lumen of the spongy urethra to remain patent.

2. *Corpus cavernosum:* Paired and lateral in position on the dorsal aspect. The corpora cavernosa are not completely separated from each other and a single tunica albuginea surrounds both corpora cavernosa, allowing blood to fill across both, creating a bilateral erectile event. The corpora cavernosa are supplied by the _deep artery_ of the penis, a branch of the internal pudendal artery.

3. *Glans of penis:* Expanded distal end of the corpus spongiosum that contains the _external urethral orifice_

4. *Corona of glans penis:* Margin of the glans penis that extends over the distal end of the corpora cavernosa

5. *Prepuce (foreskin):* At the neck of the glans, the skin and fascia leave the surface of the glans and fold back onto themselves (only present on an uncircumcised penis)

6. *Frenulum of prepuce (penis):* Median fold that passes from the prepuce to the urethral surface of the glans (only present on an uncircumcised penis)

7. *Dartos fascia:* Except at the glans of the penis, skin of the penis is loosely attached to the dartos fascia

8. *Deep fascia of penis (Buck's fascia):* Tough fascia deep to the dartos fascia that binds the corpora cavernosa and corpus spongiosum together

9. *Superficial dorsal vein of penis:* Lies within the dartos fascia of the penis and drains the skin and subcutaneous tissue of the penis to the external pudendal veins

10. *Deep dorsal vein of penis:* Lies in the midline on the dorsum of the penis deep to the deep fascia of the penis and superficial to the tunica albuginea. Drains most of the blood from the glans, prepuce, corpora cavernosa, and corpus spongiosum to the prostatic venous plexus

11. *Dorsal artery of the penis:* Paired artery lying on either side of the deep dorsal vein of the penis deep to the deep fascia of the penis and superficial to the tunica albuginea. Terminal branch of the internal pudendal artery supplying the skin and subcutaneous tissue of the penis.

12. *Dorsal nerve of the penis:* Paired nerve lateral to each dorsal artery of the penis. Terminal branch of pudendal nerve supplying the skin of the penis.

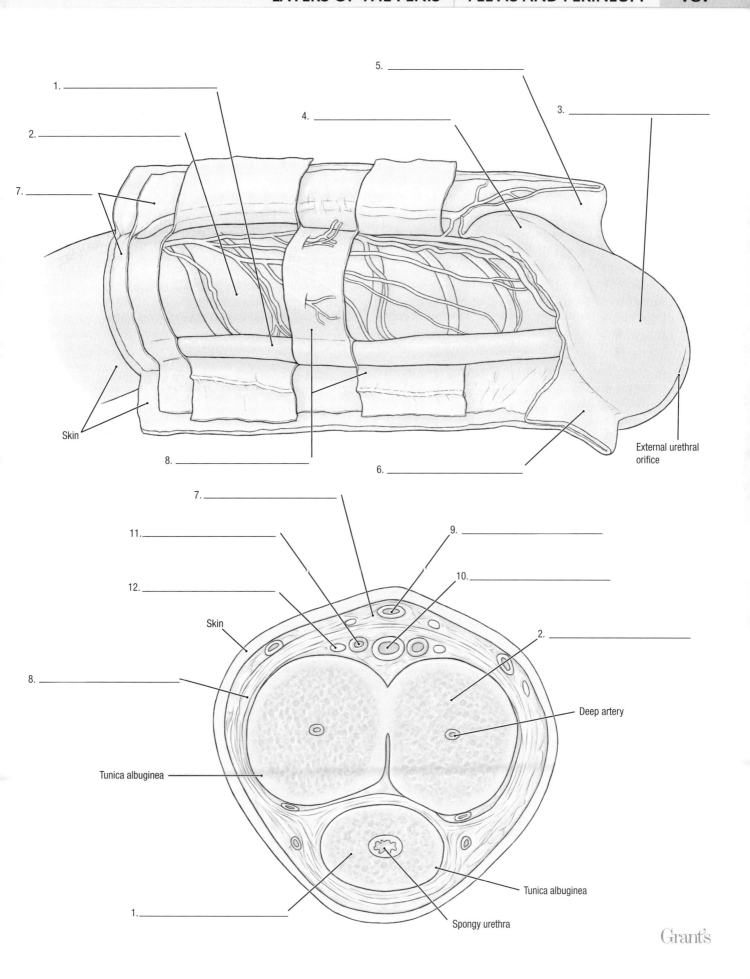

1. _____

2. _____

7. _____

5. _____

4. _____

3. _____

8. _____

6. _____

Skin

External urethral orifice

7. _____

11. _____

12. _____

Skin

8. _____

9. _____

10. _____

2. _____

Deep artery

Tunica albuginea

Tunica albuginea

1. _____

Spongy urethra

Grant's

5.9 FEMALE EXTERNAL GENITALIA

On the right side, a superficial cut through the skin and subcutaneous tissue has been performed, displaying the contents of the labium majus. On the left side, a majority of the fat within the labium majus has been removed, demonstrating the deeper neurovascular structures of the perineum.

COLOR each of the following structures using a different color for each:

○ 1. **Mons pubis:** Rounded, fatty prominence anterior to pubic symphysis

○ 2. **Labium majus (cut):** Folds of skin on either side of the pudendal cleft filled with loose connective tissue

○ 3. **Round ligament of the uterus:** Terminates in the labia majus after emerging from the superficial inguinal ring

○ 4. **Glans clitoris:** External expanded portion of the body of the clitoris

○ 5. **Labium minus:** Rounded folds of fat-free, hairless skin on either side of the **vestibule of the vagina**

　○ 6. **Frenulum of labium minus (fourchette):** Location where the labium minus of each side meets in the midline posteriorly

　○ 7. **Frenulum of clitoris:** Medial laminae of each labium minus unite midline posterior to the glans clitoris

　○ 8. **Prepuce (foreskin) of clitoris:** Lateral laminae of each labium minus unite anterior to glans of clitoris and partially covering the glans

○ 9. **Posterior labial artery:** Terminal branches of the perineal artery (branch of internal pudendal artery)

○ 10. **External pudendal artery:** Gives rise to anterior labial arteries

○ 11. **Posterior labial nerve:** Terminal branches of the perineal nerve (branch of pudendal nerve) supplying skin of labia majora, labia minora, and vestibule of vagina

○ 12. **Ilioinguinal nerve:** Gives rise to anterior labial nerves that supply the mons pubis

CLINICAL NOTE: ROUND LIGAMENT PAIN

Stretching of the round ligament of the uterus is a common source of temporary pain during the second or third trimester of pregnancy. Pain may present within the pelvic cavity, the inguinal area, or within the labia majora at the termination of the round ligament of the uterus. Changing position and rest often alleviate the pain.

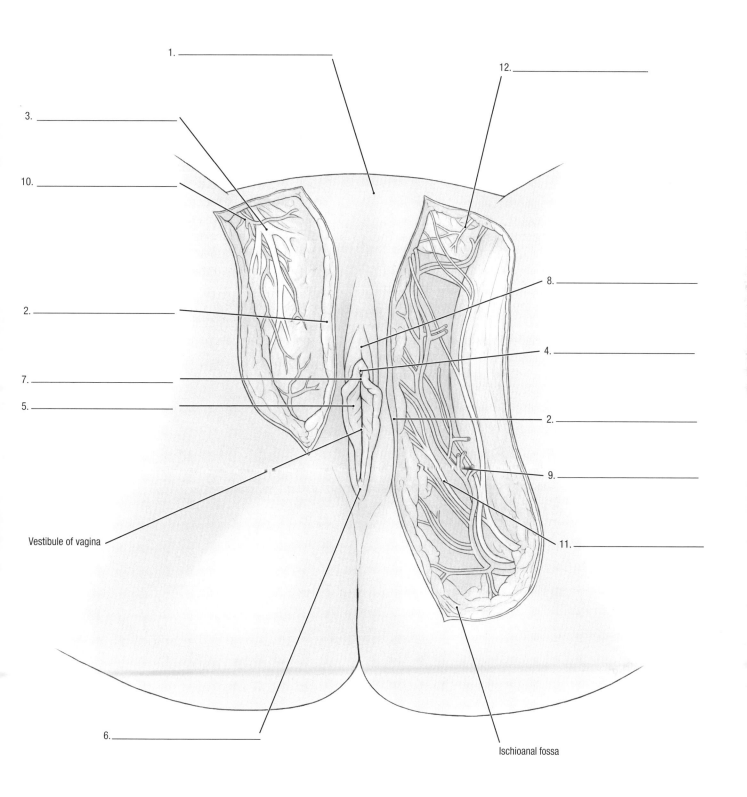

1. _____

12. _____

3. _____

10. _____

2. _____

7. _____

5. _____

8. _____

4. _____

2. _____

9. _____

11. _____

Vestibule of vagina

6. _____

Ischioanal fossa

5.10   FEMALE SUPERFICIAL PERINEAL POUCH

The labia majora have been removed along with the mons pubis. The labia minora have been removed except at the formation of the **_prepuce of clitoris_** and **_frenulum of clitoris_** in relation to the **_glans clitoris_**. The membranous layer of subcutaneous fascia (Colles fascia, the inferior boundary of the superficial perineal pouch) has been removed, revealing the muscles of the superficial perineal pouch. A string reflects the right side of the prepuce of the clitoris laterally.

The boundaries of the female perineum, contents of the anal triangle, and the layers of the superficial perineal pouch are the same as in males (see the figure in Sections 5.5 and 5.6).

COLOR each of the following structures using a different color for each:

Unlike the male urogenital triangle, the female urogenital triangle is separated by the vestibule of the vagina into distinct right and left sides. Within the space of the vestibule of the vagina, two structures are visible:

○ 1. **_Vaginal orifice:_** Opening of the vagina
○ 2. **_Urethral orifice:_** Opening of the urethra anterior to the vaginal orifice

   Unlike the male urogenital triangle, the superficial fatty layer of the subcutaneous fascia is expanded in females, forming the **_mons pubis_** and labia majora.

   The muscular contents of the female superficial perineal pouch are similar to those in men; however, the muscles are typically smaller and less pronounced because they are covering smaller erectile tissue structures.

○ 3. **_Ischiocavernous muscle:_** Paired muscles covering the crus of the clitoris and attached to the ischiopubic rami
○ 4. **_Bulbospongiosus muscle:_** Paired muscles covering the bulb of the vestibule. In females, the bulbospongiosus muscle does not meet in the midline because they are separated by the vestibule of the vagina.
○ 5. **_Superficial transverse perineal muscle:_** Paired muscles at the posterior aspect of the superficial perineal pouch, spanning between the ischial tuberosities and the perineal body
○ 6. **_Perineal membrane:_** Forms the superior boundary of the superficial perineal pouch, separating the superficial and deep perineal pouches of the urogenital triangle

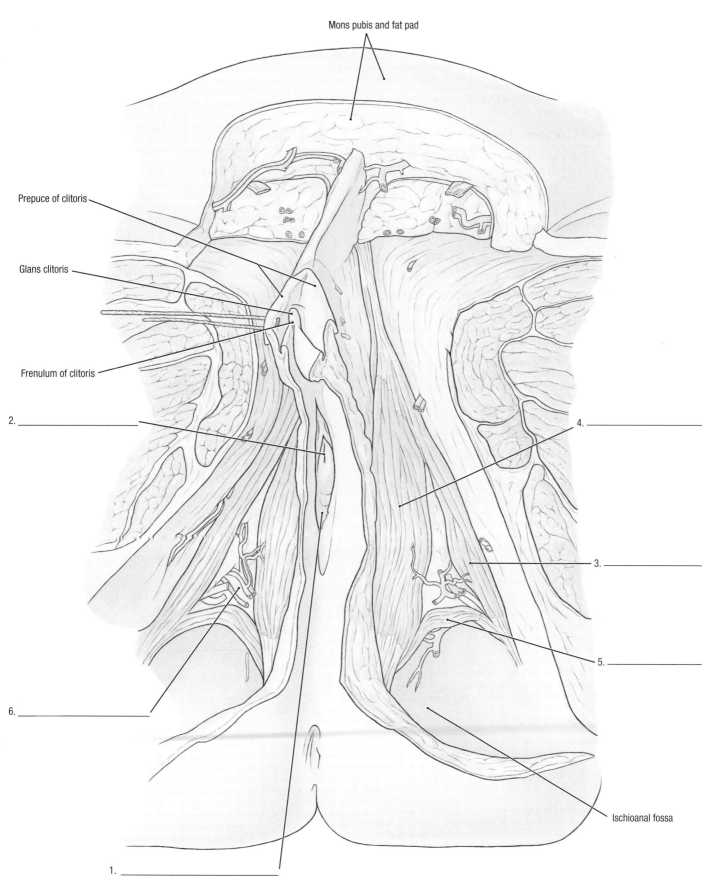

Mons pubis and fat pad

Prepuce of clitoris

Glans clitoris

Frenulum of clitoris

2. _____

4. _____

3. _____

5. _____

6. _____

Ischioanal fossa

1. _____

5.11   DEEP DISSECTION OF THE FEMALE SUPERFICIAL PERINEAL POUCH

The majority of the muscles of the superficial perineal pouch have been removed or reflected. On the left side, the posterior half of the perineal membrane, greater vestibular bulb, and bulb of vestibule have been removed.

COLOR each of the following structures using a different color for each:

Deep Structures of the Superficial Perineal Pouch

With the muscles of the superficial perineal pouch removed, the full extent of the erectile tissue and the greater vestibular gland are visible on the right side:

○ 1. *Body of clitoris:* Free, pendulous portion covered by the prepuce

○ 2. *Glans clitoris:* Expanded external portion of the body of the clitoris

○ 3. *Crus of clitoris:* Paired, lateral structures attached to the ischiopubic rami forming the root of the clitoris in the superficial perineal pouch. Covered by ischiocavernous muscles.

○ 4. *Bulb of vestibule:* Erectile tissue homologous to the bulb of the penis on either side of the vestibule of the vagina

○ 5. *Greater vestibular gland:* Located on either side of the vestibule of the vagina, posterolateral to the vaginal orifice, and partially overlapped by the bulb of the vestibule

○ 6. *Bulbospongiosus muscle (cut):* Covers the bulb of the vestibule and the greater vestibular gland

○ 7. *Perineal membrane:* Provides attachment for the bulb of vestibule and greater vestibular gland superficially

○ 8. *Perineal branches of internal pudendal vessels:* Supply the structures of superficial perineal pouch

With the perineal membrane cut away on the left side, the inferior vagina and levator ani can be viewed:

○ 9. *Vaginal wall:* The lower portion of the vagina extends inferior to the pelvic diaphragm to the vestibule of the vagina

○10. *Levator ani:* Forms the superior boundary of both the urogenital triangle and anal triangle

Neurovascular Structures of the Clitoris

○11. *Superficial dorsal vein of clitoris* (reflected): Drains skin and subcutaneous tissue of the clitoris

○12. *Dorsal artery of clitoris:* Paired arteries from the internal pudendal artery supplying the skin and subcutaneous tissue of the clitoris

○13. *Dorsal nerve of clitoris:* Paired nerves branching from the pudendal nerve supplying the skin and subcutaneous tissue of the clitoris

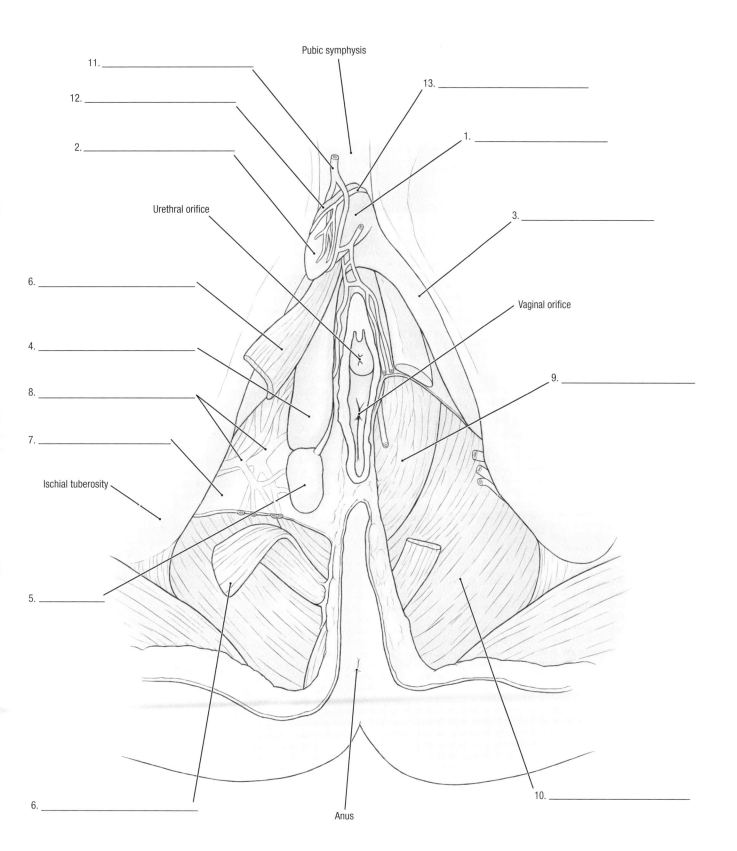

Pubic symphysis

11. _____

12. _____

13. _____

2. _____

1. _____

Urethral orifice

3. _____

Vaginal orifice

6. _____

4. _____

9. _____

8. _____

7. _____

Ischial tuberosity

5. _____

10. _____

6. _____

Anus

5.12 FEMALE DEEP PERINEAL POUCH

The perineal membrane and contents of the superficial perineal pouch have been removed.

In females, the deep transverse perineal muscle is typically replaced by a mass of smooth muscle and has also been removed in this image.

COLOR each of the following structures using a different color for each:

The external urethral sphincter is the primary structure occupying the deep perineal pouch in females. It forms a tubular portion surrounding the urethra, with some fibers extending superiorly to the neck of the bladder.

○ 1. **Urethrovaginal sphincter:** Band-like portion of external urethral sphincter that extends posteriorly encircling both the urethra and vagina

The ischioanal fossa of the anal triangle in females has the same structures and relationships as that in men (see the figure in Sections 5.5 and 5.6).

○ 2. **Levator ani:** Forms the superomedial boundary and the apex as it attaches to the tendinous arch of the levator ani

○ 3. **External anal sphincter:** Forms the remainder of the medial boundary as it surrounds the anal canal

○ 4. **Anococcygeal body:** Posterior attachment site of the external anal sphincter

○ 5. **Perineal body:** Central point of perineum with muscular fibers converging from the following:

○ 6. (Lower muscular) **wall of the vagina**
  • Lower muscular portion of the rectum
  • External anal sphincter
  • Levator ani
  • Bulbospongiosus muscle
  • Superficial transverse perineal muscle
  • External urethral sphincter (urethrovaginal sphincter)

CLINICAL NOTE: WEAKENING OF THE PELVIC FLOOR

Weakened pelvic floor muscles and ligaments can result in urinary and/or fecal incontinence or organ prolapse depending on which structure(s) are affected. The weakening may be due to direct damage to the structures or to the nerves that supply them. Females are more likely than males to develop a weakened or damaged pelvic floor, and this risk increases with the number of childbirths and after onset of menopause. Obese and overweight individuals are also at a higher risk. Nonsurgical treatments include strengthening the muscles of the pelvic floor (Kegel exercises), decreasing activities such as heavy lifting, weight loss, and the use of a pessary (a device inserted into the vagina that helps support pelvic structures). Surgical interventions are also available to repair pelvic organ prolapse.

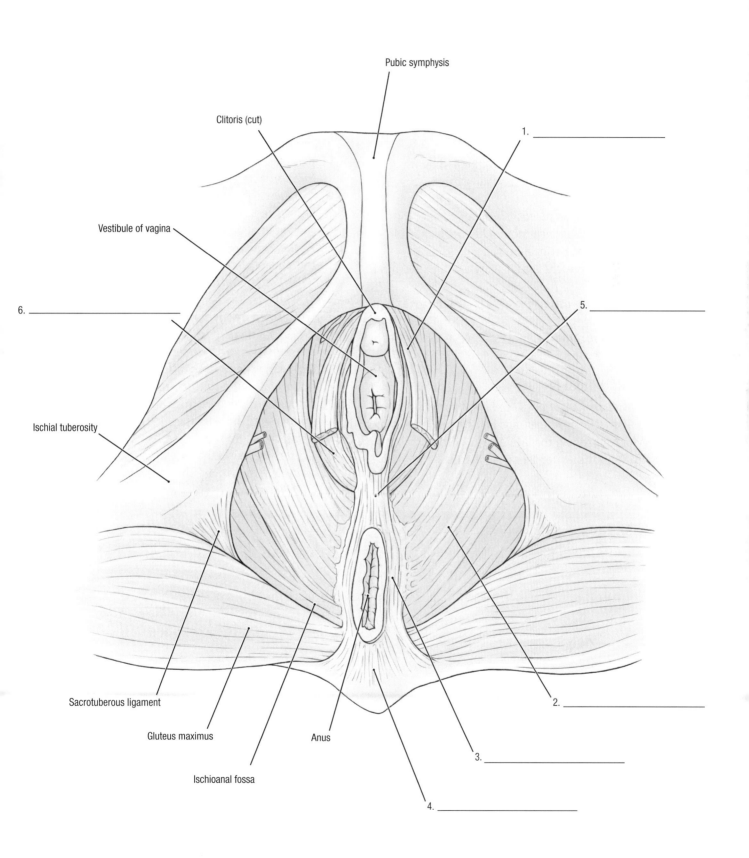

Pubic symphysis

Clitoris (cut)

1. _____

Vestibule of vagina

6. _____

5. _____

Ischial tuberosity

Sacrotuberous ligament

Gluteus maximus

Anus

Ischioanal fossa

2. _____

3. _____

4. _____

Grant's

5.13   INNERVATION OF THE PERINEUM

Branching of the pudendal nerve is shown in a female specimen, however, the male branching pattern is the same.

The pudendal nerve is the main nerve of the perineum for both males and females. Only the anterior aspect of the perineum receives anterior labial nerves derived from ilioinguinal nerve and genital branch of genitofemoral nerve.

COLOR each of the following structures using a different color for each:

Review of Boundaries and Contents of Perineum

○ 1. *Levator ani:* Superior boundary of the perineum

○ 2. *External anal sphincter:* Surrounds anal canal in the anal triangle

○ 3. *Superficial transverse perineal muscle:* Posterior muscle of the superficial perineal pouch between the ischial tuberosity and the perineal body

○ 4. *Ischiocavernous muscle:* Lateral muscle of the superficial perineal pouch

○ 5. *Bulbospongiosus muscle:* Medial muscle of the superficial perineal pouch

○ 6. *Perineal membrane:* Separates superficial and deep perineal pouches

Branching of Pudendal Nerve

○ 7. *Pudendal nerve:* Arises from S2 to S4, enters the perineum via the lesser sciatic foramen, and immediately enters the pudendal canal along the lateral wall of the ischioanal fossa. Within the pudendal canal, the pudendal nerve terminates into three main branches: inferior rectal, perineal, and dorsal nerve of clitoris/penis.

○ 8. *Inferior rectal nerve:* Arises from pudendal nerve within the pudendal canal, pierces through the obturator fascia, and traverses the fat of the ischioanal fossa to reach the external anal sphincter and perianal skin

○ 9. *Perineal nerve:* Branches from the pudendal nerve within the pudendal canal. Gives rise to the following:

  ○ 10. *Superficial perineal nerve:* Supplies the skin of the urogenital triangle by posterior labial/scrotal nerves

  ○ 11. *Deep perineal nerve:* Supplies structures of the superficial and deep perineal pouches and the inferior vagina in females

○ 12. *Dorsal nerve of clitoris/penis:* Branches from the pudendal nerve within the pudendal canal, travels through the deep perineal pouch (superior to perineal membrane), and emerges on the dorsal surface of the penis/clitoris to supply the skin of the clitoris or penis. Dotted line marks the path of the dorsal nerve of clitoris as it courses through the deep perineal pouch.

5. _____

12. _____

4. _____

6. _____

Glans clitoris

External urethral orifice

Vagina

11. _____

10. _____

12. _____

3. _____

9. _____

Anus

7. _____

Gluteus maximus

8. _____

2. _____

1. _____

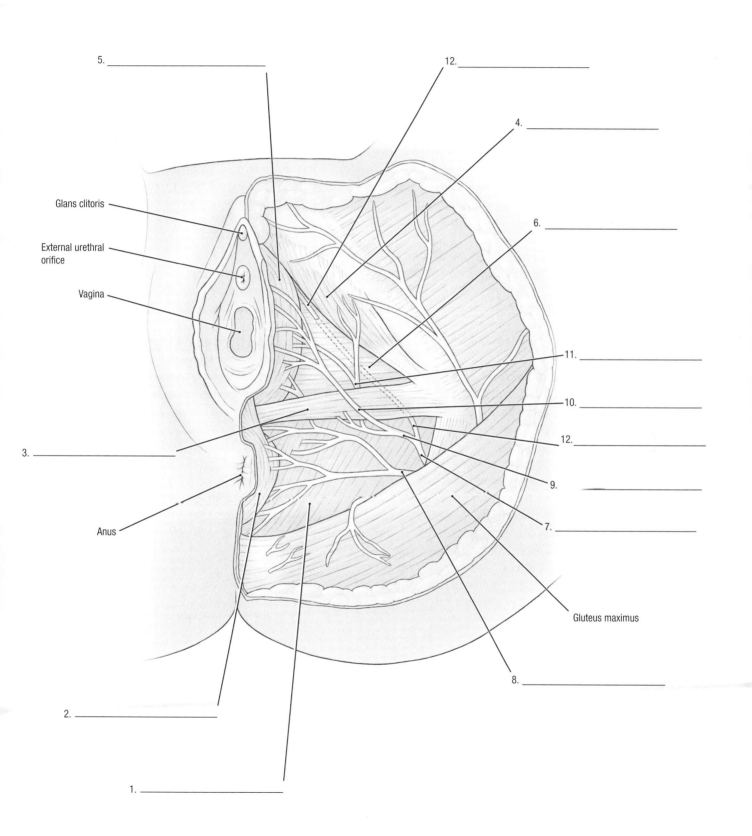

Grant's

5.14A and B MALE PELVIC ORGANS

Figure A depicts a midsagittal view of the male pelvic organs and root of the penis. Figure B depicts a posterior view of the prostate, seminal gland, ductus deferens, and bladder. The left seminal gland and ampulla of ductus deferens have been opened along with a portion of the prostate gland to reveal the formation of the ejaculatory duct. The **_peritoneum_** covering the superior aspect of the bladder is left intact along with the **_visceral pelvic fascia_** over the posterior aspect of the seminal gland and ampulla of the ductus deferens on the specimen's right side.

COLOR each of the following structures using a different color for each:

Male Pelvic Organs

◯ 1. *Urinary bladder:* In the adult, lies posterior and slightly superior to pubic bones and **_pubic symphysis_** when empty and is located subperitoneal (roof of bladder covered by peritoneum)

◯ 2. *Prostate:* Walnut-sized pyramidal organ situated inferior to the neck of the bladder, posterior to the pubic symphysis, anterior to the rectum, and superior to the urogenital hiatus of the levator ani

The prostatic urethra and ejaculatory ducts traverse the prostate gland.

　◯ 3. *External urethral sphincter:* Muscle of the deep perineal pouch located superior to the **_perineal membrane_** and inferior to the urogenital hiatus. A portion will extend superiorly along the anterior aspect of the prostate gland.

◯ 4. *Seminal gland (vesicle):* Elongated structures located posterior to the bladder, anterior to the rectum, lateral to the **_ampulla of the ductus deferens_**, superior to the prostate, and inferior to the **_ureter_**

◯ 5. *Ductus (vas) deferens:* Crosses superior to the ureter near the posterolateral aspect of the bladder, lies superior to the seminal gland, and then descends medial to the ureter and the seminal gland where it enlarges to form the ampulla of ductus deferens

◯ 6. *Ejaculatory duct:* Paired structure formed by the merging of the seminal gland and the ampulla of the ductus deferens. Traverses the prostate gland to the prostatic part of the male urethra.

Parts of the Male Urethra

◯ 7. *Intramural part:* Located in the neck of the bladder and surrounded by the internal urethral sphincter that prevents semen from flowing into the bladder during ejaculation

◯ 8. *Prostatic part:* Traverses the prostate gland and receives urine from the bladder along with sperm and secretions from the seminal vesicle and prostate

◯ 9. *Intermediate (membranous) part:* Narrowest part of the male urethra and surrounded by the external urethral sphincter

◯ 10. *Spongy part:* Longest and most mobile part of the male urethra; first traverses **_bulb of the penis_** in the superficial perineal pouch and then travels within the **_corpus spongiosum_**; receives the final component of semen from the bulbourethral glands embedded in the external urethral sphincter in the deep perineal pouch

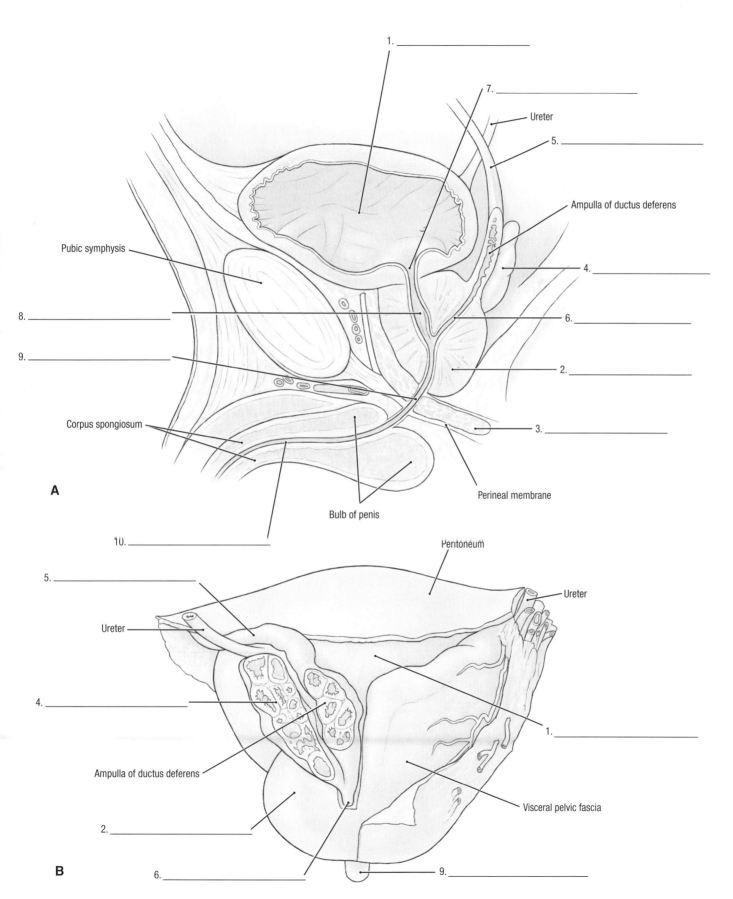

1. _____

7. _____

Ureter

5. _____

Ampulla of ductus deferens

Pubic symphysis

4. _____

8. _____

6. _____

9. _____

2. _____

Corpus spongiosum

3. _____

Perineal membrane

A

Bulb of penis

10. _____

Peritoneum

5. _____

Ureter

Ureter

4. _____

1. _____

Ampulla of ductus deferens

2. _____

Visceral pelvic fascia

B

6. _____

9. _____

Grant's

5.15 INTERIOR VIEW OF MALE BLADDER AND PROSTATIC URETHRA

Anterior walls of the *__bladder__*, *__prostate__*, and *__urethra__* are cut away. On the right side of the specimen, the superior aspect of the posterior wall of the bladder is also removed, demonstrating the *__ureter__* and *__ductus deferens__* as they travel posterior to the bladder.

COLOR each of the following structures using a different color for each:

Internal Features of the Bladder

The wall of the bladder is composed of the detrusor muscle and is typically folded in most areas especially when empty.

○ 1. *Ureteric orifices:* Right and left sites of entry of the ureter into the bladder
○ 2. *Interureteric fold:* Fold of mucosa extending between the two ureteric orifices
○ 3. *Internal urethral orifice:* Beginning of urethra in the neck of the bladder
○ 4. *Trigone:* Consistent smooth area between the two ureteric orifices, the interureteric fold, and the internal urethral orifice

Internal Features of the Prostatic Urethra

○ 5. *Urethral crest:* Midline ridge
○ 6. *Seminal colliculus:* Rounded eminence in the middle of the urethral crest
○ 7. *Prostatic utricle:* Small, blind pouch located on the seminal colliculus. The ejaculatory ducts open on either side of the prostatic utricle.

○ 8. *Prostatic sinus:* Bilateral grooves on either side of the urethral crest in which the numerous prostatic ducts open into

CLINICAL NOTE: HYPERTROPHY AND CANCER OF THE PROSTATE GLAND

The prostate gland can be divided into five lobes. The two lateral lobes are situated on either side of the prostatic urethra, and the anterior lobe is located anterior to it. The posterior lobe is located posterior to the urethra and inferior to the ejaculatory ducts, whereas the median lobe is situated between the two ejaculatory ducts and the urethra. The posterior lobe is the portion of the prostate palpated during a rectal examination. The prostate gland is also commonly referenced into zones for pathology. The central zone contains the ejaculatory ducts and the proximal prostatic urethra. The peripheral zone comprises a majority of the prostate containing the distal prostatic urethra and extending superiorly surrounding the central zone. The peripheral zone, especially posteriorly, is the most common site for prostate cancer. A transitional zone exists between the central and peripheral zones and is a common site for benign prostatic hyperplasia (BPH). This enlargement of the prostate can restrict the lumen of the urethra, resulting in increased urgency and frequency of urination, dysuria (difficulty initiating or maintaining urinary stream), and nocturia (frequent night-time urination). BPH risk increases with age but is not considered a precursor to prostate cancer.

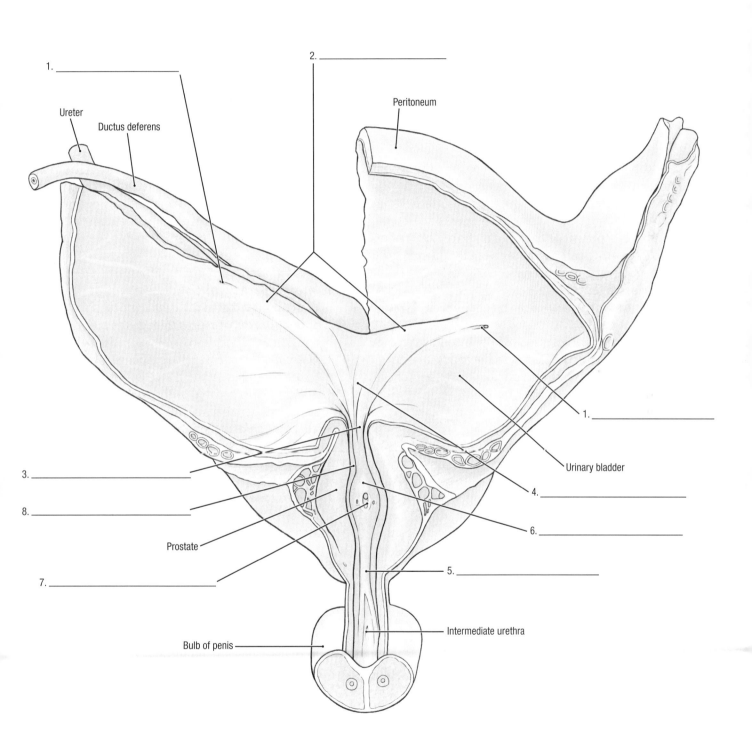

1. _____

Ureter

Ductus deferens

2. _____

Peritoneum

1. _____

Urinary bladder

3. _____

8. _____

4. _____

6. _____

Prostate

5. _____

7. _____

Intermediate urethra

Bulb of penis

Grant's

5.16 MALE PELVIC ORGANS AND PERINEUM

This image depicts the male pelvic organs and perineal structures in situ in the midsagittal plane. The bladder in this specimen is displaced and distended posteriorly from its typical location. The parietal **peritoneum** lining the abdominal walls continues inferiorly into the pelvic cavity folding over the superior or superolateral aspects of the pelvic organs. The pelvic organs are termed subperitoneal because of their inferior relationship to the peritoneum. Because of its position inferior to the bladder, the prostate gland does not have a relationship to the peritoneum. As the peritoneum transitions between the pelvic organs, peritoneal spaces, or fossas, form.

COLOR each of the following structures using a different color for each:

Male Pelvic Organs

○ 1. **Bladder:** Peritoneum covers the superior surface and descends slightly along the posterior aspect
○ 2. **Rectum:** Peritoneum covers the anterior surface of the middle one-third only and covers the anterior and lateral surfaces of the superior one-third of the rectum. There is no intervening peritoneum between the inferior one-third of the rectum and the prostate.
○ 3. **Supravesical fossa:** Reflection of peritoneum from the anterior abdominal wall to the bladder, which elevates as the bladder fills
○ 4. **Rectovesical fossa:** Reflection of peritoneum from the posterior aspect of the bladder to the middle one-third of the rectum. This is the lowest point of the peritoneal cavity in men in the standing position.

Deep Perineal Pouch of the Urogenital Triangle

○ 5. **Perineal membrane:** Inferior boundary of the deep perineal pouch separating it from the superficial perineal pouch
○ 6. **External urethral sphincter:** Lies within the deep perineal pouch superior to the perineal membrane and inferior to the urogenital hiatus of the levator ani. Surrounds the intermediate urethra and embeds the bulbourethral glands.
○ 7. **Deep transverse perineal muscle:** Paired muscle spanning the distance between the ischiopubic rami and the perineal body on each side within the deep perineal pouch

Relationships of Male Pelvic and Perineum Structures

○ 8. **Prostate:** Inferior to bladder, anterior to rectum, posterior to **pubic symphysis**, and superior to urogenital hiatus and the muscles of the deep perineal pouch
○ 9. **Internal urethral sphincter:** Located between the bladder and the prostate in men only
○ 10. **Prostatic urethra:** Courses through the prostate gland
○ 11. **Intermediate urethra:** Courses through the external urethral sphincter in the deep perineal pouch
○ 12. **Spongy urethra:** Courses through the bulb of the penis and corpus spongiosum
○ 13. **Navicular fossa:** Expansion of spongy urethra proximal to the external urethral orifice in the glans penis
○ 14. **Bulb of penis:** Located in the root of the penis in the superficial perineal pouch
○ 15. **Bulbospongiosus muscle:** Covers the bulb of the penis in the superficial perineal pouch
○ 16. **Corpus spongiosum:** Distal continuation of the bulb of the penis in the body of the penis
○ 17. **Corpus cavernosum:** Distal continuation of the crus of the penis dorsal to the corpus spongiosum
○ 18. **Anal canal:** Lies in the anal triangle of perineum surrounded on either side by ischioanal fossae
○ 19. **External anal sphincter:** Surrounds lower portion of the anal canal
○ 20. **Internal anal sphincter:** Surrounds upper portion of anal canal
○ 21. **Puborectalis:** Most medial pair of levator ani muscles forming a sling around the anorectal junction
○ 22. **Levator ani:** Forms the pelvic diaphragm with the coccygeus muscle separating the true pelvis and pelvic organs from the perineum

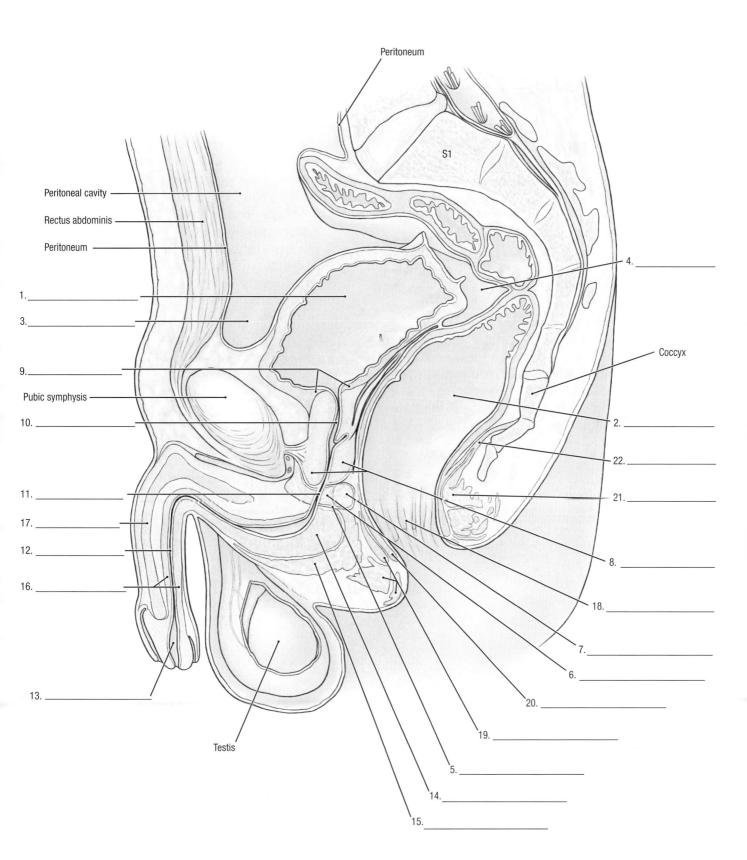

Peritoneum

S1

Peritoneal cavity

Rectus abdominis

Peritoneum

1. _____

3. _____

9. _____

Pubic symphysis

10. _____

11. _____

17. _____

12. _____

16. _____

13. _____

Testis

4. _____

Coccyx

2. _____

22. _____

21. _____

8. _____

18. _____

7. _____

6. _____

20. _____

19. _____

5. _____

14. _____

15. _____

Grant's

5.17   FEMALE PELVIC ORGANS

A portion of the pubic bones and the anterior aspect of the bladder have been removed.

On the right side, the uterine tube, ovary, broad ligament, and peritoneum have also been removed.

COLOR each of the following structures using a different color for each:

Bladder and Ureter

○ 1. **Ureter:** Descends along the posterior abdominal wall and crosses the **external iliac artery** and vein to enter the true pelvis. In females, the uterine artery and round ligament of the uterus cross the ureter as it traverses the pelvis to reach the wall of the bladder.

The bladder in females, as in males, lies posterior to the pubic bones and pubic symphysis. In females, the posterior aspect of the bladder is related to the vagina and the superior surface is related to the body and fundus of the uterus.

The internal structure of the bladder in females is the same as in males:

○ 2. **Ureteric orifice:** Two openings in the posterolateral wall of the bladder for the entry of the ureters

○ 3. **Trigone:** Smooth triangular area between the ureteric orifices and the internal urethral orifice

Uterus and Adnexa

○ 4. **Fundus of the uterus:** Typically lies superior to the roof of the bladder because the uterus is anteverted and anteflexed

○ 5. **Uterine tube:** Extends laterally from the uterus

○ 6. **Ovary:** Associated with the fimbriae of the distal end of the uterine tube

○ 7. **Round ligament of uterus:** Developmental remnant of the gubernaculum that tethers the uterus by extending from the uterus, through the inguinal canal, to the labium majus

○ 8. **Broad ligament:** Peritoneal fold over the uterus, uterine tubes, and the ovaries

○ 9. **Uterine artery:** Branch of the internal iliac artery that crosses the ureter near the level of the cervix to reach the uterus

○10. **Vaginal artery:** Branch(es) of the internal iliac artery that supply the upper vagina

---

CLINICAL NOTE: UTERINE ARTERY LIGATION

Hysterectomy (removal of the uterus with or without the adnexa) is the most common nonpregnancy-related major surgery performed on females in the United States. During the procedure, the **uterine artery** must be ligated and is typically done close to the cervix, so that **vaginal arteries** arising from the uterine artery remain intact. The **ureter** lies in close proximity (1 cm) to the cervix en route to the bladder. In addition, the uterine artery crosses the ureter superiorly ("water under the bridge"). Injury to the pelvic portion of the ureter is less common than damage to the bladder or rectum, but is often associated with significant morbidity, formation of ureterovaginal fistulas, and potential loss of kidney function.

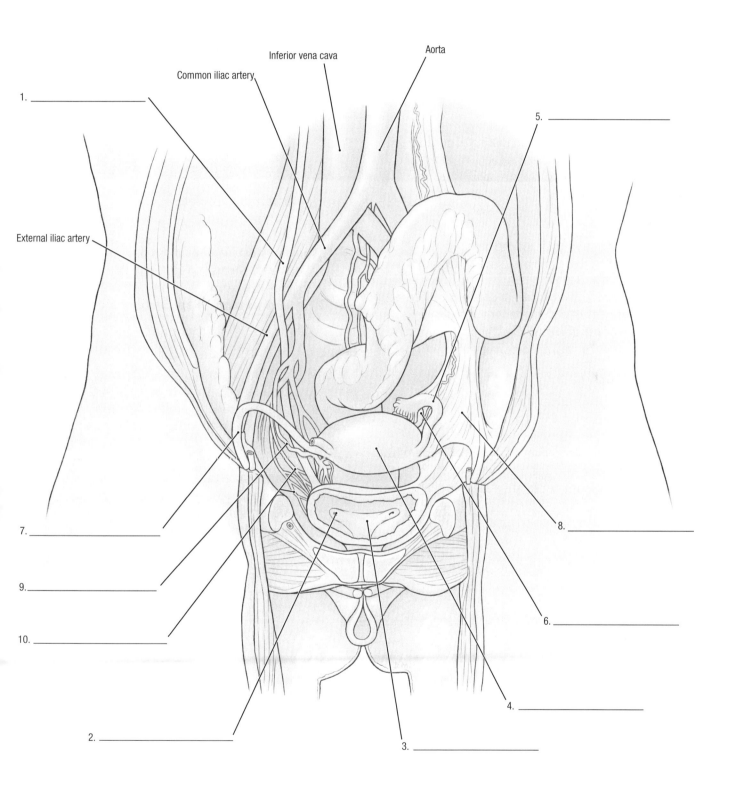

Inferior vena cava

Aorta

Common iliac artery

1. _____

5. _____

External iliac artery

7. _____

9. _____

10. _____

2. _____

3. _____

4. _____

6. _____

8. _____

Grant's

5.18A and B　UTERUS, ADNEXA, AND BROAD LIGAMENT

In Figure A, a portion of the uterine wall, round ligament, and vaginal wall have been removed on the left side. In Figure B, the uterus and adnexa have been removed. The broad ligament has been removed on the right side but is left intact along the anterior surface of the uterus and on the left side.

▋ *COLOR each of the following structures using a different color for each:*

Uterus

The wall of the uterus is composed of three layers:

○ **1.　*Perimetrium:*** Outer layer consisting of peritoneum
○ **2.　*Myometrium:*** Intermediate, smooth muscle layer
○ **3.　*Endometrium:*** Internal mucous layer

The uterus is subdivided into two main parts:

○ **4.　*Body:*** Superior two-thirds of the uterus
　○ **5.　*Fundus:*** Portion of the body superior to the openings of the uterine tubes
○ **6.　*Cervix:*** Cylindrical, narrow inferior one-third of the uterus, which protrudes into the superior vagina
　○ **7.　*External ostium of cervix:*** Opening in the central aspect of the vaginal portion of the cervix

Adnexa of Uterus

The adnexa of the uterus are composed of uterine tubes and ovaries along with associated ligaments.

○ **8.　*Uterine tubes:*** Extend laterally from each side of the uterus and open into the peritoneal cavity near the ovaries. The uterine tubes are subdivided into three parts:
　○ **9.　*Isthmus:*** Medial portion associated with the body of the uterus
　○ **10.　*Ampulla:*** Widest and longest portion and is the typical site of fertilization of the oocyte
　○ **11.　*Infundibulum:*** Funnel-shaped distal end that opens into the peritoneal cavity
　　○ **12.　*Fimbriae:*** Fingerlike processes of the infundibulum

○ **13.　*Ovary:*** Almond-shaped and almond-sized female gonad
　○ **14.　*Ligament of ovary:*** Remnant of the gubernaculum connecting the proximal (uterine) end of the ovary to the lateral aspect of the uterus immediately inferior to the entrance of the uterine tube
○ **15.　*Suspensory ligament of ovary:*** Peritoneal fold containing the ovarian vessels to the superolateral aspect of the ovary

Vagina

○ **16.　*Vagina:*** Musculomembranous tube extending from the vestibule of the vagina to the middle of the external aspect of the cervix
　○ **17.　*Vaginal fornix:*** Recess around the inferior aspect of the cervix

Broad Ligament

The broad ligament is a double layer of peritoneum that extends from the uterus to the lateral walls of the pelvis. The ligament of the ovary and the round ligament of the uterus lie between the two layers of the broad ligament. The broad ligament is subdivided into four parts. The perimetrium is the portion of the broad ligament that covers the body of the uterus and composes the outer layer. The mesovarium of the broad ligament is the small mesentery of the ovary.

○ **18.　*Mesosalpinx:*** Small mesentery of the uterine tube
○ **19.　*Mesometrium:*** Largest portion of the broad ligament forming a mesentery on either side of the uterus inferior to the mesosalpinx and mesovarium

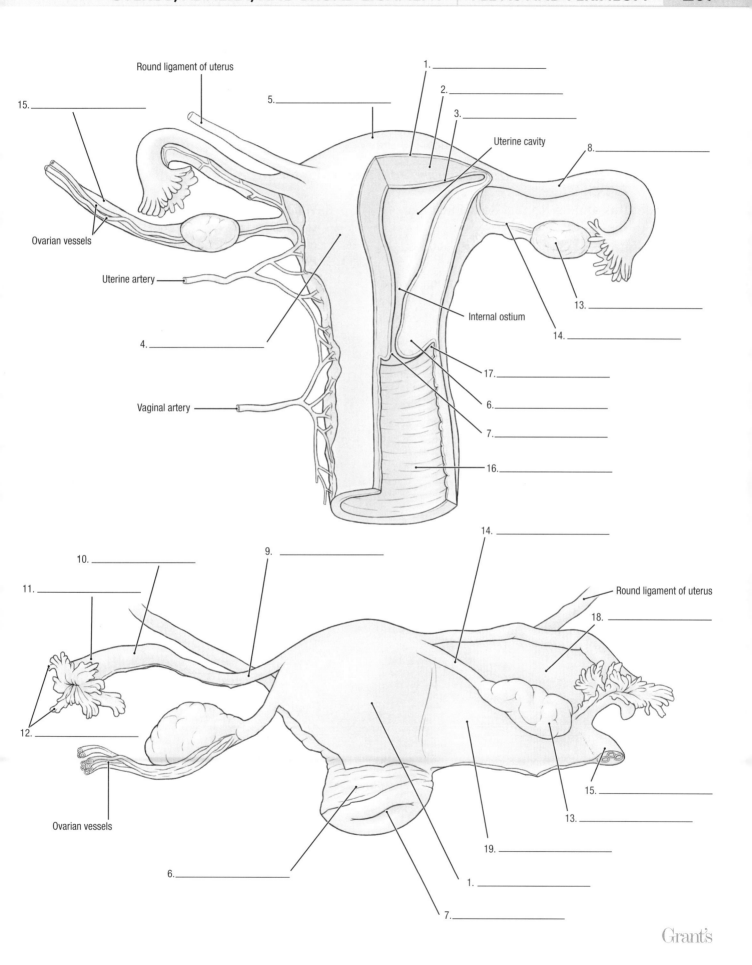

Round ligament of uterus

15. _____

Ovarian vessels

Uterine artery _____

4. _____

Vaginal artery _____

5. _____

1. _____
2. _____
3. _____

Uterine cavity

8. _____

Internal ostium

13. _____

14. _____

17. _____

6. _____

7. _____

16. _____

10. _____

11. _____

9. _____

12. _____

Ovarian vessels

6. _____

14. _____

Round ligament of uterus

18. _____

15. _____

13. _____

19. _____

1. _____

7. _____

5.19 FEMALE PELVIC ORGANS (MIDSAGITTAL VIEW)

Similar to the male pelvic organs, most of the female pelvic organs are subperitoneal (pelvic organs are inferior to the **peritoneum** and have their superior or superolateral aspects covered by peritoneum). In females, the ovaries and the uterine tubes are intraperitoneal (ensheathed in peritoneum). In addition, the uterus is positioned between the bladder and rectum, creating different peritoneal spaces than are found in males.

COLOR each of the following structures using a different color for each:

Pelvic Structures and Peritoneal Relationships

○ 1. *Bladder:* Peritoneum covers only the superior surface of the bladder
  ○ 2. *Urethra:* Much shorter in females, extending from the internal urethral orifice in the neck of the bladder to the external urethral orifice in the vestibule of the vagina
○ 3. *Uterus:* Peritoneum covers the fundus and the anterior and posterior aspects of the body of the uterus. The uterus is normally anteverted and anteflexed over the roof of the bladder.
○ 4. *Cervix:* Peritoneum descends from the posterior aspect of the body of uterus and covers the posterior aspect of the cervix
○ 5. *Vagina:* Related directly to posterior wall of the bladder and urethra anteriorly and to the rectum posteriorly with no intervening peritoneum
○ 6. *Rectum:* Peritoneum covers the anterior surface of the middle one-third only and covers the anterior and lateral surfaces of the superior one-third of the rectum. There is no intervening peritoneum between the vagina and the rectum.
○ 7. *Supravesical fossa:* Reflection of peritoneum from the anterior abdominal wall to the bladder, which elevates as the bladder fills

○ 8. *Vesicouterine pouch:* Reflection of peritoneum from the superior surface of the bladder to the anterior aspect of the body and fundus of the uterus
○ 9. *Rectouterine pouch:* Reflection of peritoneum from the posterior aspect of the body and cervix of the uterus to the middle one-third of the rectum. This pouch is the lowest point of the peritoneal cavity in females when standing.
  ○ 10. *Posterior vaginal fornix:* Space in the vagina related to the cervix as it extends into the upper vagina. The rectouterine pouch is directly related to the posterior fornix of the vagina.
○ 11. *Broad ligament:* Extends from the uterus laterally to the pelvic wall as the peritoneum folds over the fundus and body of the uterus, the uterine tubes, the round ligament, and the ovaries
  ○ 12. *Uterine tube:* Enclosed within the free edge of the broad ligament except at the lateral opening of the uterine tube to the peritoneal cavity
  ○ 13. *Ovary:* Enclosed within the broad ligament
  ○ 14. *Round ligament of uterus:* Enclosed within the two layers of the broad ligament
○ 15. *Suspensory ligament of ovary:* Peritoneum covering the ovarian vessels as they travel from/to the abdominal aorta/inferior vena cava and the ovaries

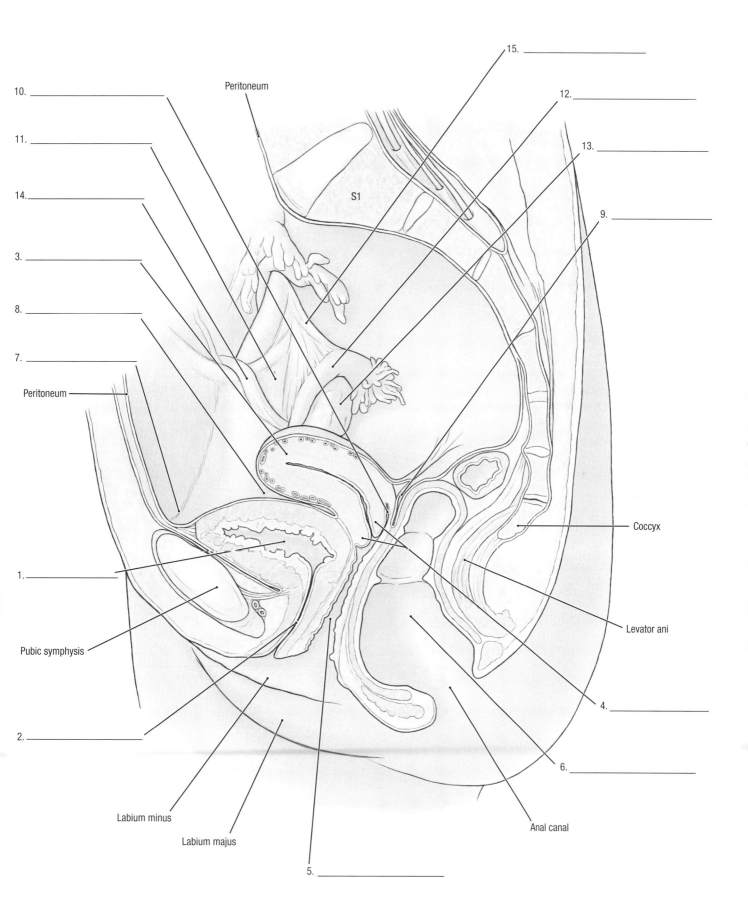

15. _____

Peritoneum

10. _____

12. _____

11. _____

13. _____

14. _____

S1

9. _____

3. _____

8. _____

7. _____

Peritoneum

Coccyx

1. _____

Levator ani

Pubic symphysis

4. _____

2. _____

6. _____

Labium minus

Anal canal

Labium majus

5. _____

Grant's

5.20 | INTERNAL ILIAC ARTERY

The internal iliac artery is the primary artery supplying the structures of the pelvic cavity but it also sends branches to the gluteal region, medial thigh, and the perineum. The branching of the internal iliac artery is shown in a male specimen, however the branching pattern is the same in the female except for specific branches to male or female pelvic organs.

COLOR each of the following structures using a different color for each:

○ 1. *Common iliac artery:* Bifurcates into the *external iliac* and internal iliac arteries at the IV disk between L5 and S1 vertebrae

○ 2. *Internal iliac artery:* Descends posteromedially into the lesser pelvis medial to the external iliac vein and *obturator nerve*

○ 3. *Superior gluteal artery:* Passes between the lumbosacral trunk and the anterior ramus of S1 to exit the pelvis superior to the piriformis muscle

○ 4. *Inferior gluteal artery:* Exits the pelvis inferior to piriformis muscle

○ 5. *Internal pudendal artery:* Exits the pelvis inferior to piriformis muscle with inferior gluteal artery

○ 6. *Middle rectal artery:* Descends within the pelvis to supply inferior rectum

○ 7. *Inferior vesical artery:* Descends within the pelvis to supply inferior bladder and prostate (typically only found in males)

○ 8. *Umbilical artery:* Courses anteriorly for a short course and then becomes obliterated as the median umbilical ligament

○ 9. *Superior vesical arteries:* Branches of the patent portion of the umbilical artery passing to the superior aspect of the bladder

○ 10. *Anomalous (aberrant) obturator artery:* Typically, the obturator arises from the internal iliac artery; however, in some individuals it arises from the inferior epigastric artery instead (anomalous), as shown in this image

In females, the uterine artery also arises from the internal iliac artery. One or more vaginal arteries also arise either directly from the internal iliac artery or from the uterine artery.

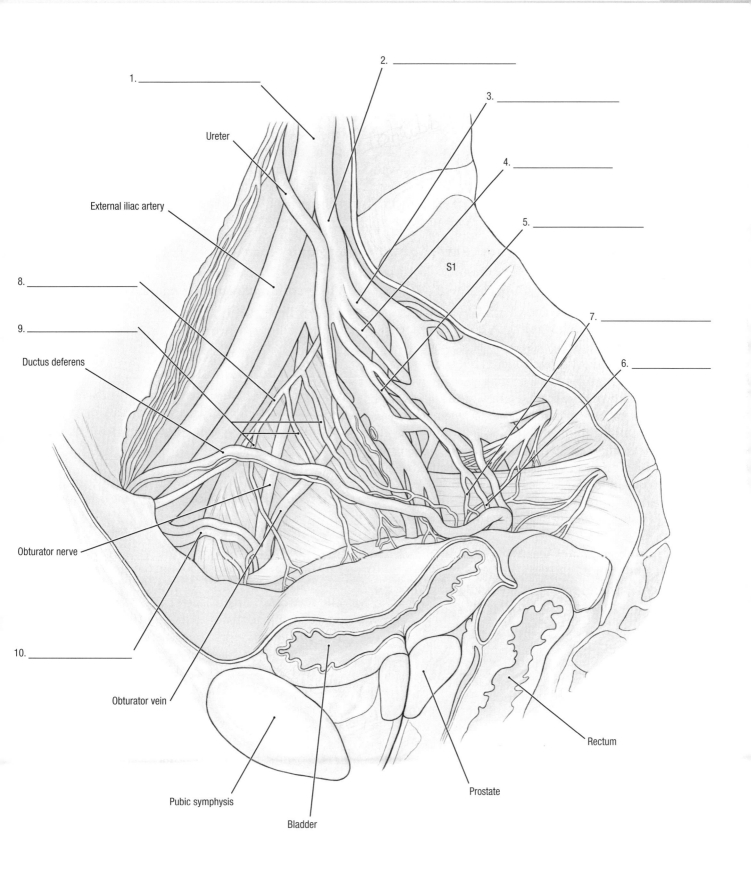

1. _____

2. _____

3. _____

4. _____

5. _____

6. _____

7. _____

8. _____

9. _____

10. _____

Ureter

External iliac artery

Ductus deferens

Obturator nerve

Obturator vein

Pubic symphysis

Bladder

Prostate

Rectum

S1

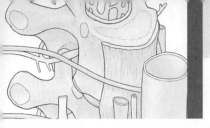

CHAPTER 6

Lower Limb

6.1A and B BONES OF THE LOWER LIMB

For the bony anatomy of the pelvic girdle, please review figure in Section 5.1A and B.

Figure A depicts the anterior view of the left lower limb; Figure B depicts the posterior view of the right lower limb with the hip joint disarticulated.

The femur is the longest and heaviest bone in the human body, transmitting weight from the *__hip bone__* to the tibia when a person is standing. The tibia and fibula are the bones of the leg, but only the tibia articulates with the femur and is responsible for transferring the weight of the body. The fibula functions as an attachment for muscles primarily. The bones of the foot include the 7 tarsal bones, 5 metatarsal bones, and 14 phalanges.

COLOR each of the following structures using a different color for each:

Femur

○ 1. *Head:* Round, medial projection of the superior end articulating with the *__acetabulum__* of hip bone

○ 2. *Neck:* Trapezoidal, inferolateral to the head and links the head to the shaft of the femur

○ 3. *Greater trochanter:* Large, laterally placed mass where the neck joins the shaft providing attachment for several muscles of the thigh

○ 4. *Lesser trochanter:* Small and rounded projection medially placed where the neck joins the shaft providing attachment for the iliopsoas muscle

○ 5. *Linea aspera* (B only): Broad, rough line located posteriorly on the shaft providing attachment for the adductors of the thigh

○ 6. *Medial femoral condyle:* Medial inferior end of the femur forming part of the knee joint

○ 7. *Lateral femoral condyle:* Lateral inferior end of the femur forming part of the knee joint

Tibia

○ 8. *Medial tibial condyle:* Medial superior end of the tibia forming part of the knee joint

○ 9. *Lateral tibial condyle:* Lateral superior end of the tibia forming part of the knee joint

○ 10. *Tibial tuberosity* (A only): Broad, oblong projection on the anterior border providing attachment of the patellar ligament from the inferior aspect of the *__patella__*

○ 11. *Medial malleolus:* Flared medial projection of the inferior end articulating with the talus bone

Fibula

○ 12. *Head:* Enlarged superior end
○ 13. *Neck:* Small, slender area inferior to the head
○ 14. *Lateral malleolus:* Enlarged lateral projection of the inferior end articulating with the talus bone

Bones of the Foot

○ 15. *Talus:* Superior surface gripped by the lateral and medial malleoli
○ 16. *Calcaneus:* Articulates with the talus superiorly and with the cuboid anteriorly
○ 17. *Cuboid:* Most lateral bone in the distal row, anterior to the calcaneus
○ 18. *Navicular:* Boat-shaped bone located anterior to the talus and posterior to the cuneiforms
○ 19. *Cuneiforms:* Three (medial, intermediate, and lateral) bones located anterior to the navicular and posterior to the appropriate metatarsal (1-3)
○ 20. *Metatarsal:* Five bones numbered from the medial side of the foot
○ 21. *Phalanx:* 14 bones in total; the first digit contains only a proximal and distal bone and the other four digits have proximal, middle, and distal bones

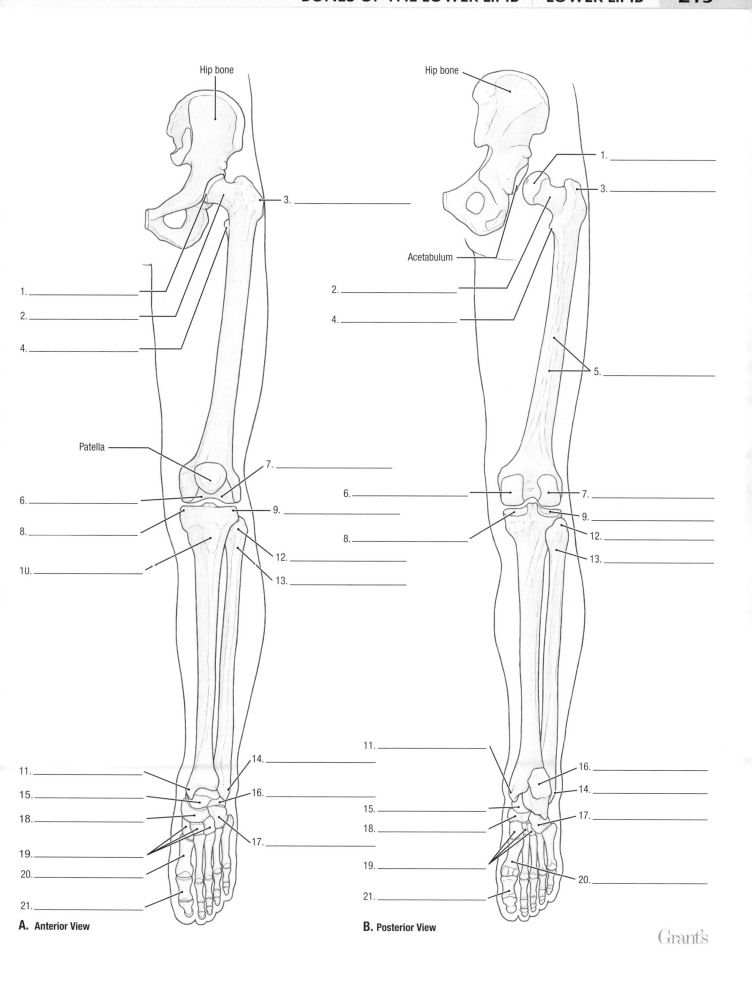

Hip bone

3. _____

1. _____
2. _____
4. _____

Patella

7. _____

6. _____
8. _____
9. _____
10. _____
12. _____
13. _____

11. _____
15. _____
18. _____
19. _____
20. _____
21. _____

14. _____
16. _____
17. _____

A. Anterior View

Hip bone

1. _____
3. _____

Acetabulum

2. _____
4. _____

5. _____

6. _____
7. _____
8. _____
9. _____
12. _____
13. _____

11. _____
15. _____
18. _____
19. _____
21. _____

16. _____
14. _____
17. _____
20. _____

B. Posterior View

Grant's

6.2A and B   FASCIA LATA AND FEMORAL TRIANGLE

Figure A depicts the thigh with the fascia lata intact except where it has been cut away from the inguinal ligament and pinned inferiorly. The *lateral border of the saphenous opening* has also been reflected inferiorly due to this incision. In Figure B, the fascia lata has been removed to reveal the contents and borders of the femoral triangle.

The deep fascia of the thigh is called the fascia lata. The fascia lata is continuous with the inguinal ligament and deep fascia of the leg and attaches to the pubis, iliac crest, sacrum, coccyx, iliopubic ramus, ischial tuberosity, sacrotuberous ligament, and bony prominences of the knee. Laterally, fascia lata thickens to form the *iliotibial tract* extending from the iliac tubercle to the anterolateral tubercle of the tibia. Inferior to the medial portion of the inguinal ligament is a gap in the fascia lata, the saphenous opening, for the passage of the great saphenous vein and superficial lymphatic vessels.

COLOR each of the following structures using a different color for each:

◯ 1. *Fascia lata* (A only): Deep fascia enclosing the thigh muscles
◯ 2. *Great saphenous vein:* Traverses the saphenous opening of the fascia lata to drain to femoral vein

The *femoral triangle* is a useful landmark for understanding neurovascular relationships in the superomedial thigh.

Boundaries of the Femoral Triangle

It is bounded by the:

◯ 3. *Adductor longus* (B only): Medial border
◯ 4. *Sartorius:* Lateral border
◯ 5. *Inguinal ligament:* Superior border
◯ 6. *Iliopsoas* (B only): Lateral portion of the floor formed by *iliacus* and *psoas major* muscles
◯ 7. *Pectineus* (B only): Medial portion of the floor

Contents of the Femoral Triangle

The contents of the femoral triangle from lateral to medial are femoral nerve, femoral artery, femoral vein, and deep lymphatic vessels. The femoral nerve is the only structure not enclosed in the femoral sheath.

◯ 8. *Femoral nerve:* Located lateral to the femoral vessels
◯ 9. *Femoral sheath* (A only): Fascial tube enclosing the femoral artery, femoral vein, and deep lymphatic vessels
◯10. *Femoral artery* (B only): Located lateral to the femoral vein and medial to the femoral nerve, continuation of the *external iliac artery* as the artery passed deep to the inguinal ligament
◯11. *Femoral vein* (B only): Located medial to the femoral artery, receives drainage from great saphenous vein and other superficial veins, and drains to *external iliac vein*

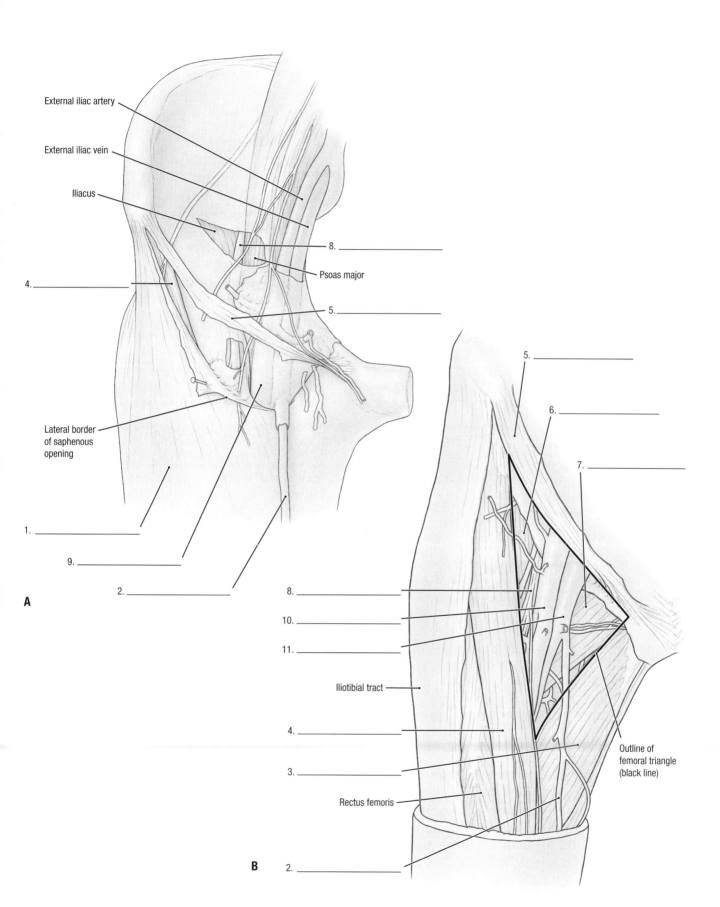

External iliac artery

External iliac vein

Iliacus

8. _____

Psoas major

4. _____

5. _____

Lateral border
of saphenous
opening

1. _____

9. _____

2. _____

A

5. _____

6. _____

7. _____

8. _____

10. _____

11. _____

Iliotibial tract

4. _____

3. _____

Rectus femoris

Outline of
femoral triangle
(black line)

B   2. _____

Grant's

6.3A and B ANTERIOR VIEW OF THE THIGH

The thigh is divided into three compartments (anterior, medial, and posterior) by intermuscular septa that extend from the fascia lata to the femur. From the anterior view of the thigh, muscles of the anterior and medial compartment along with one muscle of the gluteal region are visible.

Figure A depicts the muscles intact. In Figure B, the sartorius, rectus femoris, iliotibial tract, pectineus, and adductor longus have been incised.

COLOR each of the following structures using a different color for each:

Anterior Thigh Muscles

The anterior thigh muscles are the flexors of the hip and extensors of the knee. All anterior thigh muscles are innervated by the femoral nerve except for the iliopsoas muscle, which is innervated by the anterior rami of L1 to L3 and pectineus, which receives innervation from both femoral and obturator nerves.

Quadriceps femoris comprises most of the anterior aspect of thigh and is formed by four muscles that unite inferiorly to form the quadriceps tendon:

○ 1. *Rectus femoris:* Courses straight in the midline from the hip to the knee

○ 2. *Vastus lateralis:* Lies lateral to rectus femoris

○ 3. *Vastus medialis:* Lies medial rectus femoris

○ 4. *Vastus intermedius* (B only): Lies deep to the rectus femoris and between the vastus lateralis and the vastus medialis

○ 5. *Patellar ligament* (B only): Continuation of the quadriceps tendon from the **patella** to the tibial tuberosity

○ 6. *Sartorius* (A only): Superficial, long, and slender muscle passing from lateral to medial

○ 7. *Iliopsoas:* Medial to superior aspect of the sartorius deep to the contents of the femoral triangle; composed of the **iliacus** and **psoas major** muscles

Muscles of the Anterior Thigh

Muscle	Proximal Attachment	Distal Attachment	Action
Rectus femoris	Anterior inferior iliac spine; ilium superior to acetabulum	Via quadriceps tendon to base of patella; indirectly via patellar ligament to tibial tuberosity	Extend leg at knee joint; rectus femoris assists in hip flexion
Vastus lateralis	Greater trochanter and lateral lip of linea aspera of femur		
Vastus medialis	Intertrochanteric line and medial lip of linea aspera of femur		
Vastus intermedius	Anterior and lateral surfaces of shaft of femur		
Sartorius	Anterior superior iliac spine	Superomedial surface of tibia	Flexes, abducts, and laterally rotates the thigh at hip joint; flexes leg at knee joint
Iliopsoas	Psoas major: Lateral aspects of T12-L5 vertebrae and IV discs; transverse process of all lumbar vertebrae Psoas minor: Lateral aspects of T12-L1 vertebrae and IV discs Iliacus: Iliac crest, iliac fossa, ala of sacrum	Lesser trochanter of femur	Flexes thigh at hip joint

Medial Compartment Muscles

○ 8. *Pectineus:* Medial to iliopsoas and is a transition muscle between anterior and medial compartments due to its mixed function and innervation of both compartments

○ 9. *Obturator externus* (B only): Lateral rotator of the thigh located deep to the pectineus and innervated by the obturator nerve (muscle of the medial compartment)

○10. *Adductor longus:* Most anterior of the adductor muscles

○11. *Adductor brevis* (B only): Lies deep to the pectineus and adductor longus

○12. *Gracilis:* Most medial of the thigh muscles

Lateral Aspect of the Thigh

○13. *Tensor fasciae latae:* Medial rotator and abductor of the thigh and tensor of the iliotibial tract (muscle of the gluteal region)

○14. *Iliotibial tract:* Lateral thickening of the fascia lata extending from the iliac tubercle to the anterolateral tibia

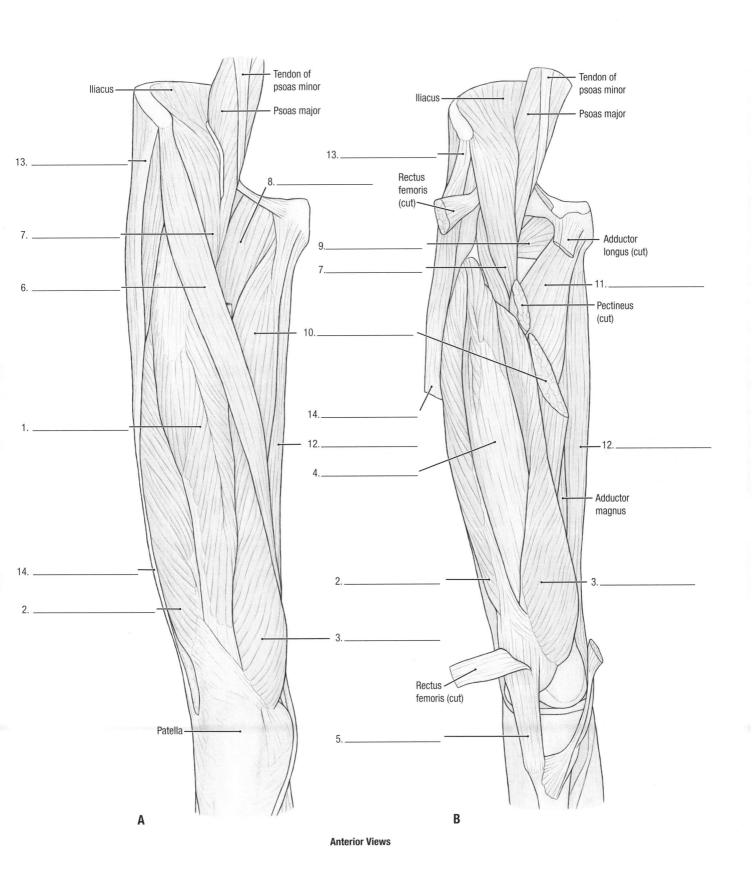

Iliacus

Tendon of
psoas minor

Psoas major

13.

8.

7.

6.

1.

14.

2.

Patella

A

Iliacus

Tendon of
psoas minor

Psoas major

13.

Rectus
femoris
(cut)

9.

7.

Adductor
longus (cut)

11.

Pectineus
(cut)

10.

14.

12.

4.

12.

Adductor
magnus

2.

3.

Rectus
femoris (cut)

5.

B

Anterior Views

Grant's

6.4 MEDIAL VIEW OF THE THIGH

From the medial view of the right thigh, the superficial muscles of the medial compartment along with some of the muscles from the anterior compartment, posterior compartment, and gluteal region are visible. The three muscles (one each from the anterior, medial, and posterior compartments) contributing to the pes anserinus are apparent as they converge into their attachment on the medial aspect of the knee.

COLOR each of the following structures using a different color for each:

Medial View of the Thigh

○ 1. *Adductor longus:* Anteriorly placed, large, fan-shaped muscle superficial to the adductor brevis and a portion of the adductor magnus

○ 2. *Adductor magnus:* Largest and posteriorly placed muscle composed of an adductor part and a hamstring part

○ 3. *Gracilis:* Superficial, medial, and strap-like muscle attaching to superomedial tibia

○ 4. *Sartorius:* Anterior thigh muscle attaching to superomedial tibia

○ 5. *Semitendinosus:* Posterior thigh muscle attaching to superomedial tibia

○ 6. *Pes anserinus:* Common tendinous insertion of the sartorius, gracilis, and semitendinosus to the superomedial tibia

○ 7. *Semimembranous:* Broad posterior compartment muscle of the thigh attaching independently to the superomedial tibia

Medial Thigh Muscles

The medial thigh muscles are the adductors of the thigh. All medial thigh muscles are innervated by the obturator nerve except for the hamstring portion of the adductor magnus, which is innervated by the tibial branch of the sciatic nerve.

Muscles of the Medial Thigh

Muscle	Proximal Attachment	Distal Attachment	Action
Adductor longus	Body of pubis inferior to pubic crest	Middle third of linea aspera of femur	Adducts thigh
Adductor brevis (See Sections 6.3 and 6.5)	Body and inferior ramus of pubis	Pectineal line and proximal linea aspera of femur	
Adductor magnus	Adductor part: inferior ramus of pubis, ischial ramus Hamstrings part: ischial tuberosity	Adductor part: gluteal tuberosity, linea aspera Hamstring part: adductor tubercle of femur	Adducts thigh Adductor part: flexes thigh Hamstrings part: extends thigh
Gracilis	Body and inferior ramus of pubis	Superomedial tibia	Adducts thigh; flexes leg; assists in medial leg rotation
Pectineus	Superior ramus of pubis	Pectineal line of femur	Adducts and flexes thigh; assists with medial rotation of thigh
Obturator externus (see figure in Section 6.3)	Margins of obturator foramen and obturator membrane	Trochanteric fossa of femur	Laterally rotates thigh

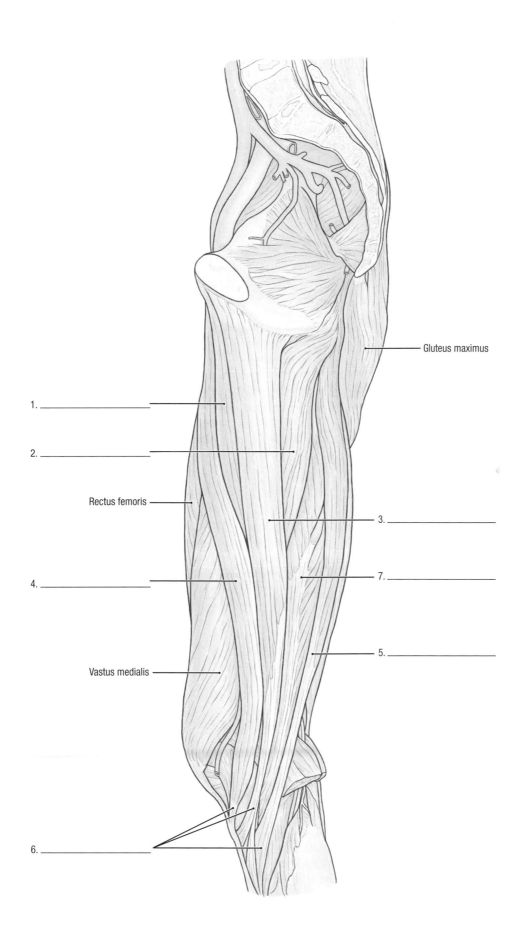

Gluteus maximus

1. _____

2. _____

Rectus femoris _____

3. _____

7. _____

4. _____

Vastus medialis _____

5. _____

6. _____

Grant's

6.5   NEUROVASCULATURE OF THE ANTERIOR AND MEDIAL THIGH

The limb is rotated laterally to demonstrate the neurovasculature pathways of the anterior and medial thigh. The **sartorius**, **rectus femoris**, and **adductor longus** have been cut in this image to reveal deeper structures. Additionally, the femoral sheath has been removed to demonstrate the neurovascular branches and the middle segments of the femoral artery and vein have been removed.

The adductor canal is a long, narrow passageway in the middle third of the thigh extending from the apex of the femoral triangle to the adductor hiatus of the tendon of the adductor magnus. The adductor canal provides passage of the femoral artery, femoral vein, nerve to vastus medialis, and saphenous nerve. Note that only two branches from the femoral nerve enter the adductor canal, not the femoral nerve itself.

COLOR each of the following structures using a different color for each:

The adductor canal is bounded by the:

○ 1. **Vastus medialis:** Anterior and lateral
○ 2. **Adductor magnus:** Posterior
    Adductor longus: Posterior
    Sartorius: Medial

The adductor hiatus is a gap between the adductor and hamstring attachments of the adductor magnus and is best visualized from a posterior view of the popliteal fossa.

○ 3. **Femoral artery:** Enters the femoral triangle lateral to the femoral vein and superficial to **iliopsoas muscle** and then courses through the adductor canal to emerge in the popliteal fossa through the adductor hiatus
○ 4. **Profunda femoris (deep artery of thigh):** Primary artery to the thigh arising from the femoral artery in the femoral triangle passing superficial to the **pectineus** and then deep to the adductor longus
○ 5. **Femoral vein:** Continuation of the popliteal vein proximal to the adductor hiatus, travels through the adductor canal with the femoral artery, and receives venous drainage from the **great saphenous vein** and deep vein of the thigh within the femoral triangle

○ 6. **Femoral nerve:** Arises from L2 to L4 ventral rami of the lumbar plexus, descends into the femoral triangle lateral to the femoral artery, and then divides into several branches to the anterior thigh muscles and the saphenous nerve
○ 7. **Saphenous nerve:** Terminal cutaneous branch of the femoral nerve accompanying the femoral artery and vein through the adductor canal; does not traverse the adductor hiatus and becomes superficial medial to the knee to supply anteromedial aspects of the knee, leg, and foot
○ 8. **Nerve to vastus medialis:** Branch of the femoral nerve that enters the adductor canal briefly before entering the muscle belly of the vastus medialis
○ 9. **Obturator nerve:** Arises from L2 to L4 ventral rami of the lumbar plexus, descends through the obturator canal within the obturator membrane, and then divides into anterior and posterior parts to supply the medial thigh muscles
○ 10. **Adductor brevis:** Lies deep to the adductor longus and is a useful landmark for the anterior and posterior divisions of the obturator nerve with the anterior division lying anterior and the posterior division coursing posteriorly

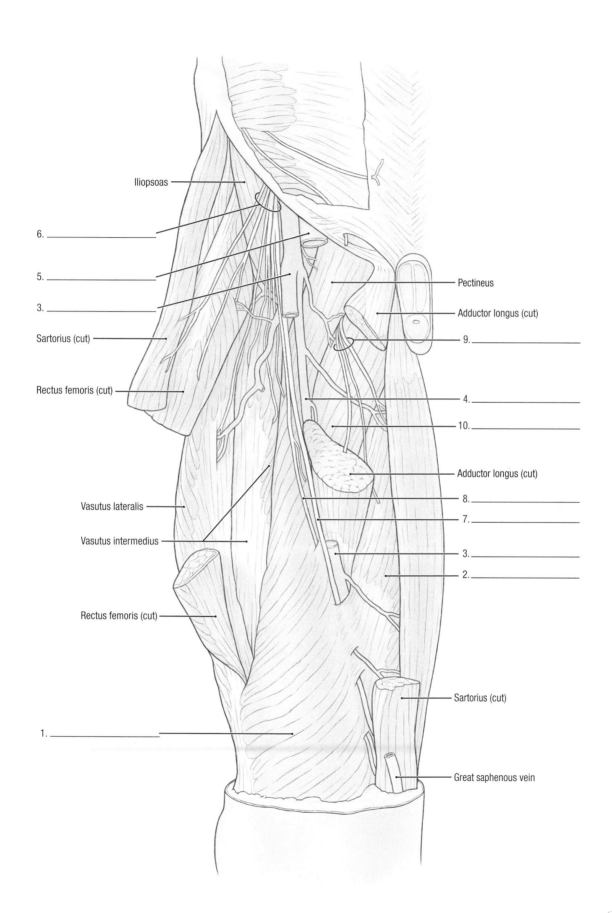

Iliopsoas

6.

5.

3.

Sartorius (cut)

Rectus femoris (cut)

Vasutus lateralis

Vasutus intermedius

Rectus femoris (cut)

1.

Pectineus

Adductor longus (cut)

9.

4.

10.

Adductor longus (cut)

8.

7.

3.

2.

Sartorius (cut)

Great saphenous vein

Grant's

6.6 LATERAL VIEW OF THE THIGH

From the lateral view, muscles of the anterior and posterior compartments of the thigh and gluteal region are visible along with the iliotibial tract.

COLOR each of the following structures using a different color for each:

Posterior Compartment Muscles

○ 1. *Gluteus maximus:* Most superficial and largest gluteal muscle

○ 2. *Tensor fasciae latae:* Enclosed between two layers of fascia lata located superiorly to the iliotibial tract

○ 3. *Iliotibial tract:* Lateral thickening of the fascia lata formed by the aponeurosis of the gluteus maximus and tensor fasciae latae extending from the iliac tubercle to the anterolateral tubercle of the tibia

○ 4. *Gluteus medius* (*covered by gluteal fascia*)*:* Fan-shaped, lying mostly deep to the gluteus maximus except at the superolateral aspects

○ 5. *Long head of biceps femoris:* Crosses the posterior thigh from medial to lateral to attach to the ***head of fibula***

○ 6. *Short head of biceps femoris:* Courses along the lateral aspect of the posterior thigh to attach to the head of fibula

Anterior Compartment Muscles

○ 7. *Vastus lateralis:* Largest component of the quadriceps lying on the lateral side of the thigh

○ 8. *Rectus femoris:* Superficial and anteriorly placed muscle of the quadriceps

○ 9. *Quadriceps tendon:* Common tendinous attachment to the patella from the quadriceps muscles

○10. *Patellar ligament:* Continuation of the quadriceps tendon from the patella to the tibia tuberosity

---

CLINICAL NOTE: ILIOTIBIAL BAND SYNDROME

Iliotibial band syndrome (ITBS) occurs as a result of inflammation and irritation of the iliotibial tract. The most frequent site of irritation is distally near the lateral femoral condyle due to repetitive extension and flexion of the knee or a lack of flexibility of the band during the stance phase of the gait cycle. ITBS is most common in endurance athletes, such as long-distance runners or cyclists. Patients typically present with pain on the lateral aspect of the knee, especially during any activity that places weight on the knee during flexion. If untreated, pain may also be present at rest. Initial treatments are aimed at reducing inflammation using RICE (rest, ice, compression, and elevation) and anti-inflammatory medications. Upon resolution of the inflammation, physical therapy is implemented, focusing on active stretching exercises of the muscles of the gluteal and thigh regions to improve the flexibility of the iliotibial tract.

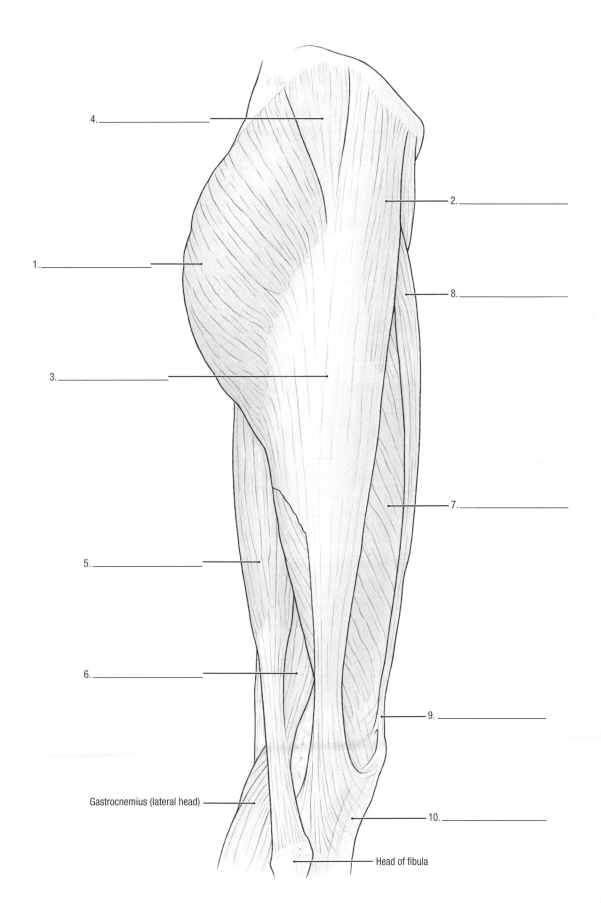

4.

2.

1.

8.

3.

7.

5.

6.

9.

Gastrocnemius (lateral head)

10.

Head of fibula

Grant's

6.7 POSTERIOR VIEW OF THE THIGH AND GLUTEAL REGION: SUPERFICIAL DISSECTION

From the posterior view of the thigh, the muscles of the gluteal region and posterior compartment of the thigh are visible, along with some of the muscles of the medial compartment.

The terminal divisions of the sciatic nerve, *tibial* and *common fibular nerves*, are visible deep within the inferior aspect of the posterior compartment.

COLOR each of the following structures using a different color for each:

Gluteal Region Muscles

The muscles of the gluteal region are organized into superficial and deep layers. The superficial layer consists of the three gluteal muscles and the tensor fascia latae. The deep layer consists of the piriformis, obturator internus, superior and inferior gemelli, and quadratus femoris.

○ 1. *Gluteus maximus:* Most superficial gluteal muscle covering at least in part all of the other gluteal muscles
○ 2. *Gluteus medius:* Fan-shaped muscle, mostly deep to the gluteus maximus except for the superolateral aspect

Posterior Compartment Muscles

Three of the four muscles of the posterior compartment comprise the hamstrings: semitendinosus, semimembranosus, and the long head of the biceps femoris. The hamstrings share common features:
  A. Proximal attachment to the ischial tuberosity
  B. Innervated by the tibial division of the sciatic nerve
  C. Act on both hip and knee joints
  The *short head of biceps femoris* does not share any of the above features of the hamstrings.

Muscles of the Posterior Thigh (Hamstring)

Muscle	Proximal Attachment	Distal Attachment	Innervation	Action
Short head of biceps femoris	Linea aspera and lateral supracondylar line of femur	Lateral surface of the fibular head; tendon split by fibular collateral ligament	Common fibular division of the sciatic nerve	Flexes leg and rotates it laterally when knee is flexed; long head also extends the thigh
○ 3. *Long head of biceps femoris*	Ischial tuberosity		Tibial division of the sciatic nerve	
○ 4. *Semitendinosus*		Superomedial tibia		Extend thigh; flex leg and rotate it medially when the knee is flexed
○ 5. *Semimembranosus*		Posterior aspect of the medial condyle of the tibia		

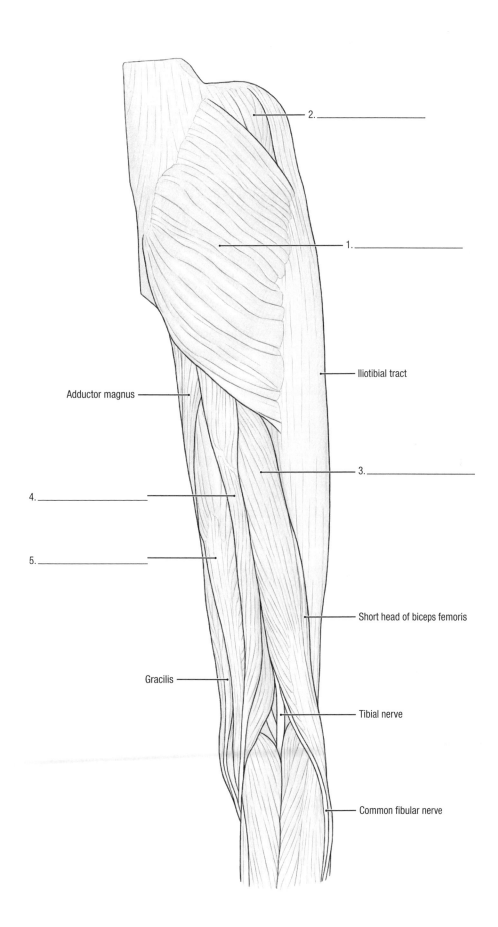

2. _____

1. _____

Iliotibial tract

Adductor magnus

3. _____

4. _____

5. _____

Short head of biceps femoris

Gracilis

Tibial nerve

Common fibular nerve

6.8 POSTERIOR VIEW OF THE THIGH AND GLUTEAL REGION—INTERMEDIATE DISSECTION

The gluteus maximus has been divided and the middle portion excised except for two small cubes to demonstrate the deeper gluteal region structures. In the posterior thigh, the long head of biceps femoris has been pulled medially to reveal the deeper muscles of the posterior compartment and the *sciatic nerve*.

COLOR each of the following structures using a different color for each:

Muscles of the Gluteal Region

Muscle	Proximal Attachment	Distal Attachment	Innervation	Action
○ 1. *Gluteus maximus*	Ilium posterior to posterior gluteal line; dorsal aspect of sacrum and coccyx; **sacrotuberous ligament**	Iliotibial tract; gluteal tuberosity	Inferior gluteal nerve	Extends the thigh and assists in lateral rotation
○ 2. *Gluteus medius*	Ilium between anterior and inferior gluteal lines	Lateral surface of the greater trochanter	Superior gluteal nerve	Abduct and medially rotate the thigh
Gluteus minimus (see Section 6.9)	Ilium between anterior and inferior gluteal lines	Anterior surface of the greater trochanter		
Tensor fasciae latae (see Section 6.6)	Anterior superior iliac spine; anterior surface of the iliac crest	Iliotibial tract		
○ 3. *Piriformis*	Anterior surface of the sacrum; sacrotuberous ligament	Superior surface of the greater trochanter	Nerve to piriformis	Laterally rotate the extended thigh and abduct the flexed thigh
○ 4. *Obturator internus*	Pelvic surface of the obturator membrane	Medial surface of greater trochanter	Nerve to obturator internus	
○ 5. *Superior gemellus*	Ischial spine			
○ 6. *Inferior gemellus*	Ischial tuberosity		Nerve to the quadratus femoris	
○ 7. *Quadratus femoris*	Lateral surface of the ischial tuberosity	Intertrochanteric crest		Laterally rotates the thigh

Posterior Compartment Muscles

○ 8. *Long head of biceps femoris:* Courses from medial to lateral to attach to the head of the fibula

○ 9. *Short head of biceps femoris:* Lies deep to the long head of the biceps femoris

○ 10. *Semitendinosus:* Medial to the long head of the biceps femoris with a long, cord-like tendon attaching to the tibia as part of the pes anserinus

○ 11. *Semimembranosus:* Medial to the semitendinosus with a broader muscle belly and tendon attaching to the tibia independent of the pes anserinus

○ 12. *Adductor magnus:* Composed of an adductor part and a hamstring part. The hamstring portion attaches to the ischial tuberosity, extends the thigh, and is innervated by the tibial division of the sciatic nerve

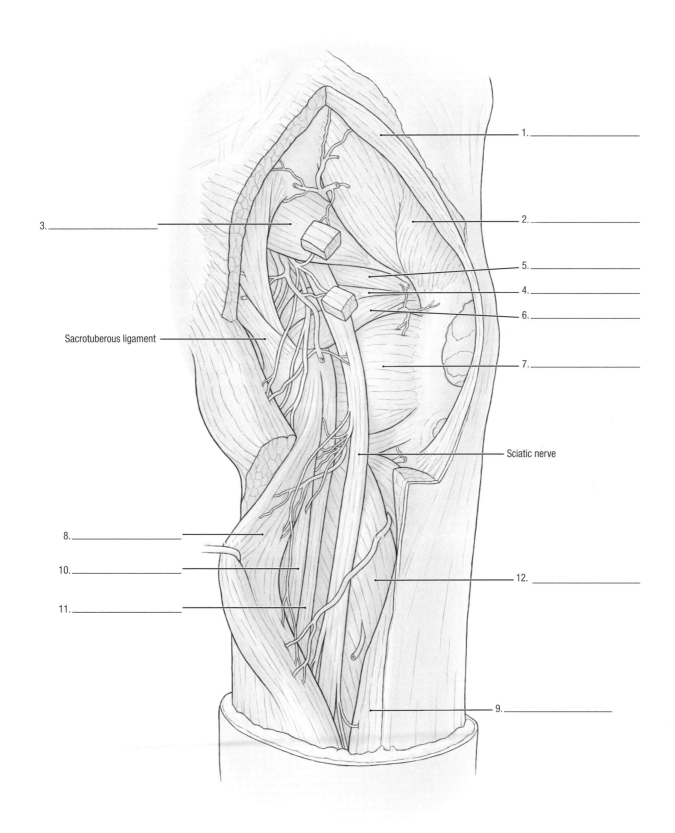

1. _____

2. _____

3. _____

5. _____

4. _____

6. _____

Sacrotuberous ligament _____

7. _____

Sciatic nerve

8. _____

10. _____

11. _____

12. _____

9. _____

Grant's

6.9 POSTERIOR VIEW OF THE THIGH AND GLUTEAL REGION—DEEP DISSECTION

The *gluteus maximus* has been divided and reflected except for the most inferior fibers. *Gluteus medius* has also been mostly removed to reveal the gluteus minimus and the extent of the superior gluteal artery and nerve. The middle portions of *semitendinosus*, *semimembranosus*, and the *long head of biceps femoris* have been removed to demonstrate the adductor magnus, sciatic nerve, and short head of biceps femoris.

COLOR each of the following structures using a different color for each:

○ 1. *Piriformis muscle:* Key landmark for neurovascular structures exiting the pelvis via the greater sciatic foramen

○ 2. *Gluteus minimus:* Deepest of the three gluteal muscles and lies deep to the superior gluteal artery and nerve

○ 3. *Superior gluteal artery:* Branch of the internal iliac artery that emerges into the gluteal region superior to the piriformis in the plane between the gluteus medius and minimus. A smaller branch of the artery extends superficially to the gluteus maximus

○ 4. *Superior gluteal nerve:* Travels with the superior gluteal artery and is composed of L4 to S1 anterior rami

○ 5. *Inferior gluteal artery and nerve:* Emerge inferior to the piriformis muscle to supply the gluteus maximus. The artery arises from the internal iliac artery and the nerve is composed of L5 to S2 anterior rami

○ 6. *Posterior cutaneous nerve of thigh:* Composed of S1 to S3 anterior rami and emerges inferior to piriformis muscles medial to the sciatic nerve and lateral to the *nerve to obturator internus*, *internal pudendal artery*, and *pudendal nerve*; then descends in the posterior thigh to supply the skin of the inferior half of the gluteal region, posterior thigh, and popliteal fossa along with the upper medial thigh and lateral perineum

○ 7. *Sciatic nerve:* Large nerve composed of L4 to S3 anterior rami and emerges inferior to the piriformis

The sciatic nerve courses posterior (superficial) to the:

○ 8. *Superior gemellus*
○ 9. *Obturator internus*
○10. *Inferior gemellus*
○11. *Quadratus femoris*
○12. *Short head of biceps femoris:* Lies lateral to the sciatic nerve
○13. *Adductor magnus, adductor part:* Courses from the ischial ramus and inferior pubic ramus to the linea aspera and gluteal tuberosity of the femur
○14. *Adductor magnus, hamstring part:* Attaches to the ischial tuberosity similar to the other hamstring muscles and courses inferiorly to attach to the adductor tubercle of the femur. The adductor hiatus is formed by the gap between the two parts of the adductor magnus and marks the location of the name change of the femoral vessels to/from popliteal vessels.

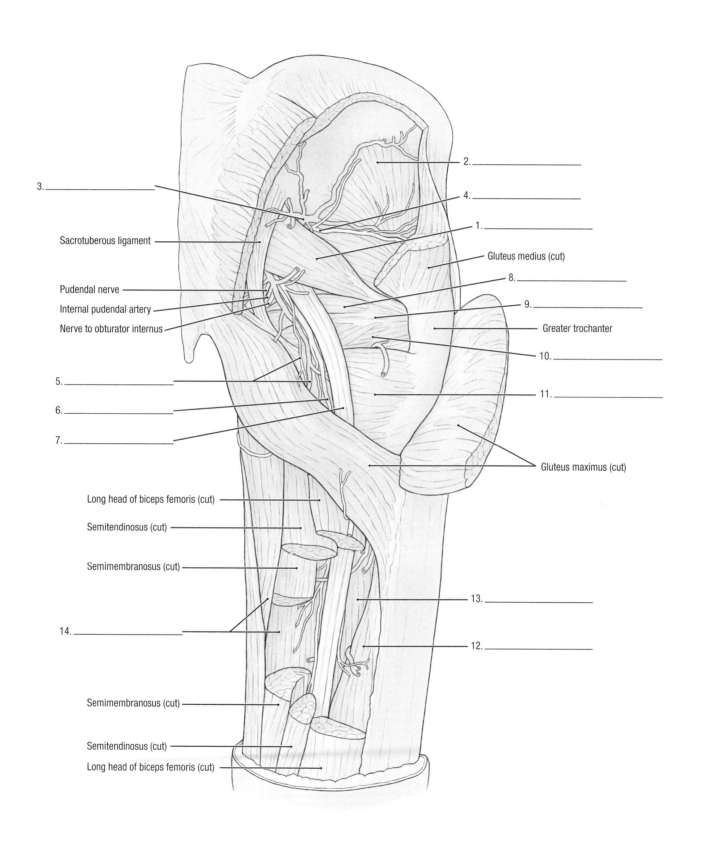

3. _____

Sacrotuberous ligament _____

Pudendal nerve _____

Internal pudendal artery _____

Nerve to obturator internus _____

5. _____

6. _____

7. _____

Long head of biceps femoris (cut) _____

Semitendinosus (cut) _____

Semimembranosus (cut) _____

14. _____

Semimembranosus (cut) _____

Semitendinosus (cut) _____

Long head of biceps femoris (cut) _____

2. _____

4. _____

1. _____

Gluteus medius (cut)

8. _____

9. _____

Greater trochanter

10. _____

11. _____

Gluteus maximus (cut)

13. _____

12. _____

Grant's

6.10   HIP JOINT

The hip joint is a multi-axial ball-and-socket type of synovial joint connecting the pelvic girdle to the femur. The hip joint is enclosed within a strong joint capsule with three intrinsic ligaments composing the external fibrous layer.

Figure A depicts the anterior view of the hip joint, whereas Figure B depicts the posterior view.

COLOR each of the following structures using a different color for each:

○ 1. *Head of femur* (A only)*:* Forms two-third of a sphere that articulates with the acetabulum of the hip bone to form the hip joint

○ 2. *Acetabular labrum* (A only)*:* Fibrocartilaginous lip-shaped rim attached to the margin of the acetabulum of the hip bone, increasing the articulating area of the acetabulum

The ligaments of the hip joint comprise the fibrous layer of the joint capsule.

○ 3. *Iliofemoral ligament:* Inverted Y-shaped ligament placed anterosuperiorly; attaches to the acetabular rim and anterior inferior iliac spine proximally and to the *intertrochanteric line* distally

○ 4. *Pubofemoral ligament* (A only)*:* Located at the antero-inferior aspect of the hip joint arising from the obturator crest of the pubic bone passing laterally to blend with the medial part of the iliofemoral ligament

○ 5. *Ischiofemoral ligament* (B only)*:* Located posteriorly arising from the ischial part of the acetabular rim passing distally to the *neck of the femur* medial to the *greater trochanter*

CLINICAL NOTE: HIP DISLOCATIONS

Two types of hip dislocations occur: congenital and acquired. Congenital dislocation of the hip (developmental dysplasia of the hip, DDH) is observed in newborns. DDH occurs in approximately 1 in 1 000 individuals and occurs with increased frequency in females and first-born children. The risk of DDH is increased in infants presenting in the breech position during childbirth and those with certain conditions such as cerebral palsy and skeletal dysplasia. In DDH, hip instability results in improper placement of the femoral head in the acetabulum, leading to the inability to abduct the thigh and a shortened limb. Acquired dislocations are typically the result of high-energy blunt trauma, such as a motor vehicle accident or a fall from a height. Most acquired dislocations occur posteriorly (80-90%) with the femoral head driven posteriorly out of the acetabulum by a force through the knee while the hip is flexed (eg, knee striking dashboard during a motor vehicle accident). Anterior and central dislocations occur less frequently. A central dislocation is more complex as it involves a fracture of the acetabulum.

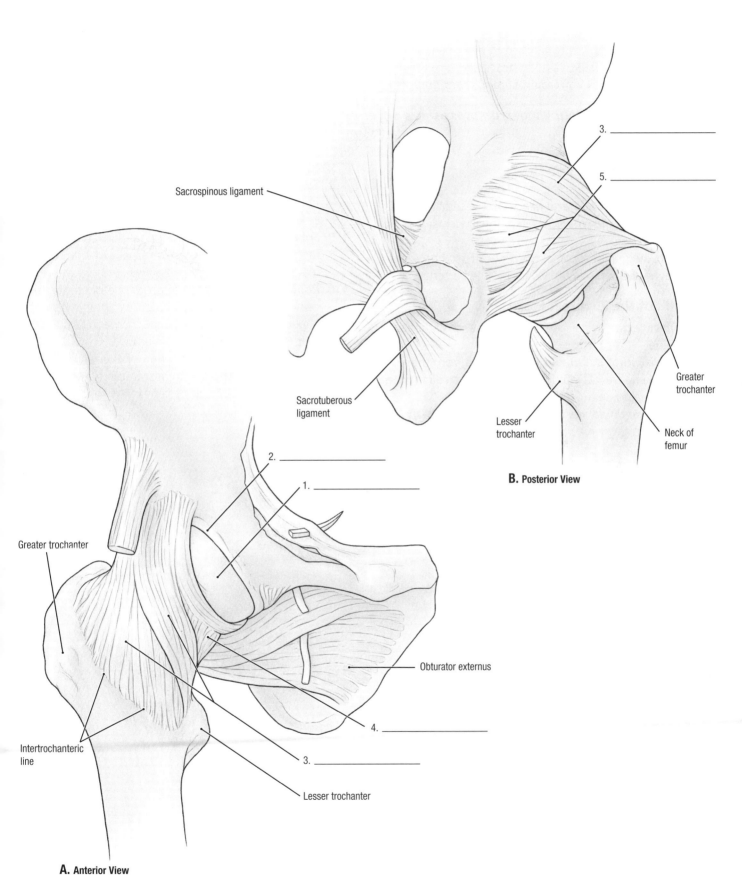

Sacrospinous ligament

3. _____

5. _____

Sacrotuberous
ligament

Greater
trochanter

Lesser
trochanter

Neck of
femur

B. Posterior View

Greater trochanter

2. _____

1. _____

Obturator externus

Intertrochanteric
line

4. _____

3. _____

Lesser trochanter

A. Anterior View

Grant's

6.11 POPLITEAL FOSSA: SUPERFICIAL DISSECTION

The popliteal fossa is a mostly fat-filled compartment allowing passage of the major neurovascular structures from the thigh to the leg. A small hook is grasping a ***branch communicating with inferior gluteal vein*** and pulling the superficial veins away from the deeper structures.

COLOR each of the following structures using a different color for each:

Boundaries of the Popliteal Fossa

○ 1. *Biceps femoris:* Superolateral

○ 2. *Semimembranosus:* Superomedial

○ 3. *Gastrocnemius, lateral head:* Inferolateral

○ 4. *Gastrocnemius, medical head:* Inferomedial

Within the popliteal fossa, the order of structures from superficial to deep are nerves, veins, and then arteries.

Contents of the Popliteal Fossa

○ 5. *Tibial nerve:* Medial, larger terminal branch of the sciatic nerve

○ 6. *Medial sural cutaneous nerve:* Arises from the tibial nerve and travels inferiorly through the midline of the popliteal fossa

○ 7. *Common fibular nerve:* Lateral, smaller terminal branch of the sciatic nerve passing medial to the biceps femoris and the head of the fibula to wrap around the neck of the fibula

○ 8. *Sural communicating branch:* Arises from the common fibular nerve and will unite inferiorly with the medial sural cutaneous nerve to form the sural nerve

○ 9. *Small saphenous vein:* Terminal portion pierces the fascia covering the posterior aspect of the popliteal fossa to drain to the popliteal vein

○ 10. *Popliteal vein:* Continuation of the posterior tibial vein; lies superficial to the popliteal artery within the popliteal fossa and then changes name to femoral vein as it traverses the adductor hiatus

○ 11. *Popliteal artery:* Continuation of the femoral artery lying close to the joint capsule of the knee; gives rise to several genicular arteries that supply the knee joint

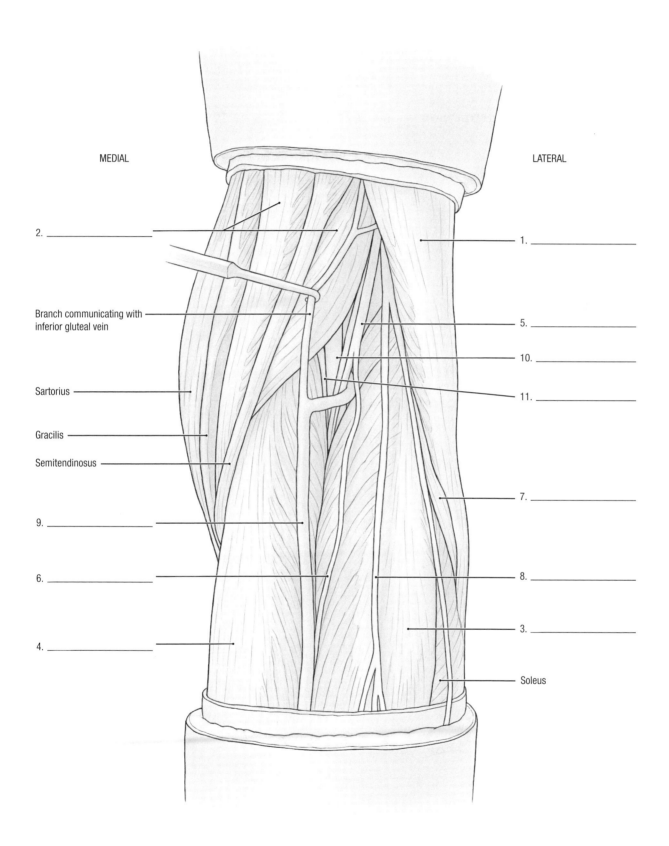

MEDIAL

LATERAL

2. _____

Branch communicating with
inferior gluteal vein

Sartorius _____

Gracilis _____

Semitendinosus _____

9. _____

6. _____

4. _____

1. _____

5. _____

10. _____

11. _____

7. _____

8. _____

3. _____

Soleus _____

Grant's

6.12   POPLITEAL FOSSA, NERVES

The *medial* and *lateral heads of the gastrocnemius muscle* are separated by two fingers. Vascular branches have been removed to demonstrate the branching of the sciatic nerve.

The formation of the sural nerve is variable: it can occur high in the popliteal fossa as it does in this image or anywhere along the length of the posterior leg to the level of the calcaneus.

COLOR each of the following structures using a different color for each:

Nerves of the Popliteal Fossa

○ 1. **Common fibular nerve:** Terminal branch of the sciatic nerve lying deep to the **biceps femoris**
○ 2. **Tibial nerve:** Terminal branch of sciatic nerve coursing through the midline of the popliteal fossa
○ 3. **Medial sural cutaneous nerve:** Branch of the tibial nerve that unites with the sural communicating branch to form the sural nerve
○ 4. **Sural communicating branch:** Branch of the common fibular nerve that joins the medial sural cutaneous nerve to form the sural nerve
○ 5. **Sural nerve:** Courses inferiorly following the small saphenous vein to enter the foot posterior to the lateral malleolus supplying the ankle joint and the skin of the lateral foot

Muscles of the Deep Popliteal Fossa

○ 6. **Plantaris:** Small muscle with a long, skinny tendon of the superficial posterior compartment of the leg
○ 7. **Popliteus:** Thin, triangular muscle of the floor of the popliteal fossa

---

CLINICAL NOTE: TIBIAL NERVE INJURIES

Injury to the tibial nerve in the popliteal fossa is rare due to its deep and protected position; however, deep lacerations or posterior dislocation of the knee may damage the tibial nerve. Damage to the tibial nerve in the popliteal fossa produces weakened plantarflexion of the ankle, weakened flexion of the toes, and loss of sensation over the sole of the foot. The tibial nerve is more frequently damaged in the tarsal tunnel as it travels into the sole of the foot, producing loss of sensation over the sole of the foot and weakening of the intrinsic muscles of the foot but does not affect the plantarflexion of the ankle.

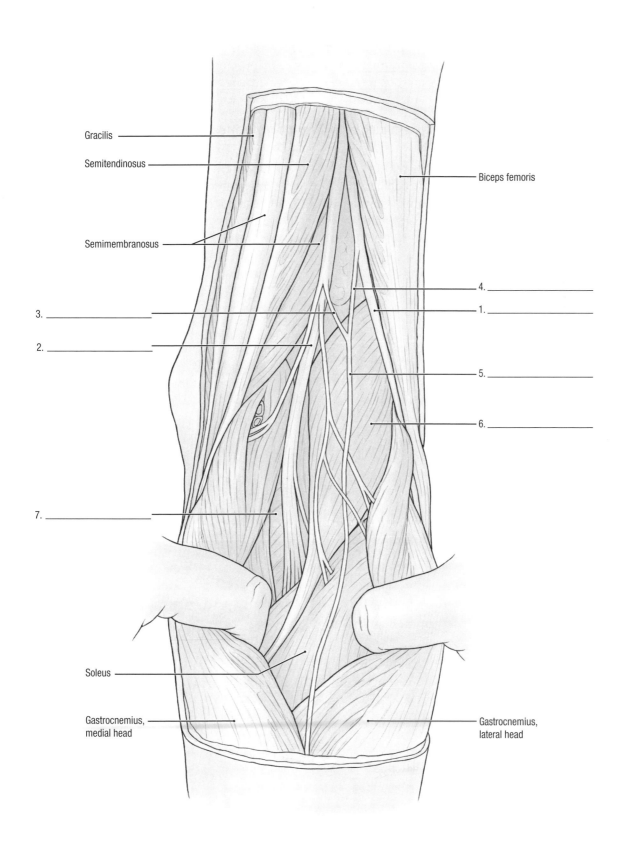

Gracilis

Semitendinosus

Semimembranosus

Biceps femoris

4. _____

3. _____

1. _____

2. _____

5. _____

6. _____

7. _____

Soleus

Gastrocnemius, medial head

Gastrocnemius, lateral head

6.13 POPLITEAL FOSSA: DEEP DISSECTION

The muscles of the posterior compartment of the thigh (*short* and *long head of biceps femoris*, *semimembranosus*, and *semitendinosus*) along with the *tibial nerve* and *popliteal vein* have been cut and their portions removed to demonstrate the course of the popliteal artery and its branches in the floor of the popliteal fossa. Inferiorly, the *lateral* and *medial heads of the gastrocnemius* and *plantaris* have been cut and partially removed as well.

COLOR each of the following structures using a different color for each:

◯ 1. **Popliteal artery:** Continuation of the femoral artery that travels inferolaterally through the popliteal fossa. Within the popliteal fossa, the popliteal artery gives rise to five genicular arteries that participate in an anastomosis around the knee:

Middle genicular artery (not shown)
◯ 2. **Superior medial genicular artery**
◯ 3. **Superior lateral genicular artery**
◯ 4. **Inferior lateral genicular artery**
◯ 5. **Inferior medial genicular artery**

◯ 6. **Popliteus:** Popliteal artery terminates at the inferior border of the popliteus by dividing into the anterior and posterior tibial arteries

◯ 7. **Soleus:** Popliteal artery passes deep to the soleus and then subsequently divides into its terminal branches. The posterior tibial artery will continue to travel deep to the soleus muscle throughout the posterior compartment of the leg.

CLINICAL NOTE: POPLITEAL ANEURYSM

The popliteal artery is the second most common aneurysm site after the abdominal aorta. A popliteal aneurysm produces edema and pain in the popliteal fossa and can be distinguished by palpable pulsations and abnormal arterial sounds (detectable by stethoscope). Although many patients are asymptomatic, some patients show signs of ischemia to the distal lower limb. The aneurysm may compress the tibial nerve, resulting in altered sensation from the posterior leg and sole of the foot.

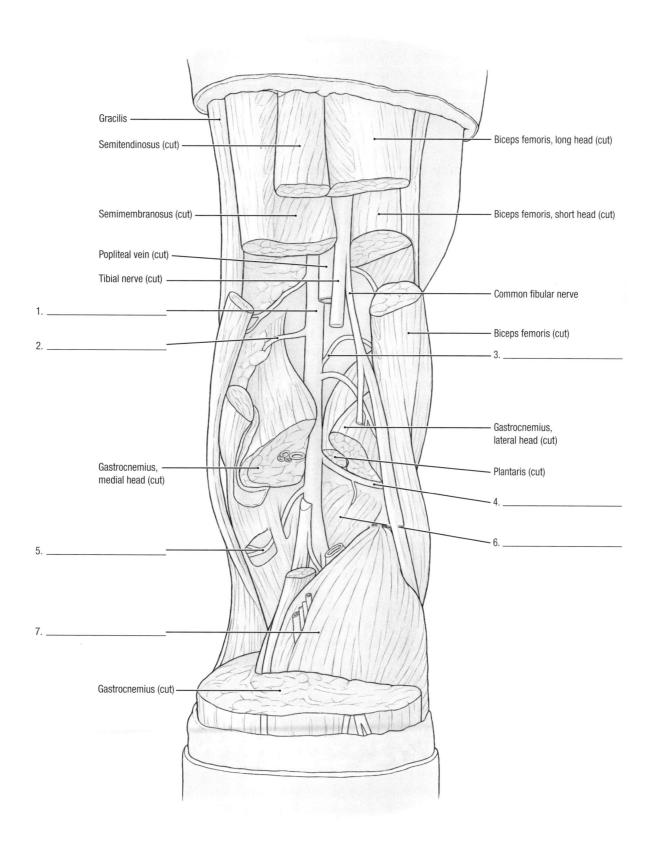

Gracilis

Semitendinosus (cut)

Semimembranosus (cut)

Popliteal vein (cut)

Tibial nerve (cut)

1. _____

2. _____

Gastrocnemius,
medial head (cut)

5. _____

7. _____

Gastrocnemius (cut)

Biceps femoris, long head (cut)

Biceps femoris, short head (cut)

Common fibular nerve

Biceps femoris (cut)

3. _____

Gastrocnemius,
lateral head (cut)

Plantaris (cut)

4. _____

6. _____

Grant's

6.14A and B   KNEE JOINT

In A, the *quadriceps tendon* has been cut and the *patella* and patellar ligament reflected inferiorly to demonstrate the anterior view of the structures of the knee joint.

In B, the oblique popliteal ligament and joint capsule have been removed to show the posterior view of the internal ligaments of the knee.

The knee joint is primarily a hinge type of synovial joint. The articulating aspects of the knee joint include the *medial and lateral femoral condyles* and the lateral and medial tibial condyles. There is also an articulation between the femur and the patella. The fibula does not participate in the articulating surfaces of the knee joint.

COLOR each of the following structures using a different color for each:

The joint capsule of the knee is strengthened by external ligaments:

◯ 1. *Patellar ligament* (A only)*:* Thick fibrous extrinsic band passing from the patella to the tibial tuberosity forming the most anterior ligament of the knee
◯ 2. *Fibular (lateral) collateral ligament:* Strong, cord-like, extrinsic ligament extending from the lateral epicondyle of the femur to the lateral surface of the *fibular head*
◯ 3. *Tibial (medial) collateral ligament:* Strong, flat, intrinsic (capsular) band extending from the medial epicondyle of femur to the medial condyle and superomedial surface of the tibia. Deep fibers are attached to the medial meniscus.

Intra-articular (internal) ligaments:

◯ 4. *Anterior cruciate ligament:* Arises from the anterior intercondylar area of the tibia just posterior to the medial meniscus. Passes superiorly, posteriorly, and laterally to attach to the posterior part of the medial side of the lateral condyle of femur.
◯ 5. *Posterior cruciate ligament:* Arises from the posterior intercondylar area of the tibia, passes superiorly and anteriorly on the medial side of the anterior cruciate ligament, and attaches to the anterior part of the lateral surface of the medial condyle of femur
◯ 6. *Medial meniscus:* C-shaped plate of the fibrocartilage on the articular surface of the medial tibia
◯ 7. *Lateral meniscus:* Nearly circular and smaller than the medial meniscus

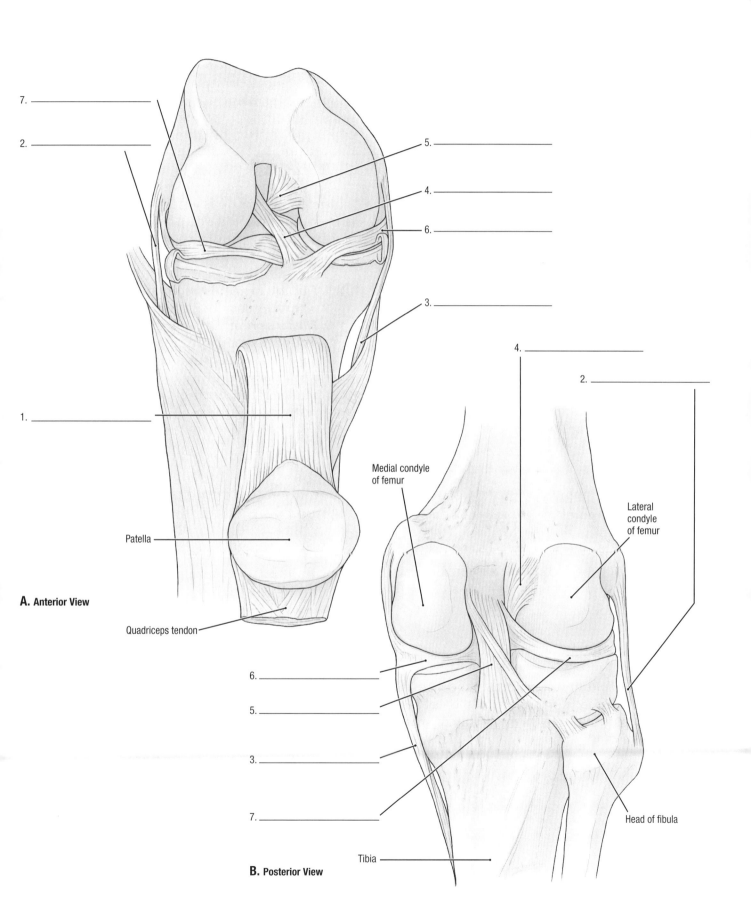

7.

2.

5.

4.

6.

3.

1.

Patella

Quadriceps tendon

A. Anterior View

Medial condyle
of femur

4.

2.

Lateral
condyle
of femur

6.

5.

3.

7.

Tibia

Head of fibula

B. Posterior View

Grant's

6.15 ANTEROLATERAL VIEW OF THE LEG AND THE DORSUM OF THE FOOT

From the anterolateral view of the leg, muscles from lateral and anterior compartments can be viewed. The three compartments of the leg (anterior, lateral, and posterior) are separated by the bones of the leg (tibia and fibula) and the anterior and posterior intermuscular septa. The leg is bounded by the _**deep fascia of the leg**_, which has been removed except for a small section in this image. Two strings are pulling on the inferior edge of the remaining section of the deep fascia of the leg.

COLOR each of the following structures using a different color for each:

Anterior Compartment Muscles

○ 1. *Tibialis anterior:* Most superficial and medial dorsiflexor lying against the lateral surface of the tibia
○ 2. *Extensor hallucis longus:* Lies between the tibialis anterior and the extensor digitorum longus in the distal leg
○ 3. *Extensor digitorum longus:* Most lateral dorsiflexor, becoming tendinous superior to the ankle forming four tendons that attach to the lateral four phalanges
○ 4. *Fibularis tertius:* Separated portion of the extensor digitorum longus with its tendon attaching to the fifth metatarsal (not always present)

Lateral Compartment Muscles

The lateral compartment of the leg is the evertor compartment and is the smallest of the leg compartments. It is bounded by the lateral surface of the fibula, the anterior and posterior intermuscular septa, and the deep fascia of the leg. The muscles of the lateral compartment are innervated by the superficial fibular nerve.

○ 5. *Fibularis longus:* More superficial and longer muscle with its tendon crossing the sole of the foot
○ 6. *Fibularis brevis:* Lies deep to the fibularis longus with its tendon attaching to the base of the fifth metatarsal
○ 7. *Superficial fibular nerve (cut):* Branch of the _**common fibular nerve**_ supplying the lateral compartment and the skin of the dorsum of the foot except between the first and second digits

Muscles of the Lateral Compartment of the Leg

Muscle	Proximal Attachment	Distal Attachment	Action
Fibularis longus	Head and superior two thirds of the lateral surface of the tibia	Base of the first metatarsal and medial cuneiform	Everts foot and weakly plantarflexes ankle
Fibularis brevis	Inferior two-thirds of lateral surface of tibia	Dorsal surface of the base of the fifth metatarsal	

Dorsum of the Foot

○ 8. *Extensor digitorum brevis:* Muscle belly lies along the lateral aspect of the dorsum of the foot deep to the tendons of the extensor digitorum longus and the fibularis tertius
○ 9. *Extensor hallucis brevis:* Muscle belly lies medial to the extensor digitorum brevis

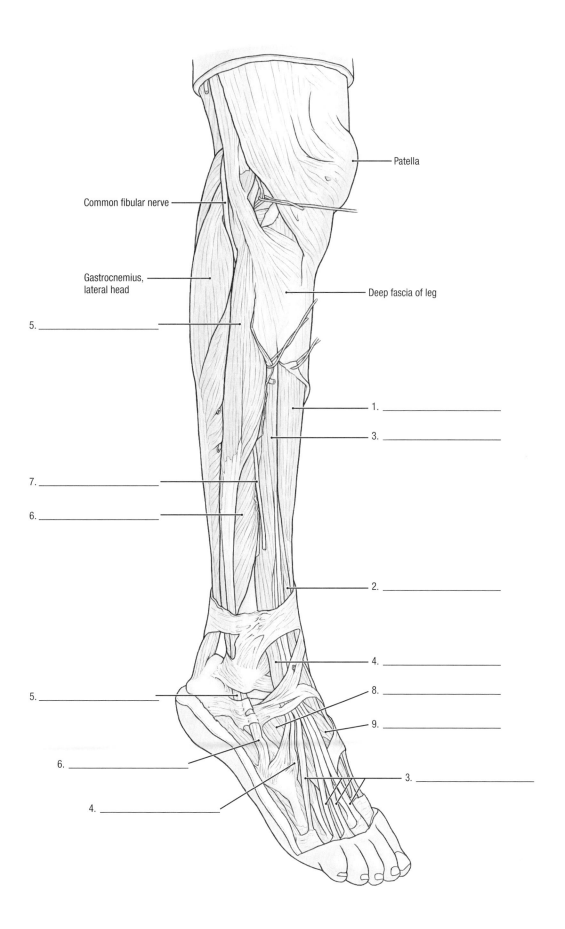

Patella

Common fibular nerve

Deep fascia of leg

Gastrocnemius,
lateral head

5. _____

1. _____

3. _____

7. _____

6. _____

2. _____

4. _____

5. _____

8. _____

9. _____

6. _____

3. _____

4. _____

Grant's

6.16   ANTERIOR COMPARTMENT OF THE LEG

The anterior compartment is the dorsiflexor (extensor) compartment. It is located anterior to the interosseous membrane between the shaft of the tibia and the medial surface of the fibula. The anterior compartment muscles are all innervated by the deep fibular nerve. The *__inferior extensor retinaculum__* has been incised and reflected.

COLOR each of the following structures using a different color for each:

Muscles of the Anterior Compartment of the Leg

Muscle	Proximal Attachment	Distal Attachment	Action
◯ 1. *Tibialis anterior*	Lateral condyle and superior half of the lateral surface of the tibia and the interosseous membrane	Medial and inferior surfaces of the medial cuneiform and base of the first metatarsal	Dorsiflexes ankle and inverts foot
◯ 2. *Extensor hallucis longus*	Middle part of the anterior surface of the fibula and the interosseous membrane	Dorsal aspects of the base of the distal phalanx of the great toe	Extends the great toe and dorsiflexes the ankle
◯ 3. *Extensor digitorum longus*	Lateral condyle of the tibia and the superior three-quarters of the medial surface of the fibula and interosseous membrane	Middle and distal phalanges of the lateral four digits	Extends the lateral four digits and dorsiflexes the ankle
◯ 4. *Fibularis tertius*	Inferior third of the anterior surface of the fibula and interosseous membrane	Dorsum of the base of the fifth metatarsal	When present, dorsiflexes the ankle and aids in the eversion of the foot

Neurovasculature of the Anterior Compartment

◯ 5. *Deep fibular nerve:* One of the two terminal branches of the common fibular nerve. Accompanies the anterior tibial artery to supply the muscles of the anterior compartment and dorsum of the foot. Superiorly, it travels between the tibialis anterior and the extensor digitorum longus and then progresses to travel between the tibialis anterior and the extensor hallucis longus.

◯ 6. *Anterior tibial artery:* Smaller terminal branch of the popliteal artery descending along the anterior aspect of the interosseous membrane between the tibialis anterior and the extensor digitorum longus muscles

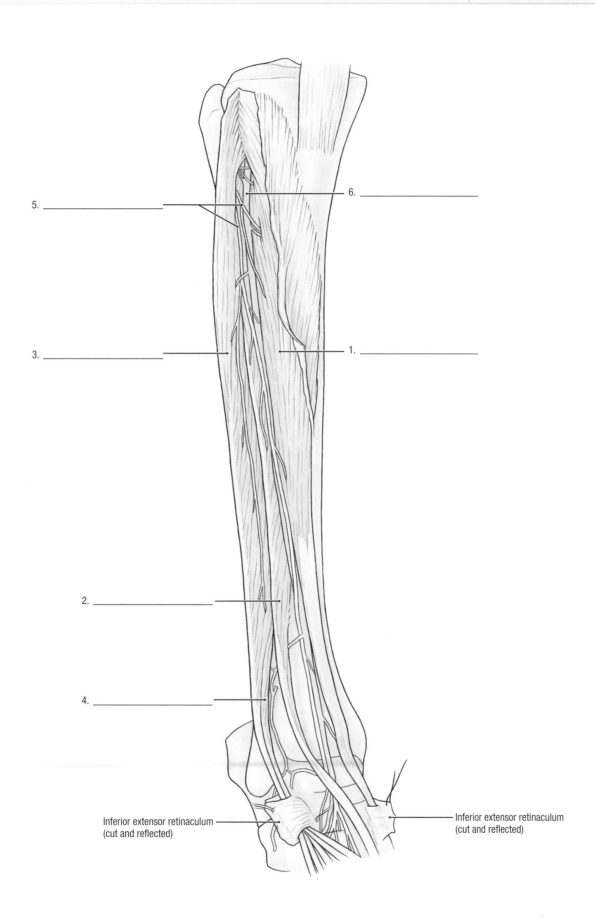

5. _____

6. _____

3. _____

1. _____

2. _____

4. _____

Inferior extensor retinaculum
(cut and reflected)

Inferior extensor retinaculum
(cut and reflected)

6.17   DORSUM OF THE FOOT

The tendons from the lateral and anterior compartments of the leg are demonstrated as they pass into the foot along with the muscles of the dorsum of the foot. The deep fibular nerve and anterior tibial vein have been cut short as they coursed into the foot.

COLOR *each of the following structures using a different color for each:*

○ 1. *Superior extensor retinaculum:* Strong, broad band of the thickened deep fascia of the leg coursing from the fibula to the tibia superior to the _**lateral and medial malleoli**_

○ 2. *Inferior extensor retinaculum:* Y-shaped band of the thickened deep fascia of the leg from the anterosuperior surface of the calcaneus to the medial malleolus and to the plantar aponeurosis. Also forms a loop around the tendons of the fibularis tertius and extensor digitorum longus.

○ 3. *Tibialis anterior:* Tendon passes deep to the superior and inferior extensor retinaculum in its own compartment to attach to the base of the fist metatarsal and the medial and inferior surfaces of the cuneiform

○ 4. *Extensor hallucis longus:* Tendon passes deep to the superior and inferior extensor retinaculum in its own compartment to then course along the dorsum of the foot to the base of the distal phalanx of the great toe

○ 5. *Extensor digitorum longus:* Tendons pass deep to the superior and inferior extensor retinaculum with the fibularis tertius (if present) to course along the dorsum of the foot to the middle and distal phalanges of the lateral four digits

○ 6. *Fibularis tertius:* Tendon passes deep to the superior and inferior extensor retinaculum with the tendons of the extensor digitorum longus to attach to the base of the fifth metatarsal superior to the attachment of the _**fibularis brevis**_

Muscles of the Dorsum of the Foot

Muscle	Proximal Attachment	Distal Attachment	Action
○ 7. *Extensor hallucis brevis*	Calcaneus; interosseous talocalcaneal ligament	Base of the proximal phalanx of the great toe	Assists the extensor hallucis longus in extending the great toe
○ 8. *Extensor digitorum brevis*		Long extensor tendons of four lateral digits	Assists the extensor hallucis longus in extending the four lateral toes

Neurovasculature of the Dorsum of the Foot

○ 9. *Dorsalis pedis artery:* Continuation of the anterior tibial artery beginning at the level of the malleoli coursing deep to the inferior extensor retinaculum. Courses between the extensor hallucis and the extensor digitorum tendons and terminates by dividing into the deep plantar artery and the first dorsal metatarsal artery (not shown)

○ 10. *Deep plantar artery:* Terminal branch of the dorsalis pedis artery that pierces between the two heads of the _**first dorsal interosseous muscle**_ to enter the sole of the foot to form the deep plantar arch

○ 11. *Deep fibular nerve (cut):* Supplies muscles of the dorsum of the foot and the area of the skin between the great toe and the second toe

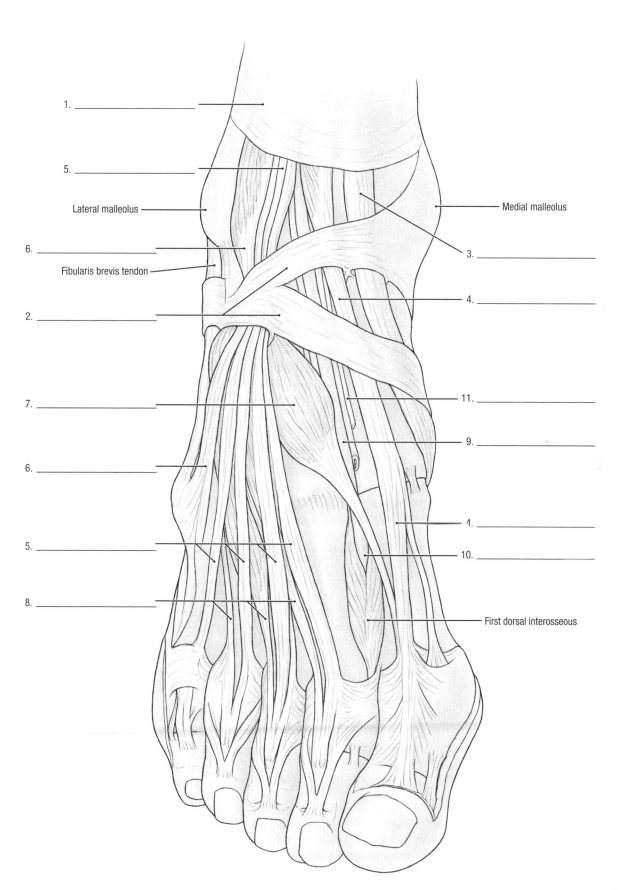

1. _____

5. _____

Lateral malleolus —

6. _____

Fibularis brevis tendon —

2. _____

7. _____

6. _____

5. _____

8. _____

Medial malleolus

3. _____

4. _____

11. _____

9. _____

1. _____

10. _____

First dorsal interosseous

Grant's

6.18A and B POSTERIOR VIEW OF THE LEG: SUPERFICIAL DISSECTION

From the posterior view, muscles of the posterior and lateral compartments are viewable. The posterior compartment of the leg is the plantarflexor compartment. The muscles of the posterior compartment are divided into superficial and deep subcompartments by the transverse intermuscular septum.

Muscles of the posterior compartment are all innervated by the *tibial nerve*.

In Figure A, the muscles of the posterior compartment are intact, whereas in Figure B the heads of the gastrocnemius muscle have been excised.

COLOR *each of the following structures using a different color for each:*

Muscles of the Superficial Posterior Compartment of the Leg

Gastrocnemius is the most superficial of the posterior compartment muscles and is composed of two heads:

○ 1. *Gastrocnemius, medial head*
○ 2. *Gastrocnemius, lateral head*

○ 3. *Soleus:* Large muscle deep to the gastrocnemius
○ 4. *Calcaneal tendon:* Shared tendon of the two heads of the gastrocnemius and the soleus muscles

Superficial Muscles of the Posterior Compartment of the Leg

Muscle	Proximal Attachment	Distal Attachment	Action
Gastrocnemius	Medial head: popliteal surface of the femur superior to the medial condyle Lateral head: lateral aspect of the lateral condyle	Posterior surface of the calcaneus via the calcaneal tendon	Plantarflexes the ankle when the knee is extended; raises the heel during walking; flexes leg at the knee joint
Soleus	Posterior surface of the head and posterosuperior surface of the fibula; soleal line and middle third of the medial border of the tibia; tendinous arch extending between the body attachments		Plantarflexes the ankle independent of the knee position; steadies the leg on foot
Plantaris (not shown)	Inferior end of the lateral supracondylar line of the femur; oblique popliteal ligament		Weakly assists the gastrocnemius in plantarflexing the ankle

The tendons of the muscles from the deep compartment become visible distally near the ankle as they pass medially to the foot:

○ 5. *Tibialis posterior:* Most anterior muscle in the posterior compartment
○ 6. *Flexor digitorum longus:* Courses immediately posterior to the tendon of the tibialis posterior near the ankle
○ 7. *Flexor hallucis longus* (B only)*:* Courses posterior to the flexor digitorum longus muscle and tendon
○ 8. *Flexor retinaculum* (A only)*:* Passes from the medial malleolus to the calcaneus with each of the tendons from the deep compartment, the tibial nerve, and posterior tibial artery passing deep to it

Lateral Compartment

○ 9. *Fibularis longus:* Longer and more superficial than the fibularis brevis
○10. *Fibularis brevis:* Shorter than and deep to the fibularis longus
○11. *Superior fibular retinaculum* (A only)*:* Passes from the fibula to the calcaneus and lies superficial to the tendons of the fibularis longus and brevis as they pass to the foot

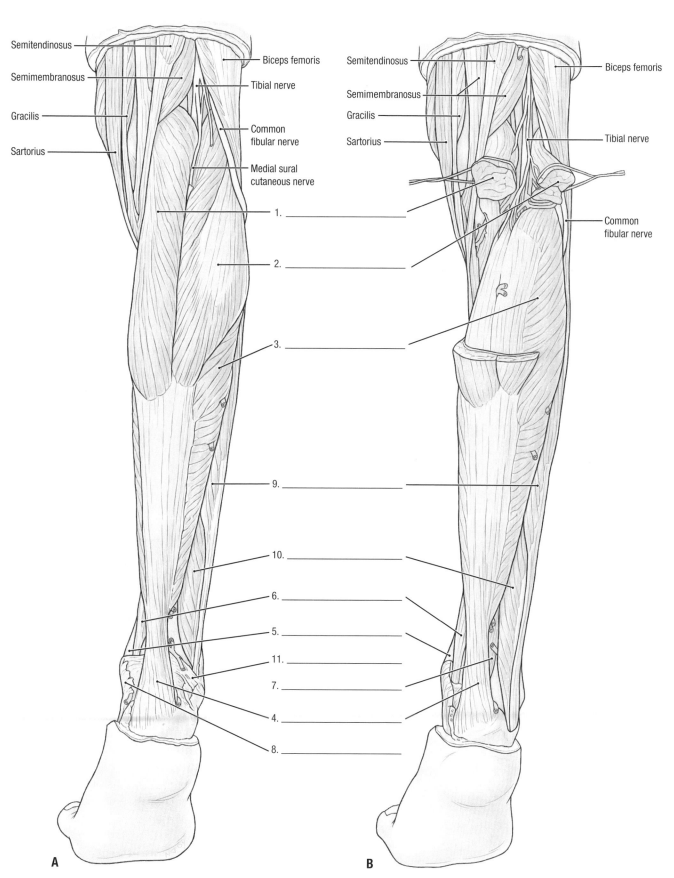

Semitendinosus

Semimembranosus

Gracilis

Sartorius

Biceps femoris

Tibial nerve

Common fibular nerve

Medial sural cutaneous nerve

1. _____

2. _____

3. _____

9. _____

10. _____

6. _____

5. _____

11. _____

7. _____

4. _____

8. _____

Semitendinosus

Semimembranosus

Gracilis

Sartorius

Biceps femoris

Tibial nerve

Common fibular nerve

A

B

Grant's

The **_calcaneal tendon_** has been cut in both A and B. The gastrocnemius muscle has been removed completely in both A and B. The **_soleus muscle_** has been excised except at proximal portions. In B, the middle portion of the posterior tibial artery and vein have also been removed. Also in B, the flexor hallucis longus and flexor digitorum longus muscles are separated from each other by two hooks to demonstrate more of the tibialis posterior.

COLOR each of the following structures using a different color for each:

Muscles of the Deep Posterior Compartment of the Leg

○ 1. *Tibialis posterior:* Deepest and most anterior muscle lying between the flexor digitorum longus and the flexor hallucis longus. Distally the tendon passes in the most anterior position deep to the flexor retinaculum to attach to the navicular bone.

○ 2. *Flexor digitorum longus:* Lies posterior to the tibialis posterior with its tendon passing immediately posterior to the tibialis posterior tendon to pass diagonally into the sole of the foot

○ 3. *Flexor hallucis longus:* Most posterior muscle with its tendon passing deep to the flexor retinaculum separated from the flexor digitorum longus tendon by the posterior tibial artery and tibial nerve

○ 4. *Popliteus:* Triangular muscle in the inferior popliteal fossa, which is covered by the popliteal fascia as it attaches to the tibia

Deep Muscles of the Posterior Compartment of the Leg

Muscle	Proximal Attachment	Distal Attachment	Action
Tibialis posterior	Interosseous membrane; posterior surface of the tibia inferior to the soleal line; posterior surface of the fibula	Tuberosity of the navicular, cuneiform, cuboid, and sustentaculum tali of calcaneus; bases of the second to fourth metatarsals	Plantarflexes the ankle, inverts the foot
Flexor digitorum longus	Medial part of the posterior surface of the tibia inferior to the soleal line; by a broad tendon to the fibula	Bases of distal phalanges of the lateral four digits	Flexes the lateral four digits; plantarflexes the ankle; supports the longitudinal arches of the foot
Flexor hallucis longus	Interior two-thirds of the posterior surface of the fibula; inferior part of the interosseous membrane	Base of the distal phalanx of the great toe	Flexes the great toe at all joints; weakly plantarflexes the ankle; supports the medial longitudinal arch of the foot
Popliteus	Lateral surface of the lateral condyle of the femur and lateral meniscus	Posterior surface of the tibia superior to the soleal line	Weakly flexes the knee and unlocks it by rotating the femur on fixed tibia; medially rotates the tibia of the unplanted limb

Neurovascular Structures of the Deep Posterior Compartment of the Leg

○ 5. *Posterior tibial artery* (A only): Larger and more direct terminal branch of the **_popliteal artery_** accompanied by the tibial nerve. Passes posterior to the medial malleolus with the tendons of the muscles of the deep compartment to the sole of the foot.

○ 6. *Anterior tibial artery* (B only): Terminal branch of the popliteal artery passing anteriorly superior to the interosseous membrane to the anterior compartment

○ 7. *Fibular artery:* Branch of the posterior tibial artery arising inferior to the popliteus muscle and courses inferiorly along the medial side of the fibula supplying posterior and lateral compartments

○ 8. *Tibial nerve:* Terminal branch of the sciatic nerve supplying the posterior compartment and descending with the posterior tibial artery to the sole of the foot

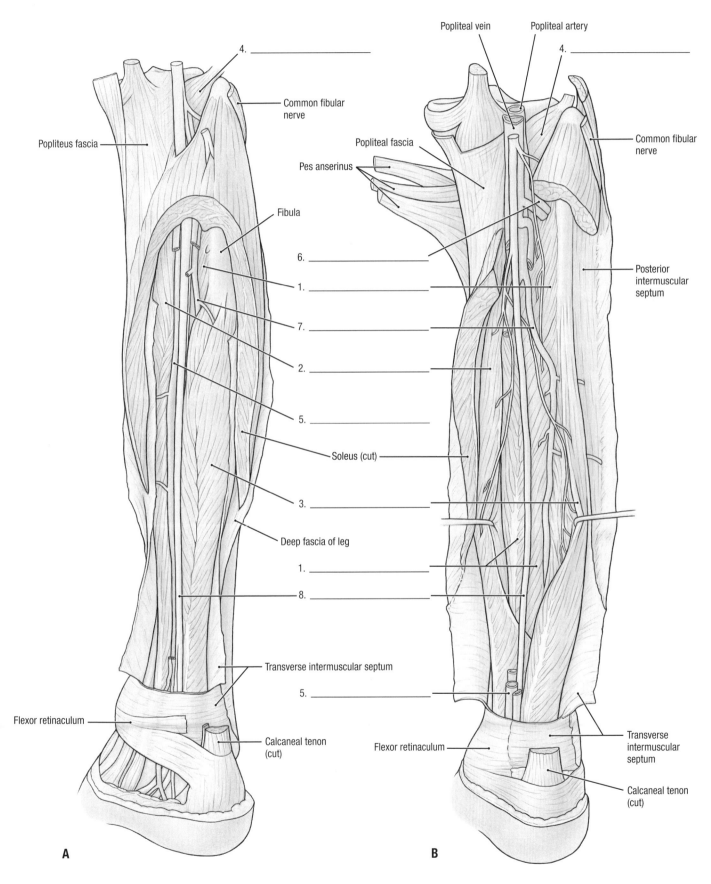

A

4. _____

Common fibular nerve

Popliteus fascia

Fibula

6. _____

1. _____

7. _____

2. _____

5. _____

Soleus (cut)

3. _____

Deep fascia of leg

1. _____

8. _____

Transverse intermuscular septum

5. _____

Flexor retinaculum

Calcaneal tenon (cut)

B

Popliteal vein

Popliteal artery

4. _____

Popliteal fascia

Pes anserinus

Common fibular nerve

Posterior intermuscular septum

Flexor retinaculum

Transverse intermuscular septum

Calcaneal tenon (cut)

Grant's

6.20   SOLE OF THE FOOT: SUPERFICIAL DISCUSSION

The sole of the foot is divided into three muscular compartments by vertical intermuscular septa at the first and fifth metatarsals: the medial, central, and lateral compartments of the sole. The sole of the foot is also arranged into four layers (1st-4th). The great toe (1st toe) is located on the medial side of the foot.

COLOR each of the following structures using a different color for each:

Superficial Foot

○ 1. *Plantar fascia:* Deep fascia of the sole of the foot that is thin and weaker medially and laterally

○ 2. *Plantar aponeurosis:* Thick, central portion of the plantar fascia arising posteriorly from the calcaneus to distally divide into five bands that are continuous with the *fibrous digital sheaths*

○ 3. *Superficial transverse metatarsal ligament:* Transverse fibers reinforcing the plantar aponeurosis inferior to the heads of the metatarsals

○ 4. *Flexor digitorum longus:* The tendons emerge from the fibrous digital sheaths to attach to the distal phalanx of digits 2 to 5

○ 5. *Flexor hallucis longus:* Tendon emerges from the fibrous digital sheaths to attach to the distal phalanx of digit 1

○ 6. *Plantar digital nerves and arteries:* Branches from the lateral and medial plantar arteries and nerves

CLINICAL NOTE: PLANTAR FASCIITIS

Plantar fasciitis is a common cause of heel pain, especially with the first steps after long periods of inactivity or after standing for significant periods of time. Plantar fasciitis presents commonly in runners and other high-impact aerobic athletes or from wearing inappropriate footwear. Inflammation and irritation of the plantar aponeurosis result in pain along the sole of the foot, particularly at the attachment to the calcaneus. The pain is typically heightened when the plantar aponeurosis is stretched such as during dorsiflexion of the ankle, extension of the great toe, and weight-bearing activities. Initial treatment includes anti-inflammatory medications, physical therapy to stretch the plantar fascia and stabilize the ankle and foot joints, night splints, and orthotics.

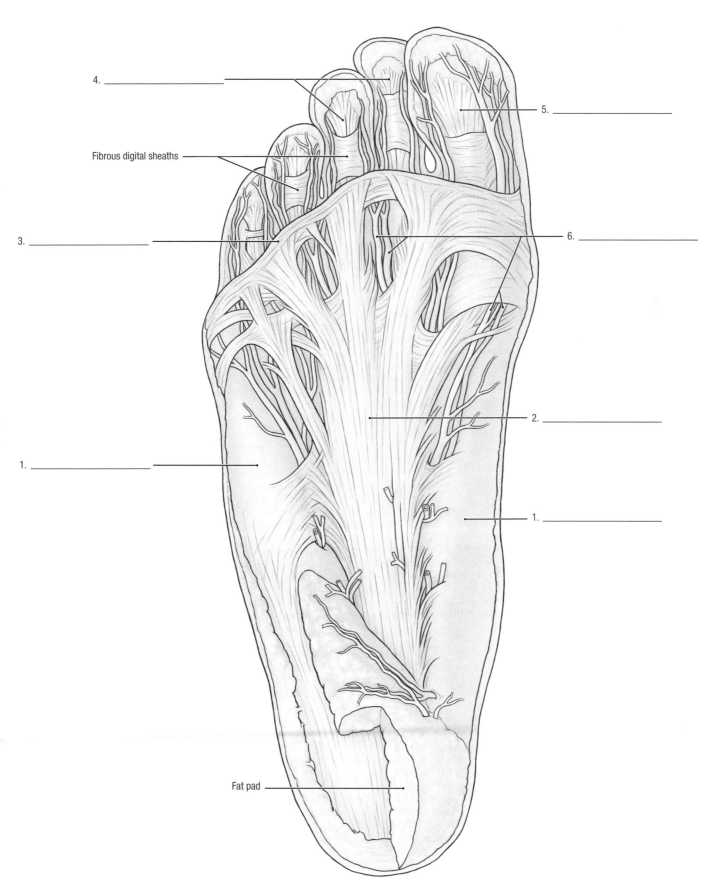

4. _____

Fibrous digital sheaths _____

5. _____

3. _____

6. _____

2. _____

1. _____

1. _____

Fat pad _____

6.21   SOLE OF THE FOOT, FIRST LAYER

The plantar fascia has been mostly removed and the *__plantar aponeurosis__* has been cut and reflected to reveal the underlying musculature. A small portion from the middle of the flexor digitorum brevis has also been excised.

First Layer of the Sole

○ 1. *Flexor digitorum brevis:* Centrally located deep to the plantar aponeurosis

○ 2. *Abductor hallucis:* Covered by the plantar fascia superficially on the medial side of the sole

○ 3. *Abductor digiti minimi:* Covered by the plantar fascia superficially on the lateral side of the sole

Muscles of the Sole of the Foot: First Layer

Muscle	Proximal Attachment	Distal Attachment	Innervation	Action
Flexor digitorum brevis	Medial tubercle of tuberosity of the calcaneus; flexor retinaculum; intermuscular septa	Both sides of middle phalanges of the lateral four digits	Medial plantar nerve	Flexes the lateral four digits
Abductor hallucis	Medial tubercle of tuberosity of the calcaneus; flexor retinaculum; plantar aponeurosis	Medial side of the base of the proximal phalanx of the first digit		Abducts and flexes the first digit
Abductor digiti minimi	Medial and lateral tubercles of tuberosity of the calcaneus; plantar aponeurosis; intermuscular septa	Lateral side of the base of the proximal phalanx of the fifth digit	Lateral plantar nerve	Abducts and flexes the fifth digit

Neurovasculature of the Sole

○ 4. *Common plantar digital nerves:* Sensory branches from the lateral and medial plantar nerves. Each common plantar digital nerve will divide into two proper plantar nerves near the base of the toes.

○ 5. *Proper plantar digital nerves:* Arise distally from the common plantar digital nerves

○ 6. *Proper plantar digital arteries:* Accompany nerve branches of the same name and arise from common plantar digital arteries. The common plantar digital arteries arise from the posterior tibial artery.

○ 7. *Plantar metatarsal artery:* Arise from the deep plantar arch and travel distally at the level of the metatarsal bones. The deep plantar arch arises from the dorsalis pedis artery after it travels through the heads of the first dorsal interosseous muscle.

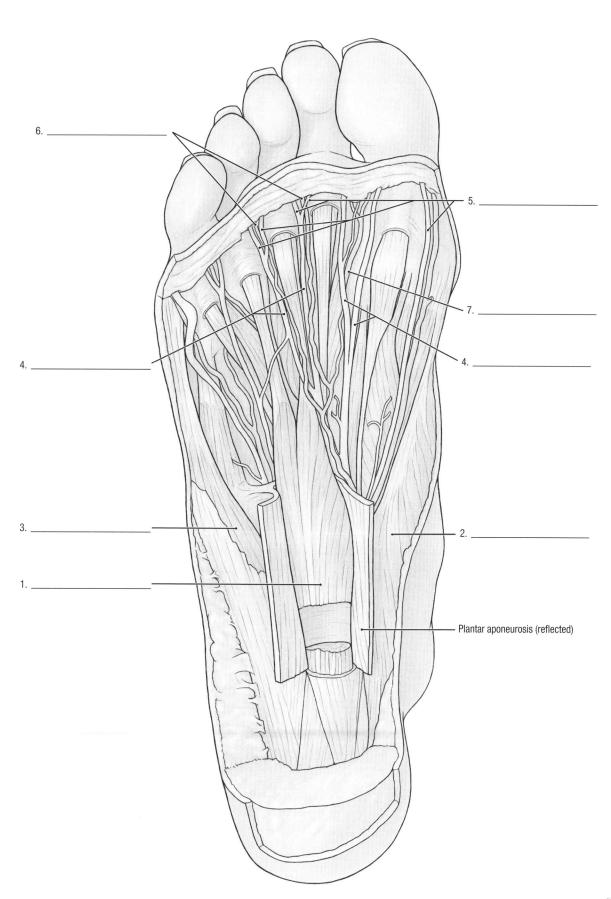

6.

5.

7.

4.

4.

3.

2.

1.

Plantar aponeurosis (reflected)

6.22 SOLE OF THE FOOT, SECOND LAYER

The *flexor digitorum brevis* muscle has been cut and reflected with its four tendons removed to demonstrate the muscles of the second layer. *Abductor digiti minimi* and *abductor hallucis* muscles remain intact laterally and medially, respectively.

COLOR each of the following structures using a different color for each:

○ 1. *Tendon of flexor hallucis longus:* Located medial to the abductor hallucis traveling to its attachment at the distal phalanx of the great toe

○ 2. *Tendons of flexor digitorum longus:* Emerges from the medial side of the sole of the foot giving rise to four tendons to the lateral four digits

○ 3. *Lumbricals 1 to 4:* Arise from the each of the four tendons of the flexor digitorum longus

○ 4. *Quadratus plantae:* Courses from the *calcaneus* anteriorly to attach to the tendon of the flexor digitorum longus

CLINICAL NOTE: SESAMOIDITIS

Sesamoid bones are embedded in tendon and not directly connected to other bones. The patella is the largest sesamoid bone in the body. In the foot, two small sesamoid bones typically develop in the tendon of the flexor hallucis longus tendon. During the stance phase of the gait cycle, these bones bear the weight of the body. Sesamoiditis is marked by pain in the ball of the foot due to inflammation and irritation of the flexor hallucis longus tendon and the sesamoid bones. Sesamoiditis presents commonly in runners and dancers. Decreased activity and a modified shoe pad to reduce pressure on the affected area typically reduce the inflammation.

Muscles in the Sole of the Foot: Second Layer

Muscle	Proximal Attachment	Distal Attachment	Innervation	Action
Lumbricals	Tendons of the flexor digitorum longus	Medial aspect of the extensor expansion over the lateral four digits	Lateral planter nerve (except the first lumbrical, which is innervated by the medial plantar nerve)	Flex the proximal phalanges and extend the middle and distal phalanges of the lateral four digits
Quadratus plantae	Medial surface and lateral margin of the plantar surface of the calcaneus	Posterolateral margin of the flexor digitorum longus tendon		Assists the flexor digitorum longus in flexing the lateral four digits

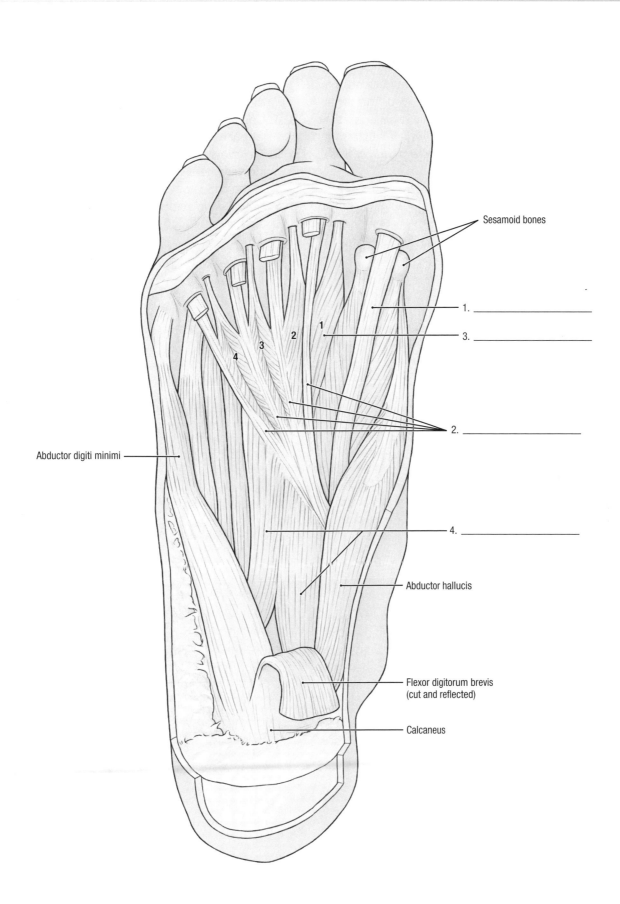

Sesamoid bones

1. _____

3. _____

2. _____

Abductor digiti minimi

4. _____

Abductor hallucis

Flexor digitorum brevis
(cut and reflected)

Calcaneus

Grant's

6.23   SOLE OF THE FOOT, THIRD LAYER

The ***flexor digitorum longus*** tendon has been cut and the four tendons along with the lumbricals removed. The distal end of the quadratus plantae has also been cut away from the flexor digitorum longus tendon. Four hooks are separating the ***abductor digiti minimi*** and the ***abductor hallucis*** from the deeper structures.

Third Layer of the Sole

○ 1. ***Tendon of flexor hallucis longus:*** Travels superficial to the flexor hallucis brevis

○ 2. ***Medial head, flexor hallucis brevis:*** Located lateral to the tendon of the abductor hallucis

○ 3. ***Lateral head, flexor hallucis brevis:*** Located deep to the flexor digitorum longus tendon

○ 4. ***Oblique head, adductor hallucis:*** Located lateral to the lateral head of the flexor hallucis brevis

○ 5. ***Transverse head, adductor hallucis:*** Transverse fibers located lateral to the distal portion of the oblique head of the adductor hallucis

○ 6. ***Flexor digiti minimi:*** Located medial to the abductor digiti minimi

Muscles in the Sole of the Foot: Third Layer

Muscle	Proximal Attachment	Distal Attachment	Innervation	Action
Flexor hallucis brevis	Plantar surfaces of cuboid and lateral cuneiforms	Both sides of the base of the proximal phalanx of the first digit	Medial plantar nerve	Flexes the proximal phalanx of the first digit
Adductor hallucis	Oblique head: bases of metatarsals 2-4 Transverse head: plantar ligaments of metatarsophalangeal joints	Tendons of both heads attach to the lateral side of the proximal phalanx of the first digit	Deep branch of the lateral plantar nerve	Adducts the first digit; assists in maintaining the transverse arch of the foot
Flexor digiti minimi brevis	Base of the fifth metatarsal	Base of the proximal phalanx of the fifth digit	Superficial branch of the lateral plantar nerve	Flexes the proximal phalanx of the fifth digit

Neurovasculature of the Sole

○ 7. ***Lateral plantar nerve:*** Smaller of the two terminal branches of the tibial nerve supplying the skin over the plantar aspects of the lateral one and a half digits and the intrinsic muscles of the foot except the abductor hallucis, flexor digitorum brevis, flexor hallucis brevis, and the first lumbrical. Gives rise to the ***deep plantar nerve***.

○ 8. ***Lateral plantar artery:*** Accompanies the lateral plantar nerve and arches medially to meet the deep plantar arch forming the ***deep plantar arch***. The deep plantar arch gives rise to the plantar metatarsal arteries.

○ 9. ***Medial plantar nerve:*** Larger terminal branch of the tibial nerve supplying the skin of the plantar aspect of the medial three and a half digits and motor innervation to the adductor hallucis, flexor digitorum brevis, flexor hallucis brevis, and the first lumbrical.

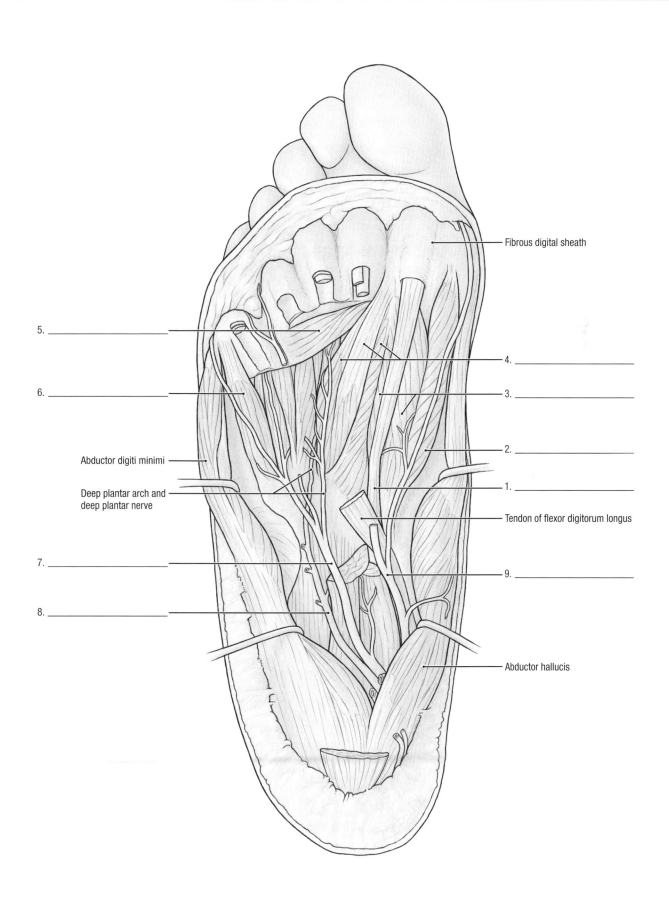

Fibrous digital sheath

5. _____

6. _____

4. _____

3. _____

2. _____

1. _____

Abductor digiti minimi

Deep plantar arch and
deep plantar nerve

Tendon of flexor digitorum longus

7. _____

8. _____

9. _____

Abductor hallucis

Grant's

6.24A and B   SOLE OF THE FOOT, FOURTH LAYER AND LIGAMENTS

In A, muscles and tendons from the superficial three layers have been removed except for the **abductor hallucis**, **flexor hallucis brevis**, **abductor digiti minimi**, and **flexor digiti minimi brevis**.

In B, the **metatarsals** have been cut and all muscles have been removed to demonstrate the ligaments of the foot.

COLOR each of the following structures using a different color for each:

○ 1. **Plantar interossei (1-3)** (A only): Three muscles located on the medial aspects of metatarsals 3 to 5

○ 2. **Dorsal interossei (1-4)** (A only): Four muscles located on adjacent sides of metatarsals 1 to 5

Muscles in the Sole of the Foot: Fourth Layer

Muscle	Proximal Attachment	Distal Attachment	Innervation	Action
Plantar interossei	Plantar aspect of medial sides of metatarsals 3-5	Medial sides of bases of phalanges of third to fifth digits	Lateral plantar nerve	Adduct digits 3-5 and flex metatarsophalangeal joints
Dorsal interossei	Adjacent sides of metatarsals 1-5	1st: medial side of the proximal phalanx of the second digit 2nd-4th: lateral sides of 2nd-4th digits		Abduct digits 2-4 and flex metatarsophalangeal joints

○ 3. **Fibularis longus tendon:** Assists in maintaining the transverse arch of the foot as it crosses from lateral to medial to attach to the 1st metatarsal

○ 4. **Tibialis posterior tendon:** Assists in maintaining the transverse arch of the foot with the fibularis longus tendon. Enters the sole of the foot inferior to the **medial malleolus**.

○ 5. **Long plantar ligament:** Passes from the plantar surface of the **calcaneus** to the **cuboid** with some fibers extending anteriorly to the bases of metatarsals, forming a tunnel over fibularis longus tendon

○ 6. **Plantar calcaneocuboid (short plantar) ligament:** Located between the long plantar and plantar calcaneonavicular ligaments extending from the antero-inferior surface of the calcaneus to the inferior surface of the cuboid. Assists in maintaining the longitudinal arch of the foot.

○ 7. **Plantar calcaneonavicular (spring) ligament:** Extends from plantar aspects and the **sustentaculum tali** of the calcaneus to the **navicular bone**. Supports the head of the **talus**, the keystone of the longitudinal arch of the foot.

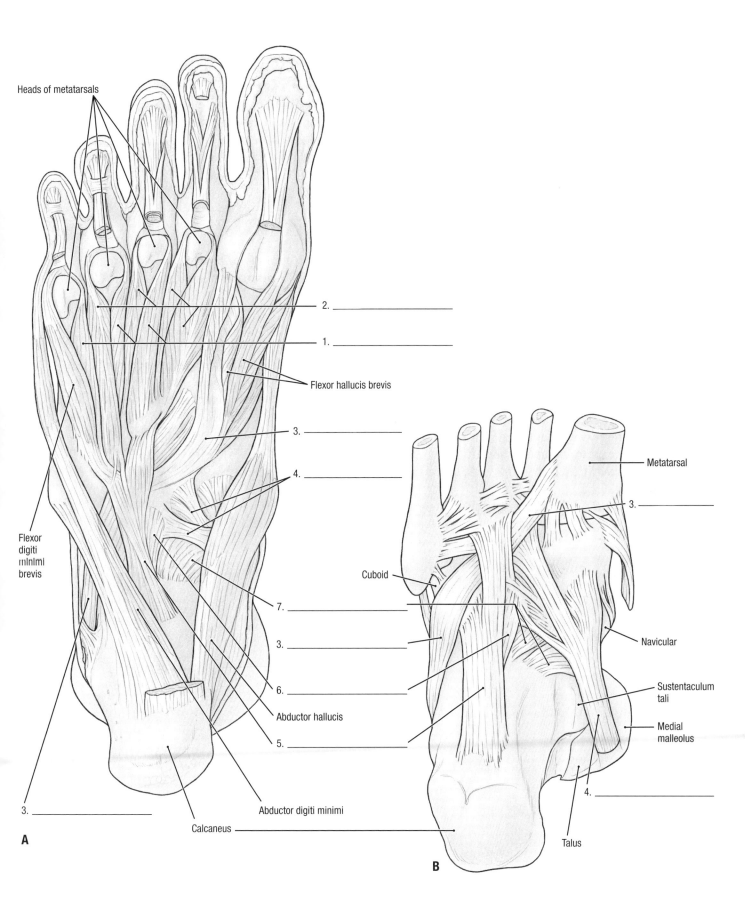

Heads of metatarsals

2. _____

1. _____

Flexor hallucis brevis

3. _____

4. _____

Flexor
digiti
minimi
brevis

7. _____

3. _____

6. _____

Abductor hallucis

5. _____

Abductor digiti minimi

3. _____

Calcaneus _____

A

Metatarsal

3. _____

Cuboid

Navicular

Sustentaculum
tali

Medial
malleolus

4. _____

Talus

B

6.25A and B ANKLE AND FOOT JOINTS

The ankle joint is a hinge-type synovial joint located between the distal ends of the tibia and fibula and the superior portion of the talus. The main movements of the ankle joint are plantarflexion and dorsiflexion of the foot. The foot is composed of many joints between the tarsals, *metatarsals*, and phalanges. The subtalar joint occurs between the *talus* and the *calcaneus*, whereas the transverse tarsal joint occurs between the calcaneus and *cuboid* bones. Both joints are involved in inversion and eversion of the foot. Movement between the tarsals and metatarsals at the tarsometatarsal joints is minimal due to the tight binding of numerous ligaments. Flexion and extension of the toes occurs at the metatarsophalangeal and interphalangeal joints.

In Figure A, the foot is plantarflexed. Figure B depicts the posterior view of the ankle joint.

COLOR each of the following structures using a different color for each:

Ankle
Ligaments of the ankle joint:

○ 1. *Medial (deltoid) ligament of the ankle:* Reinforces the ankle joint medially by attaching to the *medial malleolus*

The lateral ligament of the ankle reinforces the ankle joint laterally and is composed of three ligaments:

○ 2. *Anterior talofibular ligament* (A only)*:* Extends from the *lateral malleolus* to the neck of the talus
○ 3. *Posterior talofibular ligament* (B only)*:* Extends horizontally from malleolar fossa to lateral tubercle of the talus
○ 4. *Calcaneofibular ligament* (B only)*:* Extends from the tip of the lateral malleolus to the lateral surface of the calcaneus

○ 5. *Posterior tibiofibular ligament* (B only)*:* Horizontal fibers reinforce posterior aspect of ankle joint

Foot
Important ligaments of the foot joints:

○ 6. *Talocalcaneal (interosseous) ligament* (A only)*:* Binds the talus and calcaneus together at the subtalar joint
○ 7. *Dorsal talonavicular ligament* (A only)*:* Broad band connecting the neck of talus to the navicular bone supporting the transverse tarsal joint
○ 8. *Bifurcate (calcaneocuboid) ligament* (A only)*:* Binds the calcaneus and the cuboid together, supporting the transverse tarsal joint
○ 9. *Dorsal tarsometatarsal ligaments:* Tightly bind the *cuneiforms* to the metatarsal bones

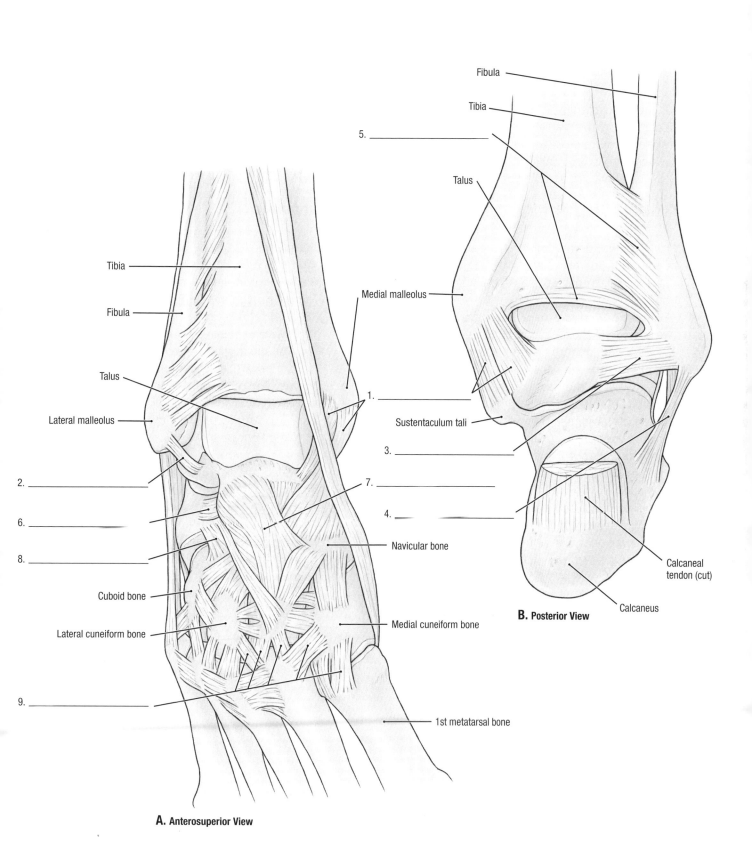

Fibula

Tibia

5. _____

Talus

Tibia

Fibula

Talus

Lateral malleolus

Medial malleolus

1. _____

Sustentaculum tali

2. _____

3. _____

6. _____

7. _____

8. _____

4. _____

Cuboid bone

Navicular bone

Lateral cuneiform bone

Calcaneal tendon (cut)

Medial cuneiform bone

Calcaneus

B. Posterior View

9. _____

1st metatarsal bone

A. Anterosuperior View

Grant's

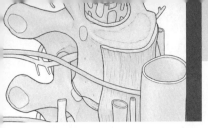

CHAPTER 7

Head

7.1 ANTERIOR ASPECT OF THE CRANIUM

The cranium, or skull, is composed of bones that form the neurocranium and the viscerocranium. The neurocranium surrounds the brain, meninges, vasculature of the brain, and proximal portions of the cranial nerves. The viscerocranium, or facial skeleton, surrounds the oral, nasal, and most of the orbital cavities. The viscerocranium is composed of 15 irregular bones, 3 singular bones (mandible, vomer, and ethmoid), and 6 paired bones (maxillae, inferior nasal concha, zygomatic, palatine, nasal, and lacrimal).

From the anterior aspect, the frontal bone contributing to the neurocranium and superior aspect of the orbit, along with many of the bones contributing to the viscerocranium, can be observed.

COLOR each of the following structures using a different color for each:

○ 1. **Frontal bone:** Forms the forehead and superior wall of the orbit and articulates with the nasal, maxillae, zygomatic, lacrimal, ethmoid, sphenoid, and parietal bones

  ○ 2. **Supraorbital foramen/notch:** Small opening for passage of the supraorbital nerve and vessels
    Glabella: Smooth area superior to nasal bones

○ 3. **Maxillae:** Form the upper jaw and contribute to the lateral walls of the nasal cavity and inferior wall of the orbits. Articulates with zygomatic, lacrimal, nasal, frontal, ethmoid, palatine, vomer, and inferior nasal concha bones.
    Intermaxillary suture: Marks the union of the two maxillae bones in the median plane inferior to the nasal aperture

  ○ 4. **Infraorbital foramen:** Opening inferior to each orbit for passage of the infraorbital nerve and vessels

○ 5. **Zygomatic bones:** Form the prominences of the cheeks and contribute to the inferior and lateral wall of the orbits. Each zygomatic bone articulates with frontal, maxilla, temporal, and sphenoid bones.

○ 6. **Nasal bones:** Form the bony portion of the nose and articulate with frontal, maxillae, and ethmoid bones

○ 7. **Mandible:** U-shaped bone that forms the lower jaw
    Ramus: Vertical portion
    Body: Horizontal portion
    Mental protuberance: Prominence of the chin

  ○ 8. **Mental foramen:** Opening inferior to premolar teeth for passage of the mental nerve and vessels. The supraorbital, infraorbital, and mental foramina are in vertical alignment with one another.

○ 9. **Vomer:** Forms the posteroinferior portion of the nasal septum that divides the nasal cavity into right and left portions. Articulates with the maxillae, palatine, and ethmoid bones.

○10. **Ethmoid bone:** Irregular, midline bone that forms a portion of the neurocranium and viscerocranium
    Perpendicular plate: Contributes to the nasal septum
    Middle conchae: Lie along the lateral walls of the nasal cavity

○11. **Inferior nasal conchae:** Lie along the lateral wall of the nasal cavity

○12. **Lacrimal bones:** Contribute to the medial wall of the orbit and articulate with the maxillae, ethmoid, and frontal bones

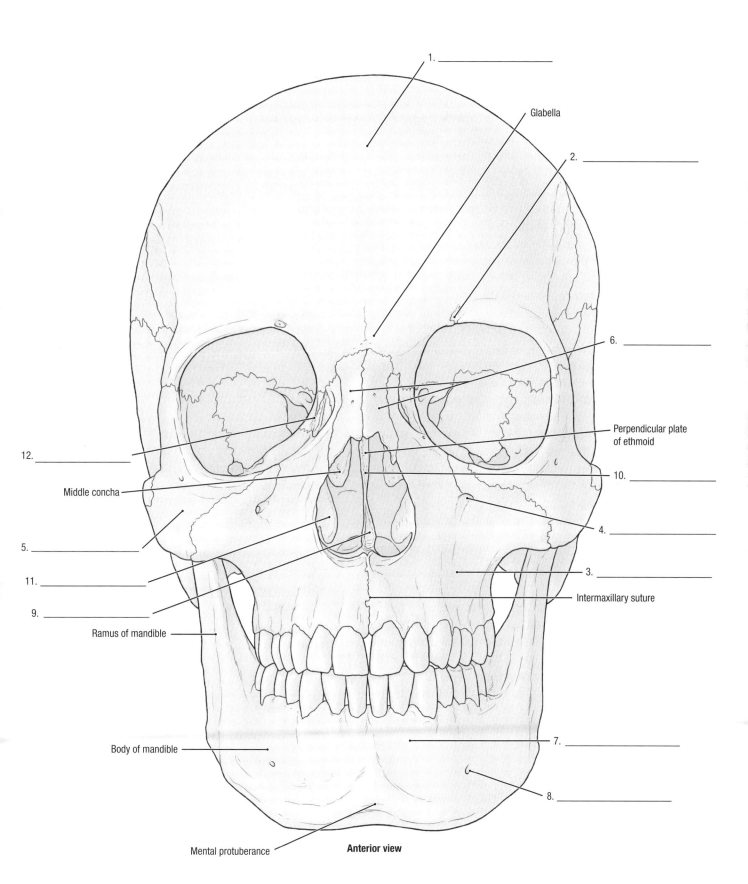

1. _____

Glabella

2. _____

6. _____

Perpendicular plate
of ethmoid

12. _____

Middle concha

10. _____

5. _____

4. _____

11. _____

3. _____

9. _____

Intermaxillary suture

Ramus of mandible

Body of mandible

7. _____

8. _____

Mental protuberance   **Anterior view**

7.2 LATERAL ASPECT OF THE CRANIUM

The lateral view of the cranium reveals aspects of both the neurocranium and the viscerocranium. The bones contributing to the lateral aspect of the cranium are the temporal, parietal, frontal, occipital, and sphenoid. Several of the sutures created between the bones of the neurocranium are named and are useful landmarks anatomically and clinically.

COLOR each of the following structures using a different color for each:

○ 1. **Parietal**: Contributes primarily to the calvaria, the dome-like roof of the neurocranium. Articulates with the occipital, frontal, sphenoid, and temporal bones.

○ 2. **Occipital:** Contributes to the occiput, the convex, posterior protuberance of the neurocranium and articulates with temporal, parietal, and sphenoid bones. The external occipital protuberance is typically prominent (especially in males) at the posterior pole.

   ○ 3. **Lambdoid suture:** Forms at the articulation of the occipital and parietal bones
     Lambda: Junction of the lambdoid suture with the sagittal suture (not shown) that courses in the midsagittal plane between the two parietal bones

○ 4. **Frontal:** Contributes to the calvaria

   ○ 5. **Coronal suture:** Forms at the articulation of the frontal and parietal bones
     Superciliary arch: Prominence between the squamous (flat, forehead) portion and orbital plate
     Bregma: Junction of the coronal and sagittal sutures

○ 6. **Temporal:** Forms the inferolateral walls of the neurocranium and a portion of the cranial base

   ○ 7. **External acoustic meatus:** Canal that leads to the tympanic membrane
     Mastoid process: Large protuberance (especially in males) posteroinferior to the external acoustic meatus
     Styloid process: Slender, pointed projection anteromedial to the mastoid process
     Zygomatic process: Articulates with the temporal process of zygomatic bone to form the zygomatic arch

   ○ 8. **Superior and inferior temporal lines:** Course on the temporal, parietal, and frontal bones and form the border of the **temporal fossa** superiorly and posteriorly

○ 9. **Sphenoid:** Irregular, singular bone that consists of a body and three pairs of processes and contributes to the inferolateral wall of the neurocranium, cranial base, and orbit
   Pterion: H-shaped formation of sutures formed from the union of the frontal, parietal, temporal, and sphenoid bones

○10. **Zygomatic:** Contributes to the lateral and inferior walls of the orbit and zygomatic arch
   Temporal process: Articulates with the zygomatic process of the temporal bone to form the zygomatic arch

○11. **Maxilla:** Contributes to lateral nasal wall, inferior wall of orbit, and alveolar process that supports the upper teeth

○12. **Nasal:** Contributes to bony aspect of the nose and bridge of the nose
   Nasion: Intersection of the frontal and nasal bones typically marked by a palpable depressed area

○13. **Lacrimal:** Contributes to medial wall of the orbit

○14. **Mandible:** Articulates with the temporal bone at the **temporomandibular joint** (TMJ)
   Condylar process: Arises posteriorly from the superior aspect of the **ramus**
   Coronoid process: Arises anteriorly from the superior aspect of the ramus
   Mental protuberance: Anterior, midline projection forming the chin

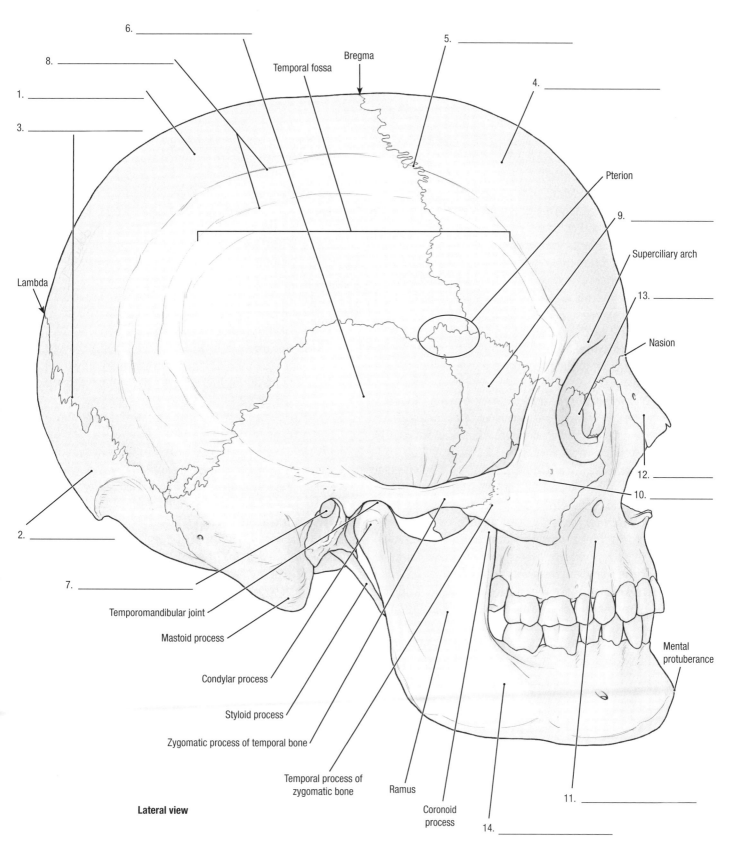

6. _____

8. _____

1. _____

3. _____

Bregma

Temporal fossa

5. _____

4. _____

Pterion

9. _____

Superciliary arch

13. _____

Nasion

Lambda

12. _____

10. _____

2. _____

7. _____

Temporomandibular joint

Mastoid process

Condylar process

Styloid process

Zygomatic process of temporal bone

Temporal process of
zygomatic bone

Ramus

Coronoid
process

Mental
protuberance

11. _____

14. _____

Lateral view

Grant's

7.3 INFERIOR ASPECT OF THE CRANIUM

The cranial base is the inferior portion of the neurocranium and the viscerocranium except for the mandible. Portions of the occipital, temporal, sphenoid, maxillae, palatine, and vomer bones compose the cranial base.

COLOR each of the following structures using a different color for each:

○ 1. *Occipital:* Forms most of the posterior aspect of the cranial base
Foramen magnum: Large foramen for the passage of the spinal cord, meninges, vertebral arteries, and spinal accessory nerve (CN XI)

  ○ 2. *Occipital condyles:* Two large protuberances located lateral to the foramen magnum that articulate with the vertebral column

○ 3. *Temporal:* Lies anterior and lateral to the occipital bone

  ○ 4. *Jugular foramen:* Irregular opening located between the temporal and occipital bones for the passage of the internal jugular vein, glossopharyngeal nerve (CN IX), vagus nerve (CN X), and spinal acessory nerve (CN XI)

  ○ 5. *Carotid canal:* Inferior opening located anterior to the jugular foramen for the passage of the internal carotid artery

  ○ 6. *Stylomastoid foramen:* Small opening located between the **styloid** and **mastoid processes** for the passage of the portion of the facial nerve (CN VII) that emerges onto the face

  ○ 7. *Digastric (mastoid) notch:* Groove located medial to the mastoid process for the attachment of the posterior belly of the digastric

  ○ 8. *Mandibular fossa:* Depression located anterior to the external acoustic meatus and posteromedial to the **zygomatic process** that the condylar head of the mandible rests within the TMJ

○ 9. *Sphenoid:* Lies anterior to the occipital bone in the midline and anterior to the temporal bones laterally. The pterygoid processes lie in the midline and are each composed of the **medial** and **lateral pterygoid plates**. Both the **greater wings** lie lateral to their respective pterygoid process.

Pterygoid fossa: Space between the medial and lateral pterygoid plates
Hamulus of medial pterygoid plate: Slender process extending from the inferior aspect of the medial pterygoid plate

○ 10. *Foramen ovale:* Oval-shaped opening within the greater wing for the passage of mandibular division of the trigeminal nerve (CN V$_3$)

○ 11. *Foramen spinosum:* Small opening located posterolateral to foramen ovale for the passage of the middle meningeal artery

○ 12. *Petrotympanic fissure:* Small fissure located posterolateral to the foramen spinosum for the passage of the chorda tympani nerve from CN VII

○ 13. *Foramen lacerum:* Space between the temporal and sphenoid bones that is covered by a cartilage plate during life. Only small meningeal vasculature passes vertically through the space.

○ 14. *Palatine bones:* Form the posterior one-third of the hard palate

  ○ 15. *Greater palatine foramen:* Small foramen for the passage of the greater palatine nerve and vessels
Lesser palatine foramen: Smaller foramen posterior to the greater palatine foramen for the passage of the lesser palatine nerve
Posterior nasal spine: Posterior, midline extension

○ 16. *Palatine process of maxilla:* Paired processes that form the anterior two-thirds of the hard palate
Incisive foramen: Midline opening for the passage of the nasopalatine nerve

○ 17. *Vomer:* Forms the posteroinferior aspect of the nasal septum

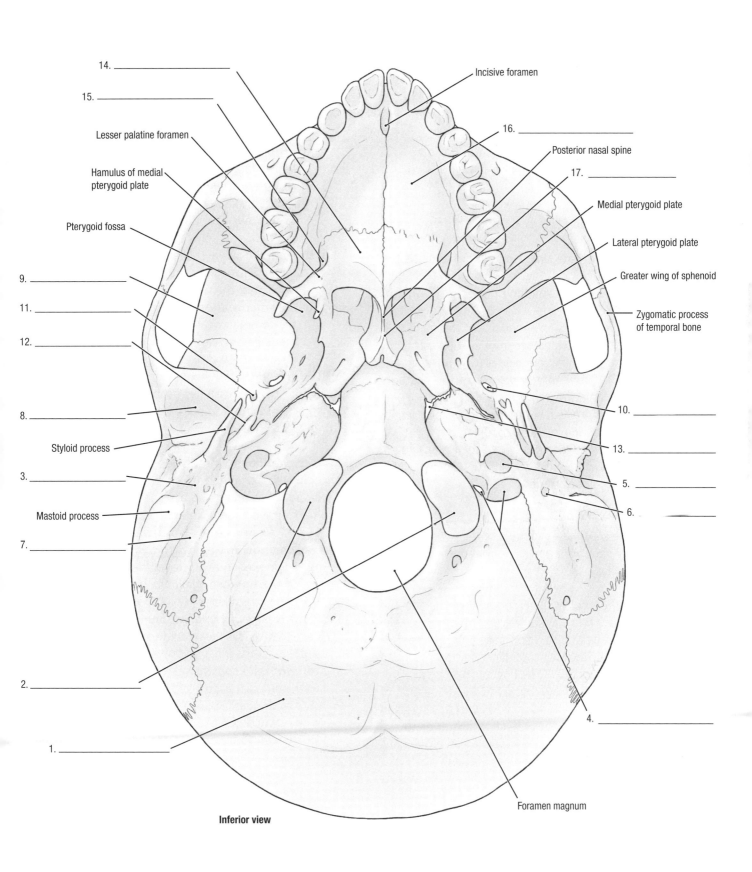

14. _____

15. _____

Lesser palatine foramen

Hamulus of medial pterygoid plate

Pterygoid fossa

9. _____

11. _____

12. _____

8. _____

Styloid process

3. _____

Mastoid process

7. _____

2. _____

1. _____

Incisive foramen

16. _____

Posterior nasal spine

17. _____

Medial pterygoid plate

Lateral pterygoid plate

Greater wing of sphenoid

Zygomatic process of temporal bone

10. _____

13. _____

5. _____

6. _____

4. _____

Foramen magnum

Inferior view

Grant's

7.4 INTERNAL VIEW OF THE CRANIAL BASE

The internal aspect of the cranial base is subdivided into three depressions: anterior, middle, and posterior cranial fossae. Each of the fossa lies at different levels, with the posterior edge of the lesser wing of the sphenoid separating the anterior and middle cranial fossae and the petrous ridge of the temporal bone separating the middle and posterior cranial fossae.

COLOR each of the following structures using a different color for each:

Anterior Cranial Fossa

The anterior cranial fossa is formed by the frontal, ethmoid, and sphenoid bones.

◯ 1. *Orbital part of frontal bone:* Forms most of the anterior cranial fossa

◯ 2. *Ethmoid bone:* Located in the middle between the two frontal bones
Crista galli: Superior, midline projection from the ethmoid bone
Cribriform plate: Lies on either side of the crista galli. Numerous, tiny foramina occupy the cribriform plate for the passage of olfactory nerves (CN I).

◯ 3. *Lesser wing of sphenoid bone:* Forms the posterior aspect of the anterior cranial fossa
Anterior clinoid process: Posteriorly directed projections from the lesser wing of the sphenoid

◯ 4. *Optic canals:* Openings within the lesser wing of the sphenoid for passage of the optic nerve (CN II) and ophthalmic arteries

Middle Cranial Fossa

The sphenoid bone contributes to most of the middle cranial fossa, with the temporal bone and its petrous portion forming the posterior boundary.

◯ 5. *Body of sphenoid:* Midline component that on the superior aspect forms a saddle-like formation, the sella turcica. The sella turcica is composed of three parts:
Tuberculum sellae: Slight, midline elevation forming the anterior boundary of the hypophyseal fossa
Hypophyseal (pituitary) fossa: Midline depression of the body of the sphenoid occupied by the pituitary gland
Dorsum sellae: Superior projection posterior to the hypophyseal fossa, with two superolateral projections composing the posterior clinoid processes

◯ 6. *Greater wing of sphenoid:* Paired lateral extensions from the body of the sphenoid

◯ 7. *Superior orbital fissure:* Located between the lesser wing and greater wing of the sphenoid for the passage of the oculomotor nerve (CN III), trochlear nerve (CN IV), ophthalmic division of the trigeminal nerve (CN V$_1$), abducens nerve (CN VI), and ophthalmic veins

◯ 8. *Foramen rotundum:* Located posterior to the medial aspect of the superior orbital fissure for the passage of the maxillary division of the trigeminal nerve (CN V$_2$)

◯ 9. *Foramen ovale:* Located posterolateral to the foramen rotundum for the passage of the mandibular division of the trigeminal nerve (CN V$_3$)

◯10. *Foramen spinosum:* Located posterolateral to the foramen ovale for the passage of the middle meningeal artery

Posterior Cranial Fossa

The posterior cranial fossa lies posterior to the ridge of the petrous portion of the temporal bone and is the deepest of the three cranial fossa.

◯11. *Occipital bone:* Contributes to most of the posterior cranial fossa, with temporal bone forming the anterolateral walls and dorsum sellae of the sphenoid bone marking the midline anterior boundary
Clivus: Sloped area posteroinferior to the dorsum sellae leading to the *foramen magnum*

◯12. *Hypoglossal canal:* Lies at the anterolateral margin of the foramen magnum for the passage of the hypoglossal nerve (CN XII)

◯13. *Petrous part of temporal bone:* Forms a prominent ridge that divides the middle and posterior cranial fossa and houses the inner and middle ear

◯14. *Internal acoustic meatus:* Opening in the posteromedial aspect of the petrous temporal bone for the passage of the facial nerve (CN VII) and vestibulocochlear nerve (CN VIII)

◯15. *Jugular foramen:* Located between the posterior aspect of the petrous temporal bone and the occipital bone inferior to the internal acoustic meatus for the passage of internal jugular vein, glossopharyngeal nerve (CN IX), vagus nerve (CN X), and spinal accessory nerve (CN XI)

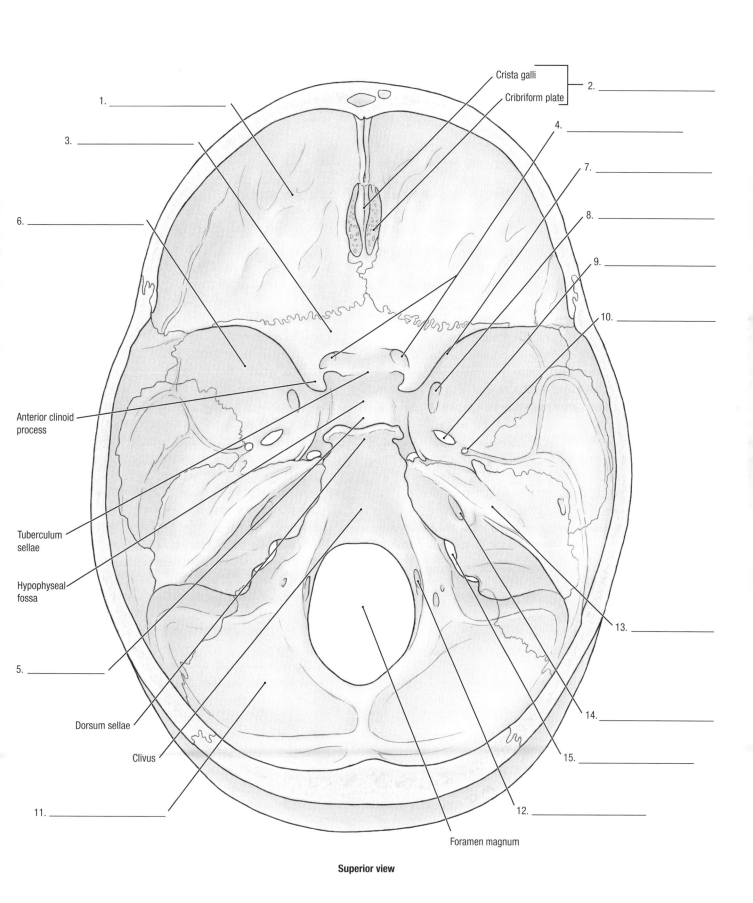

Crista galli

Cribriform plate

1. _____

3. _____

6. _____

2. _____

4. _____

7. _____

8. _____

9. _____

10. _____

Anterior clinoid
process

Tuberculum
sellae

Hypophyseal
fossa

5. _____

Dorsum sellae

Clivus

11. _____

13. _____

14. _____

15. _____

12. _____

Foramen magnum

Superior view

Grant's

7.5 CRANIAL NERVES

There are 12 pairs of cranial nerves numbered I-XII from rostral to caudal. Cranial nerves course through foramina or fissures of the cranium to reach their peripheral targets. Cranial nerves carry one or more fiber types.

On the right side, the dura mater and its formations have been left intact. On the left side, the dura mater covering the trigeminal (Meckel) cave has been cut away to expose the trigeminal ganglion and its divisions. The cerebellar tentorium has also been cut away to reveal components of the dural venous sinus system.

COLOR each of the following structures using a different color for each:

○ 1. **Olfactory nerve (CN I):** Composed of special sensory fibers for smell. Courses through the cribriform plate as multiple olfactory nerves to synapse on the **olfactory bulb**.

○ 2. **Optic nerve (CN II):** Composed of axons of retinal ganglion cells passing from the orbit through the optic canals carrying visual information from the retina

○ 3. **Oculomotor nerve (CN III):** Pierces the dura mater lateral to **sellar diaphragm** and enters the orbit via superior orbital fissure. CN III is composed of somatic motor fibers to almost all the extraocular muscles and presynaptic parasympathetic fibers to intraocular muscles.

○ 4. **Trochlear nerve (CN IV):** Pierces the dura mater at the margin of the **cerebellar tentorium** and enters the orbit via the superior orbital fissure. CN IV is composed of somatic motor fibers to one extraocular muscle.

○ 5. **Trigeminal nerve (CN V):** Composed of a large sensory root containing central processes from the trigeminal ganglion and a small motor root containing somatic motor fibers

○ 6. **Trigeminal ganglion:** Composed of somatic sensory cell bodies. The peripheral processes carry somatic sensory information from targets in the head while the central processes compose the trigeminal nerve. Somatic motor fibers bypass the ganglion and travel exclusively as a component of CN V_3.

○ 7. **Ophthalmic nerve (CN V_1):** Composed of peripheral processes carrying sensation from the cornea, skin of forehead, anterior scalp, eyelids, frontal sinus, sphenoid sinus, and mucosa of nasal cavity. Courses through superior orbital fissure.

○ 8. **Maxillary nerve (CN V_2):** Composed of peripheral processes carrying sensation from skin of face over maxilla, upper lip, maxillary teeth, mucosa of nasal cavity, maxillary sinuses, and palate. Courses through the foramen rotundum.

○ 9. **Mandibular nerve (CN V_3):** Composed of somatic motor fibers to the muscles of mastication and pharyngeal arch I muscles and peripheral processes carrying sensation from skin of face overlying the mandible, lower lip, mandibular teeth, TMJ, mucosa of oral cavity, and anterior two-thirds of the tongue. Courses through the foramen ovale.

○ 10. **Abducens nerve (CN VI):** Pierces the dura mater covering the clivus and enters the superior orbital fissure. Composed of somatic motor fibers to one extraocular muscle.

○ 11. **Facial nerve (CN VII):** Composed of facial nerve proper and the intermediate nerve. Facial nerve proper contains somatic motor fibers that supply the muscles of facial expression and the 2nd pharyngeal arch. The intermediate nerve contains special sensory for taste, presynaptic parasympathetic to most of the major glands of the head, and somatic sensory fibers to portions of the external ear. Courses through the internal acoustic meatus.

○ 12. **Vestibulocochlear nerve (CN VIII):** Composed of the vestibular nerve for balance and the cochlear nerve for hearing. Courses through the internal acoustic meatus.

○ 13. **Glossopharyngeal nerve (CN IX):** Composed of somatic sensory from the external ear, visceral sensory from the carotid sinus and body, middle ear, and mucosa of the oropharynx, special sensory for taste, somatic motor to the 3rd pharyngeal arch, and presynaptic parasympathetic to the parotid gland. Courses through the jugular foramen.

○ 14. **Vagus nerve (CN X):** Composed of somatic sensory from the external ear, special sensory for taste, visceral sensory from the base of tongue, pharynx, larynx, thoracic and abdominal organs, presynaptic parasympathetic to thoracic and abdominal organs, and somatic motor to intrinsic laryngeal muscles and most of the pharyngeal and palate muscles. Courses through the jugular foramen.

○ 15. **Spinal accessory nerve (CN XI):** Composed of somatic motor fibers to the sternocleidomastoid and trapezius muscles. Originates from the upper spinal cord, traverses the foramen magnum, and exits cranium through the jugular foramen.

○ 16. **Hypoglossal nerve (CN XII):** Composed of somatic motor fibers to most muscles of the tongue. Courses through the hypoglossal canal.

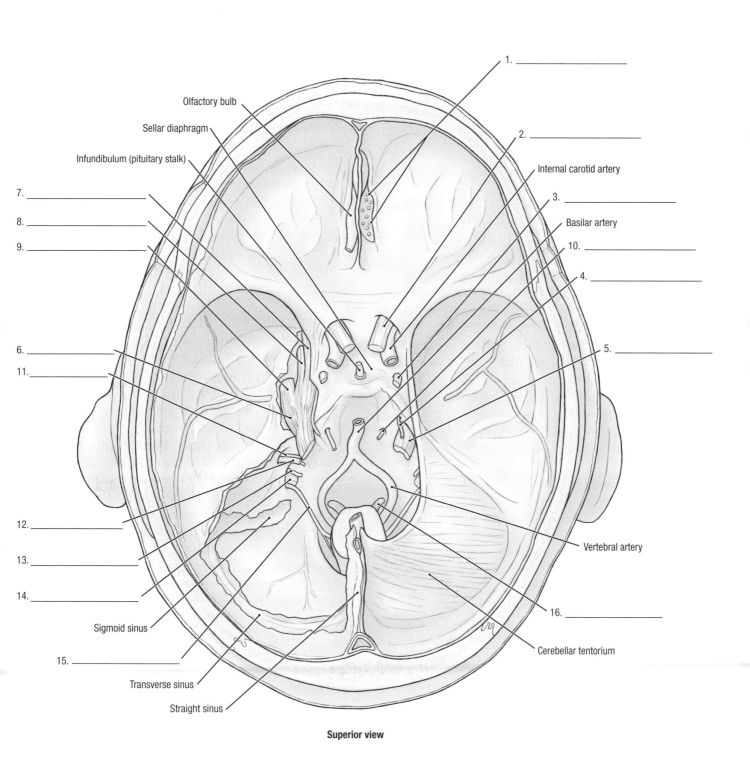

Olfactory bulb

Sellar diaphragm

Infundibulum (pituitary stalk)

7. _____

8. _____

9. _____

6. _____

11. _____

12. _____

13. _____

14. _____

Sigmoid sinus

15. _____

Transverse sinus

Straight sinus

1. _____

2. _____

Internal carotid artery

3. _____

Basilar artery

10. _____

4. _____

5. _____

Vertebral artery

16. _____

Cerebellar tentorium

Superior view

Grant's

7.6   DURAL REFLECTIONS AND DURAL VENOUS SINUSES

Dura mater is composed of two layers: the external periosteal and the internal meningeal. The external periosteal layer adheres to the internal aspect of the calvaria and cranial base. The internal meningeal layer is fused to the external periosteal layer except where dural reflections and dural sinuses occur. Dural reflections are infoldings of the meningeal layer that subdivide the cranial cavity into compartments. Dural venous sinuses are venous-filled spaces between layers of the dura that receive venous drainage from cerebral veins.

A midsagittal view of the head is shown with the brain and spinal cord removed. The midline and left-sided dural reflections and venous sinuses remain along with the left half of the arterial supply to the brain.

COLOR each of the following structures using a different color for each:

Dural Reflections

○ 1. **Cerebral falx:** Largest of the dural infoldings separating the cerebral hemispheres. Runs from the **crista galli** to the internal occipital protuberance where it becomes continuous with the cerebellar tentorium.

○ 2. **Cerebellar tentorium:** Separates the cerebellum from the cerebral hemispheres. Attaches to the clinoid processes, petrous part of the temporal bone, and internal surfaces of the occipital and parietal bones.

○ 3. **Cerebellar falx:** Vertical fold that lies inferior to the cerebellar tentorium and partially separates the cerebellar hemispheres.

○ 4. **Sellar diaphragm:** Circular sheet suspended between the clinoid processes forming a roof over the **hypophyseal fossa** except for a small opening in the middle for the infundibulum (pituitary stalk) (see figure in Section 7.5)

Dural Venous Sinuses

○ 5. **Superior sagittal sinus:** Lies in the attached border of the cerebral falx beginning at the crista galli and ending posteriorly at the confluence of sinuses near the internal occipital protuberance. Receives venous drainage from the **superior cerebral veins**.

○ 6. **Inferior sagittal sinus:** Lies in the inferior free border of the cerebral falx and ends at the straight sinus

○ 7. **Great cerebral vein:** Single midline vein that unites with the inferior sagittal sinus to form the straight sinus

○ 8. **Straight sinus:** Courses along the attachment of the cerebral falx to the cerebellar tentorium and ends at the confluence of sinuses

From the confluence of sinuses, venous blood passes laterally to the transverse sinuses that drain to the sigmoid sinuses (see figure in Section 7.5). Each sigmoid sinus drains to the internal jugular vein.

Arterial Supply to the Brain

○ 9. **Vertebral arteries:** Enter the cranial cavity via the foramen magnum and unite to form the basilar artery

○ 10. **Basilar artery:** Ascends the clivus

○ 11. **Posterior cerebral artery** (paired): Terminal branches of the basilar artery

○ 12. **Internal carotid artery** (paired): Enters cranial cavity through the carotid canal, courses along the lateral aspect of the **body of the sphenoid**, and makes a 180° turn inferior to the anterior clinoid process to course superiorly to the base of the brain

○ 13. **Anterior cerebral artery** (paired): Terminal branch of the internal carotid artery. Each anterior cerebral artery is connected to each other via an anterior communicating artery.

○ 14. **Middle cerebral artery** (paired): Terminal branch of the internal carotid artery

○ 15. **Posterior communicating artery** (paired): Unites the internal carotid artery with the posterior cerebral artery

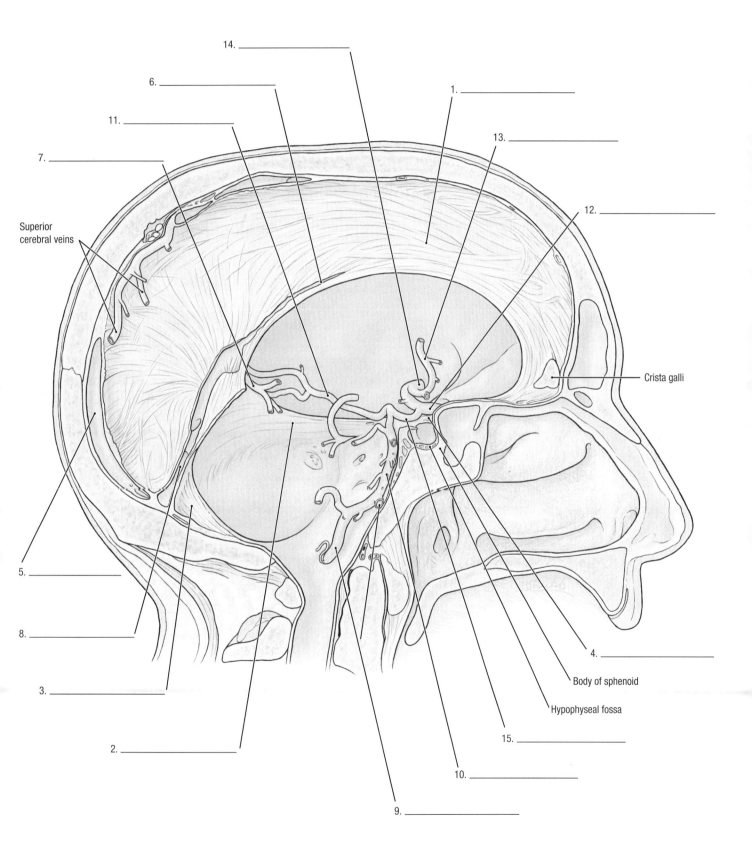

14. _____

6. _____

11. _____

7. _____

1. _____

13. _____

12. _____

Superior
cerebral veins

Crista galli

5. _____

8. _____

3. _____

2. _____

4. _____

Body of sphenoid

Hypophyseal fossa

15. _____

10. _____

9. _____

Grant's

7.7 | MUSCLES OF FACIAL EXPRESSION

The muscles of facial expression originate from skeletal or fascial structures of the cranium and insert into skin of the face, scalp, and neck. All muscles of facial expression develop from the 2nd pharyngeal arch and are innervated by the facial nerve (CN VII).

The skin and subcutaneous tissue have been removed from the right side of the face to reveal the muscles of facial expression, **_parotid gland_** and **_duct_**, and vasculature of the face. One muscle of mastication, the **_masseter_**, is also displayed along with the **_temporalis fascia_** covering the temporalis muscle. A small section of the orbicularis oculi has been removed to reveal the corrugator supercilii.

> *COLOR each of the following structures using a different color for each:*

Muscles of the Scalp, Forehead, Eyelids, and Eyebrows

Muscle	Proximal Attachment	Distal Attachment	Action
◯ 1. *Frontal belly of occipitofrontalis*	Epicranial aponeurosis	Skin and subcutaneous tissue of the eyebrows and forehead	Elevates the eyebrows and wrinkles skin of the forehead
◯ 2. *Orbicularis oculi*	Medial orbital margin; medial palpebral ligament; lacrimal bone	Skin around the margin of the orbit; superior and inferior tarsal plates	Closes the eyelids
◯ 3. *Procerus*	Lateral nasal cartilage; fascia covering the nasal bone	Skin of the inferior forehead between the eyebrows	Depresses medial end of the eyebrows; wrinkles skin over dorsum of the nose
◯ 4. *Corrugator supercilii*	Medial end of the superciliary arch	Skin superior to the middle supra-orbital margin	Draws the eyebrows medially and inferiorly

Muscles of Mouth, Lips, and Cheeks

Muscle	Proximal Attachment	Distal Attachment	Action
◯ 5. *Orbicularis oris*	Medial maxilla and mandible; deep surface of the perioral skin; angle of the mouth (modiolus)	Mucous membrane of the lips	Closes the oral fissure; compresses and protrudes the lips; resists distension
◯ 6. *Levator labii superioris*	Infraorbital margin and frontal process of the maxilla	Skin of upper lip	Elevates the upper lip; dilator of the mouth
◯ 7. *Levator anguli oris*	Infraorbital margin of the maxilla	Angle of the mouth (modiolus)	Widens the oral fissure; dilator of the mouth
◯ 8. *Zygomaticus major*	Lateral aspect of the **_zygomatic arch_**		Elevates angle of the mouth; dilator of the mouth
◯ 9. *Depressor anguli oris*	Anterolateral base of the mandible		Depresses angle of the mouth; dilator of the mouth
◯ 10. *Depressor labii inferioris*	Anterolateral body of the mandible	Skin of the lower lip	Depresses the lower lip; dilator of the mouth
◯ 11. *Mentalis*	Body of the mandible	Skin of the chin	Elevates and protrudes the lower lip; elevates skin of the chin
◯ 12. *Buccinator*	Mandible, alveolar processes of the maxilla and mandible, pterygomandibular raphe	Angle of the mouth (modiolus); orbicularis oris	Presses the cheek against the teeth; resists distension
◯ 13. *Platysma*	Subcutaneous tissue of the neck	Base of the mandible; skin of the cheek and lower lip; angle of the mouth; orbicularis oris	Depresses the mandible (against resistance); tenses the skin over the neck

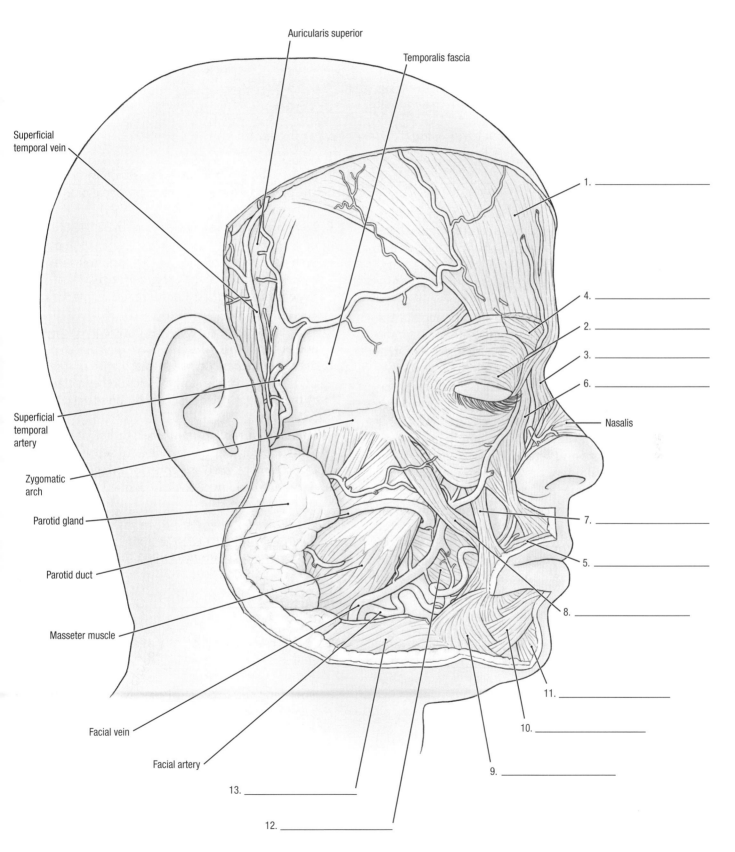

Auricularis superior

Temporalis fascia

Superficial
temporal vein

Superficial
temporal
artery

Zygomatic
arch

Parotid gland

Parotid duct

Masseter muscle

Facial vein

Facial artery

Nasalis

1. _____

4. _____

2. _____

3. _____

6. _____

7. _____

5. _____

8. _____

11. _____

10. _____

9. _____

13. _____

12. _____

Somatic motor fibers of the facial nerve (CN VII) emerge onto the face via the stylomastoid foramen. Immediately after coursing through the stylomastoid foramen, the facial nerve divides into six main branches within the parotid gland. These branches communicate with each other forming a plexus across the face.

The skin and subcutaneous tissue along with the parotid sheath have been removed over the right side of the face and neck. A pin is holding the lobule of the ear superiorly and the superior aspect of the platysma is reflected inferiorly by a string.

COLOR each of the following structures using a different color for each:

Parotid Gland and Duct

○ 1. *Parotid gland:* Largest of the salivary glands and lies anteroinferior to the external acoustic meatus. The gland fills the space between the mastoid process and ramus of the mandible, extending variably onto the lateral surface of the ***masseter***. The facial nerve branches course through the gland, but do not innervate it.

○ 2. *Parotid duct:* Extends from the anterior edge of the gland, courses superficial to the masseter muscle, and then turns medially to pierce the ***buccinator muscle*** and enter the oral cavity

○ 3. *Great auricular nerve:* Arises from the cervical plexus (C2, C3) to supply the parotid sheath that surrounds the parotid gland and the skin overlying the angle of the mandible. Travels with the ***external jugular vein***.

○ 4. *Superficial temporal artery:* Terminal branch of the external carotid artery traveling with the ***superficial temporal vein***. Emerges from the parotid gland onto the face between the TMJ and the external ear to supply the scalp.

○ 5. *Transverse facial artery:* Arises from the superficial temporal artery within the parotid gland and crosses the face superficial to the masseter and inferior to the zygomatic arch

Facial Nerve Branches

The six main branches of the facial nerve that supply the muscles of the face and scalp can be distinguished on the basis of their relationships to facial structures. Each branch divides as it courses across the face giving rise to multiple branches that supply facial expression muscles within its vicinity. Overlap of innervation to some of the facial expression muscles occurs due to the plexus formation of the facial nerve branches.

○ 6. *Temporal branches:* Pass toward the angle of the eye or superior to it to supply muscles of the upper face, such as the frontal belly of the occipitofrontalis and superior portions of the ***orbicularis oculi***

○ 7. *Zygomatic branches:* Course medially inferior to the angle of eye and superior to the parotid duct to supply muscles of the midface, such as the ***zygomaticus major*** and buccinator

○ 8. *Buccal branches:* Course medially with or inferior to the parotid duct to supply muscles of the midface, such as the buccinator and superior portion of the orbicularis oris

○ 9. *(Marginal) mandibular branches:* Course inferomedially along the angle of the mandible to supply muscles of the lower face, such as ***depressor anguli oris***

○ 10. *Cervical branches:* Course inferiorly into the neck to supply the ***platysma***

○ 11. *Posterior auricular nerve:* Courses posteriorly with the ***posterior auricular artery*** and ***vein*** to supply the ***posterior auricular muscle*** and the occipital belly of the occipitofrontalis

Facial Artery

○ 12. *Facial artery:* Branch of the external carotid artery that enters the face along the inferior border of the mandible anterior to the masseter muscle. Courses tortuously along modiolus to the angle of the nose, with the ***facial vein*** located laterally.

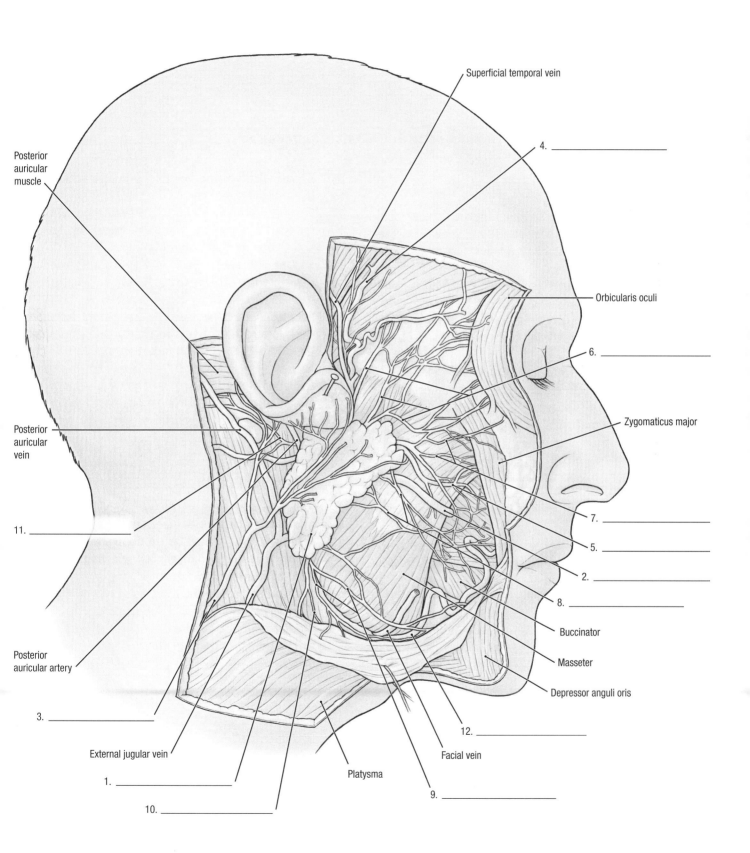

Superficial temporal vein

Posterior
auricular
muscle

4. _____

Orbicularis oculi

6. _____

Posterior
auricular
vein

Zygomaticus major

11. _____

7. _____

5. _____

2. _____

8. _____

Buccinator

Posterior
auricular artery

Masseter

Depressor anguli oris

3. _____

12. _____

External jugular vein

Facial vein

1. _____

Platysma

10. _____

9. _____

Grant's

7.9 SENSORY NERVES TO THE FACE, MUSCLES OF FACIAL EXPRESSION, AND EYELID

Sensory innervation of the face is supplied by branches of the trigeminal nerve (CN V). Unlike the facial nerve branches that cross over the face from lateral to medial, the branches of the trigeminal nerve emerge directly onto the face via many foramina to reach the skin of the face. Many of the facial expression muscles have been incised, removed, or reflected to reveal the branches of the trigeminal nerve as they emerge from their respective foramina.

The eyelids along with the lacrimal fluid protect the eyeballs from injury and irritation. The orbital septum has been removed in the left orbit.

COLOR each of the following structures using a different color for each:

Facial Expression Muscles

○ 1. **Orbicularis oris:** Fibers surround the oral fissure. Many of the other muscles that act on the upper lip, lower lip, or angle of the mouth (modiolus) blend with fibers of the orbicularis oris.

○ 2. **Zygomaticus major:** Fibers blend into and act on the modiolus

○ 3. **Levator anguli oris:** Fibers originate inferior to the infraorbital foramen and blend into and act on the modiolus

○ 4. **Levator labii superioris (cut):** Fibers originate superior to the infraorbital foramen and blend into the orbicularis oris fibers of the upper lip

○ 5. **Depressor anguli oris:** Fibers blend into and act on the modiolus

○ 6. **Mentalis:** Fibers blend with orbicularis oris fibers of the lower lip and insert into the skin of the chin

Trigeminal Nerve Branches

○ 7. **Mental nerve** (CN V_3): Emerges from the mental foramen of the mandible to supply the skin of the chin and skin and oral mucosa of lower lip

○ 8. **(Long) buccal nerve** (CN V_3): Supplies the skin and oral mucosa cheek and the buccal gingivae of the second and third mandibular molars

○ 9. **Infraorbital nerve** (CN V_2): Emerges from the infraorbital foramen of the maxilla to supply the skin over the maxilla, maxillary sinus, maxillary teeth except molars, lower eyelid, lateral nose, and skin and oral mucosa of upper lip

○ 10. **Zygomaticofacial nerve** (CN V_2): Supplies the skin over the prominence of cheek

○ 11. **Supraorbital nerve** (CN V_1): Emerges via the supraorbital foramen to supply the skin of the lateral forehead and scalp, superior eyelid, and frontal sinus

○ 12. **Supratrochlear nerve** (CN V_1): Emerges medial to the supraorbital nerve to supply the skin of the medial forehead and medial portion of eyelids

○ 13. **Infratrochlear nerve** (CN V_1): Emerges inferomedial to the supratrochlear nerve to supply the skin lateral to the bridge of the nose and over medial portion of the eyelids

○ 14. **Lacrimal nerve** (CN V_1): Emerges near the _lacrimal gland_, supplying the skin superolateral to the orbit and lateral portions of the eyelids

Eyelids

○ 15. **Superior tarsal plate:** Dense connective tissue that forms the foundation of the upper eyelid and an insertion point for the _levator palpebrae superioris muscle_

○ 16. **Inferior tarsal plate:** Dense connective tissue that forms the foundation of the lower eyelid

○ 17. **Orbital septum:** Fibrous membrane that spans from the tarsal plates to the margins of the orbit where it becomes continuous with the periosteum

○ 18. **Medial palpebral ligament:** Connects the tarsal plates to the medial margin of the orbit and provides the attachment points of the orbicularis oculi

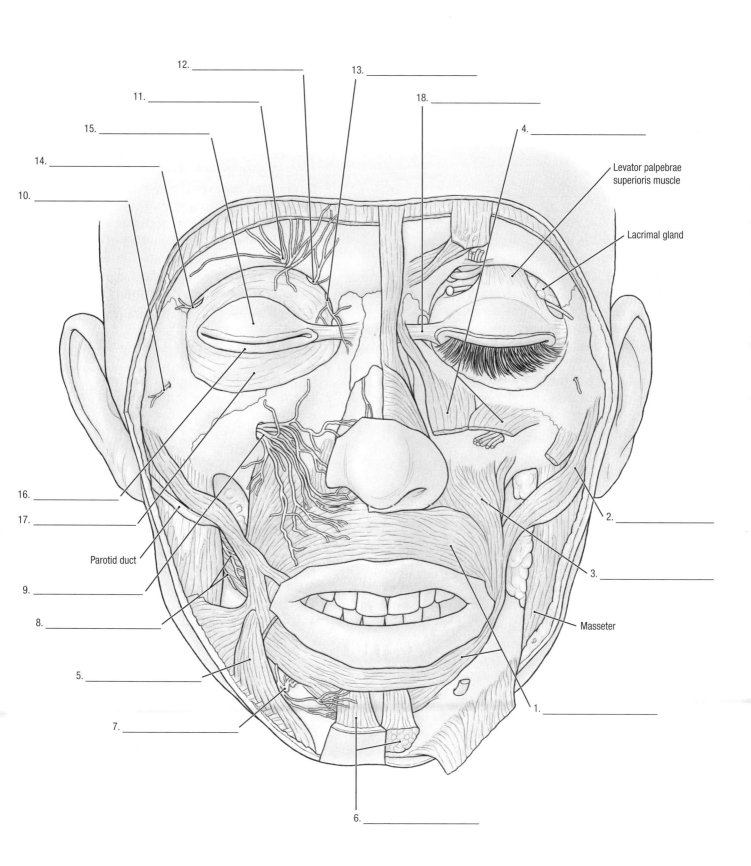

12. _____

13. _____

11. _____

18. _____

15. _____

4. _____

14. _____

Levator palpebrae
superioris muscle

10. _____

Lacrimal gland

16. _____

17. _____

2. _____

Parotid duct

3. _____

9. _____

Masseter

8. _____

5. _____

1. _____

7. _____

6. _____

7.10 ORBITAL CAVITY

The orbits are bilateral bony cavities of the facial skeleton with their bases anterolaterally directed and the apices placed posteromedially. The medial walls of each orbit are almost parallel and only separated by the ethmoidal sinuses and superior portion of the nasal cavity. The lateral walls, however, are almost at right angles (90°) to each other.

COLOR each of the following structures using a different color for each:

○ 1. *Orbital portion of the frontal bone:* Separates the orbital cavity from the anterior cranial fossa and forms most of the superior wall
Supraorbital notch/foramen: Located along the medial aspect of the frontal bone along the orbital rim for the passage of the supraorbital nerve and vessels

○ 2. *Lesser wing of sphenoid:* Forms the apex and a small portion of the superior wall of the orbit
Optic canal: Located within the lesser wing of the sphenoid at the apex of the orbit for the passage of the optic nerve (CN II) and ophthalmic artery

○ 3. *Greater wing of sphenoid:* forms the posterior aspect of the lateral wall
Superior orbital fissure: Located between the greater and lesser wings of the sphenoid for the passage of the ophthalmic veins, oculomotor nerve (CN III), trochlear nerve (CN IV), ophthalmic division of the trigeminal nerve (CN V$_1$), and abducens nerve (CN VI)

○ 4. *Zygomatic bone:* Forms most of the lateral wall and the lateral portion of the inferior wall. The lateral wall is the thickest wall of the orbit.
Zygomaticofacial foramen: Small foramen located inferolateral to the orbital rim for the passage of the zygomaticofacial nerve (CN V$_2$)

○ 5. *Maxillary bone:* Forms most of the inferior wall
Inferior orbital fissure: Space between the maxilla and greater wing of the sphenoid that demarcates the inferior wall from the lateral wall. The infraorbital nerve (CN V$_2$) and vessels begin their path from the pterygopalatine fossa through the inferior orbital fissure.
Infraorbital groove: Located in the inferior wall of the orbit for the passage of the infraorbital nerve and vessels; superior aspect is open (not covered by bone)
Infraorbital canal: Continuation of the infraorbital groove; surrounded by bone
Infraorbital foramen: Superficial opening of the infraorbital canal located inferior to the medial aspect of the inferior orbital rim. Site of emergence of the infraorbital nerve and vessels onto the face.

○ 6. *Lacrimal bone:* Forms the anterior aspect of the medial wall
Lacrimal groove: Indentation for the lacrimal sac

○ 7. *Orbital process of ethmoid bone:* Paper-thin bone forming most of the medial wall
Anterior and posterior ethmoidal foramina: Small foramina located along the suture between the frontal and ethmoid bones (or superior to the suture) for the passage of the anterior and posterior ethmoidal nerves and vessels, respectively

○ 8. *Orbital process of palatine bone:* Contributes to a minor portion of the posterior aspect of the inferior wall

1. _____

2. _____

3. _____

4. _____

8. _____

5. _____

6. _____

7. _____

Optic canal

Posterior
ethmoidal
foramen

Anterior
ethmoidal
foramen

Supraorbital
notch

Nasal bone

Superior
orbital fissure

Inferior
orbital fissure

Zygomaticofacial foramen

Infraorbital
groove

Infraorbital
foramen

Infraorbital canal

Lacrimal groove

Grant's

7.11 ANTERIOR VIEW OF THE EYEBALL AND LACRIMAL APPARATUS

The orbit houses not only the eyeball, but also the accessory visual structures, which include the eyelids, extraocular muscles, neurovasculature, orbital fat, orbital fascia surrounding the eyeballs and muscles, and conjunctiva.

The eyelids, orbital septum, levator palpebrae superioris muscle, and some of the orbital fat have been removed to reveal the eyeball within the orbit.

COLOR each of the following structures using a different color for each:

Lacrimal Apparatus

The lacrimal apparatus produces lacrimal fluid laterally and drains it medially after it is blinked across the eyeball.

○ 1. *Lacrimal gland:* Located in the superolateral aspect of the orbit; secretes lacrimal fluid that is swept across the anterior eyeball from lateral to medial during blinking through the conjunctival sac

○ 2. *Bulbar conjunctiva:* Thin, transparent mucous membrane that lines the sclera (white portion) of the anterior eyeball. Continuous with the palpebral conjunctiva that lines the internal aspect of eyelids forming the conjunctival sac, which is a closed space when the eyelids are closed.

○ 3. *Lacrimal sac:* Dilated superior part of the *nasolacrimal duct* located medially in the lacrimal groove. Lacrimal fluid is drained to the lacrimal sac via the *lacrimal canaliculi*.

Extraocular Muscles

All four of the rectus muscles insert into the anterior half of the eyeball, whereas the two oblique muscles insert into the posterior half of the eyeball.

○ 4. *Inferior oblique:* Originates from the anterior aspect of the orbital floor and courses posterolateral to insert into the sclera of the posterolateral aspect of the eyeball deep to the lateral rectus muscle

○ 5. *Inferior rectus:* Inserts into the sclera on the anteroinferior aspect of the eyeball superior to the inferior oblique

○ 6. *Lateral rectus:* Courses along the lateral aspect of the orbit and inserts into the sclera on the anterolateral aspect of the eyeball

○ 7. *Superior rectus:* Inserts into the sclera of the anterosuperior aspect of the eyeball superior to the tendon of the superior oblique

○ 8. *Superior oblique:* Courses along the superomedial aspect of the orbit with its tendon passing through the *trochlea*, a fibrous ring. At the trochlea, the tendon changes direction and inserts into the sclera on the posterolateral aspect of the eyeball deep to the superior rectus muscle.

○ 9. *Medial rectus:* Courses along the medial aspect of the orbit and inserts into the sclera on the anterolateral aspect of the eyeball

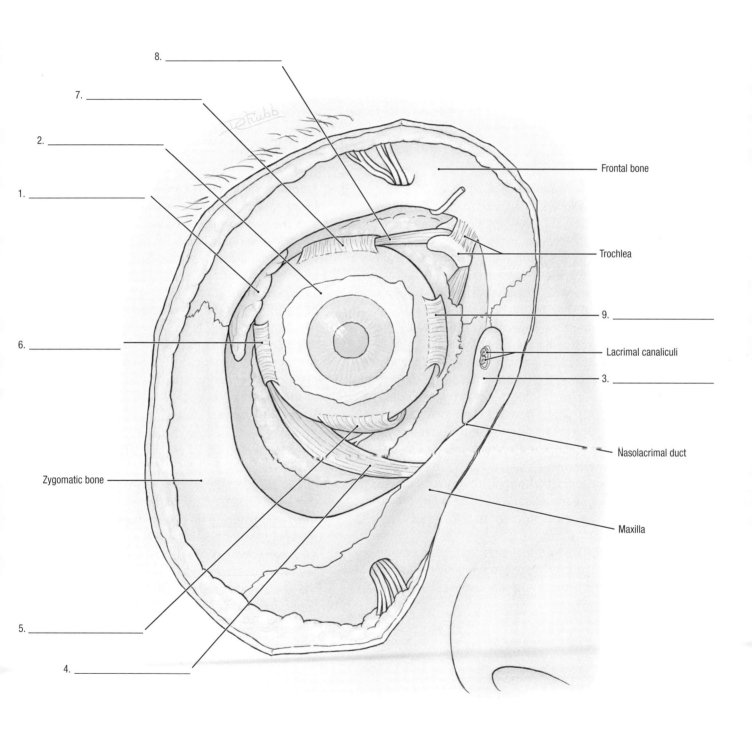

8. _____

7. _____

2. _____

1. _____

6. _____

Zygomatic bone _____

5. _____

4. _____

Frontal bone

Trochlea

9. _____

Lacrimal canaliculi

3. _____

Nasolacrimal duct

Maxilla

Grant's

7.12A and B   SUPERIOR VIEW OF ORBITAL CAVITY

The orbital plate of the frontal bone has been removed in both A and B. On the left side of A, the levator palpebrae superioris and superior rectus have been cut and reflected. On the left side of B, the levator palpebrae superioris, superior rectus, superior oblique, and many of the superiorly placed nerves and arteries have been removed. On the right side of B, the optic nerve has also been cut and resected.

All the arteries of the orbit arise from the ophthalmic artery (branch of the ***internal carotid artery***). The ***supraorbital***, ***lacrimal***, and ***anterior and posterior ethmoidal arteries*** all travel with nerves of the same name. The central artery of the retina pierces the optic nerve and provides the primary arterial supply to the eyeball.

COLOR each of the following structures using a different color for each:

Extraocular Muscles

○ 1. *Levator palpebrae superioris* (A only): Originates from the lesser wing of sphenoid superior to optic canal and inserts into the superior tarsus and skin of the superior eyelid. Elevates the superior eyelid.

○ 2. *Superior rectus* (A only): Originates from the common tendinous ring, courses deep to the levator palpebrae superioris, and inserts into the sclera just posterior to the corneoscleral junction

○ 3. *Superior oblique:* Originates from the body of the sphenoid, courses along the superomedial aspect of the orbit, with its tendon passing through the ***trochlea*** and changing course. The tendon then passes deep to superior rectus to insert into the posterolateral sclera.

○ 4. *Medial rectus:* Originates from the common tendinous ring, courses along the medial wall of the orbit inferior to the superior oblique, and inserts into sclera just posterior to the corneoscleral junction

○ 5. *Lateral rectus:* Originates from the common tendinous ring, courses along the lateral wall of the orbit, and inserts into the sclera just posterior to the corneoscleral junction

○ 6. *Inferior rectus* (B only): Originates from the common tendinous ring, courses inferior to the optic nerve, and inserts into the sclera just posterior to the corneoscleral junction

Nerves of the Orbit

○ 7. *Frontal nerve* (CN V_1) (A only): Courses superficial to the levator palpebrae superioris and terminates by dividing into the ***supraorbital*** and ***supratrochlear nerves***

○ 8. *Trochlear nerve (CN IV):* Passes into orbit superior to the levator palpebrae superioris and immediately dives into the superior oblique muscle to innervate it

○ 9. *Lacrimal nerve* (CN V_1): Travels along the superior border of the lateral rectus muscle

○ 10. *Nasociliary nerve* (CN V_1): Travels deep to the superior rectus, crosses the optic nerve, and travels medial to the medial rectus. It gives rise to the following:
Infratrochlear nerve: Emerges onto the face inferior to the trochlea
Long ciliary nerves: Pierce the posterior aspect of the eyeball
Anterior and posterior ethmoidal nerves: Supply the ***ethmoidal cells***

○ 11. *Ciliary ganglion:* Collection of postsynaptic parasympathetic cell bodies. Fibers exit the ciliary ganglion via the ***short ciliary nerves*** that pierce the back of the eyeball to supply the intraocular muscles.

○ 12. *Abducens nerve (CN VI):* Passes into orbit medial to the lateral rectus muscle and immediately dives into the lateral rectus to innervate it

○ 13. *Superior division of oculomotor nerve (CN III)* (A only): Upon entering the orbit, CN III divides into the superior and inferior divisions. The superior division pierces the inferior aspect of the superior rectus, innervating it, and then passes onto the levator palpebrae superioris to innervate it.

○ 14. *Inferior division of oculomotor nerve (CN III)* (B only): Travels deep to the optic nerve innervating the inferior rectus, medial rectus, and inferior oblique

○ 15. *Optic nerve (CN II):* Courses inferior to the superior rectus muscle and pierces the posterior aspect of the eyeball

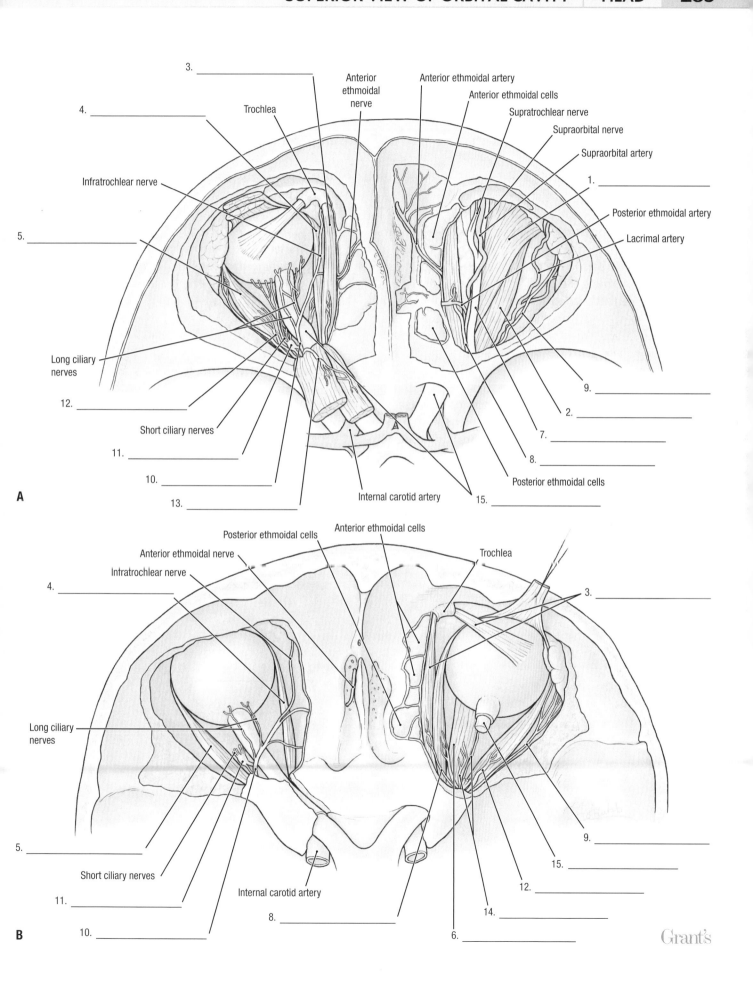

A

3. _____

4. _____

Trochlea

Anterior ethmoidal nerve

Anterior ethmoidal artery

Anterior ethmoidal cells

Supratrochlear nerve

Supraorbital nerve

Supraorbital artery

Infratrochlear nerve

1. _____

Posterior ethmoidal artery

Lacrimal artery

5. _____

Long ciliary nerves

12. _____

Short ciliary nerves

11. _____

10. _____

13. _____

Internal carotid artery

9. _____

2. _____

7. _____

8. _____

Posterior ethmoidal cells

15. _____

B

Posterior ethmoidal cells

Anterior ethmoidal cells

Anterior ethmoidal nerve

Intratrochlear nerve

Trochlea

4. _____

3. _____

Long ciliary nerves

5. _____

Short ciliary nerves

11. _____

10. _____

Internal carotid artery

8. _____

6. _____

14. _____

12. _____

15. _____

9. _____

7.13A and B MANDIBLE

Figure A depicts a lateral view of the mandible, whereas Figure B depicts a medial view.

COLOR each of the following structures using a different color for each:

○ 1. **Coronoid process:** Anteriorly placed superior projection from the ramus for the attachment of the temporalis muscle

○ 2. **Condylar process:** Posteriorly directed superior projection from the ramus
Head: Articulates with the mandibular fossa and articular tubercle forming the TMJ
Neck: Slender portion inferior to the head
Pterygoid fovea (B only): Small pit on the neck marking one of the attachment sites of the lateral pterygoid muscle
Mandibular notch: Curved section between the coronoid and condylar processes

○ 3. **Oblique line** (A only): Continuation of the **anterior border** onto the external surface of the mandible leading to mental protuberance

○ 4. **Mental protuberance** (A only): Triangular eminence forming the chin with paired lateral prominences, the **mental tubercles**

○ 5. **Mental foramen** (A only): Located inferior to the premolar teeth for the passage of the mental artery and nerve

○ 6. **Lingula** (B only): Projection, typically triangular, which marks the location of the **mandibular foramen** and provides attachment for the sphenomandibular ligament

○ 7. **Mylohyoid groove** (B only): Courses inferomedially from the mandibular foramen and lingula, marking the path of the nerve to the mylohyoid muscle

○ 8. **Mylohyoid line** (B only): Slight ridge marking the attachment site of the mylohyoid muscle
Submandibular fossa (B only): Located inferior to the mylohyoid line posteriorly marking the location of the submandibular gland
Sublingual fossa (B only): Located superior to the mylohyoid line anteriorly marking the location of the sublingual gland

○ 9. **Digastric fossa** (B only): Anterior, bilateral depressions along the inferior aspect, marking the attachment site of the anterior belly of the digastric muscle
Superior and inferior mental (genial) spines (B only): Typically two to four small projections immediately superior to the digastric fossae, marking the attachment sites of the geniohyoid and genioglossus muscles

○ 10. **Retromolar fossa** (B only): Triangular depression located posterior to the third mandibular molar

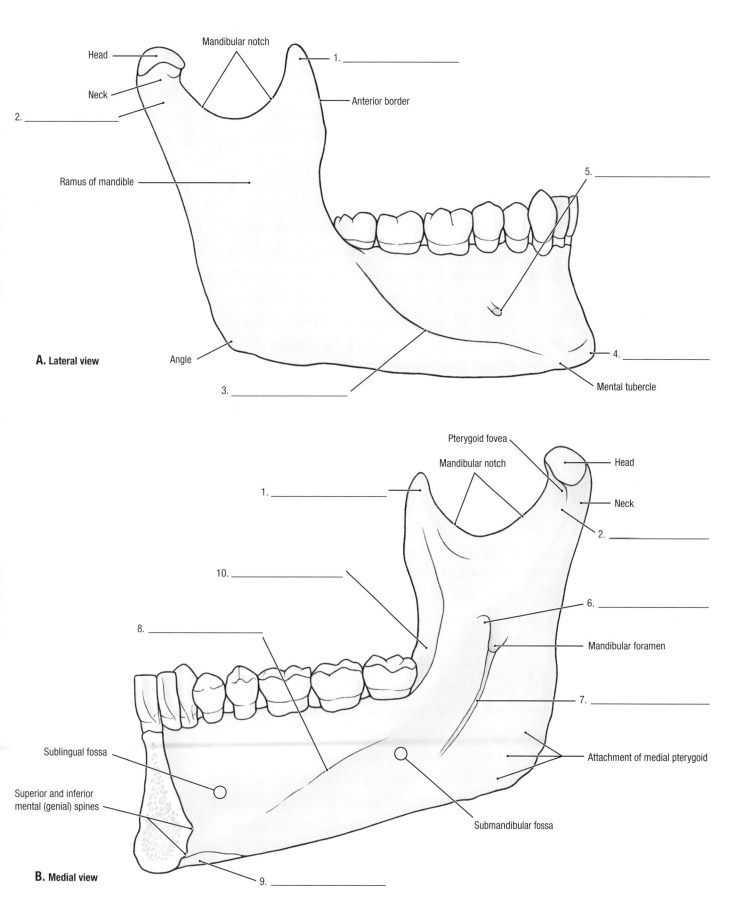

Head

Mandibular notch

Neck

2. _____

Ramus of mandible

1. _____

Anterior border

5. _____

A. Lateral view

Angle

3. _____

4. _____

Mental tubercle

Pterygoid fovea

Mandibular notch

Head

Neck

1. _____

2. _____

10. _____

6. _____

Mandibular foramen

8. _____

7. _____

Sublingual fossa

Superior and inferior
mental (genial) spines

Attachment of medial pterygoid

Submandibular fossa

B. Medial view

9. _____

Grant's

7.14 BONES OF INFRATEMPORAL AND TEMPORAL FOSSAE AND TMJ

The temporal and infratemporal fossae communicate with each other via the space between the zygomatic arch and the deeper cranial bones. In this image, the mandible and the zygomatic arch have been removed to demonstrate the superior and medial walls of the infratemporal fossa.

COLOR each of the following structures using a different color for each:

○ 1. *Temporal fossa:* Space filled by the temporalis muscle superior to the infratemporal crest and bounded medially by the bones that form the pterion: *frontal*, *parietal*, *temporal*, and *greater wing of sphenoid*

○ 2. *Infratemporal crest:* Line marking the boundary between the infratemporal and temporal fossae. Created as the greater wing of the sphenoid changes from horizontal to vertical.

○ 3. *Infratemporal surface of greater wing of sphenoid:* Horizontal portion inferior to the infratemporal crest and is the location of the following:
  Foramen ovale: Passage of the mandibular division of the trigeminal nerve (CN V₃)

  $Foramen ovale$: Passage of the mandibular division of the trigeminal nerve (CN V_3)

  Foramen spinosum: Passage of the middle meningeal artery
  Spine of sphenoid: Superior attachment of the sphenomandibular ligament

○ 4. *Lateral pterygoid plate:* Medial boundary of the infratemporal fossa and attachment site for both the lateral and medial pterygoid muscles

○ 5. *Pterygoid hamulus of medial pterygoid plate:* Does not participate in formations of the infratemporal fossa. The medial pterygoid plate structures are involved with the muscles and structures of the palate. The *pyramidal process of palatine bone* fills in the small gap between the lateral and medial pterygoid plates inferiorly.

○ 6. *Infratemporal surface of maxilla:* Posterior aspect of the maxilla that forms the anterior boundary of the infratemporal fossa
  Posterior superior alveolar foramina: One or more small openings marking the passage of the posterior superior alveolar nerves and vessels

Pterygomaxillary fissure: Space between the infratemporal surface of the maxilla and the lateral pterygoid plate that leads into the *pterygopalatine fossa*. The *sphenopalatine foramen* is located within the medial wall of the pterygopalatine fossa and leads into the nasal cavity.

Inferior orbital fissure: Located between the superior aspect of the infratemporal surface of the maxilla, orbital portion of maxilla, and the greater wing of the sphenoid

Temporomandibular Joint

The TMJ is a modified hinge joint surrounded by a joint capsule and supported by ligaments. The condylar head (see figure in Section 7.13) is separated by an articular disc from the two articular surfaces of the temporal bone.

○ 7. *Mandibular fossa:* Depressed articulating surface where the condylar head sits during rest

○ 8. *Articular tubercle:* Anterior articulating prominence that prevents anterior dislocation

○ 9. *Postglenoid tubercle:* Does not participate in the TMJ, but prevents posterior dislocation

CLINICAL NOTE: TMJ DISLOCATIONS
The TMJ dislocates anteriorly most commonly during dental procedures when the mouth is held open for an extended period of time. The condylar head lies anterior to the articular tubercle and cannot be pulled back into the mandibular fossa. The individual cannot close their mouth until the mandible is pulled inferiorly (typically by another person) and the condylar head can then return back into its normal position. The postglenoid tubercle and lateral ligament of the TMJ resist posterior and lateral dislocations; fractures of the mandible often occur before a dislocation occurs.

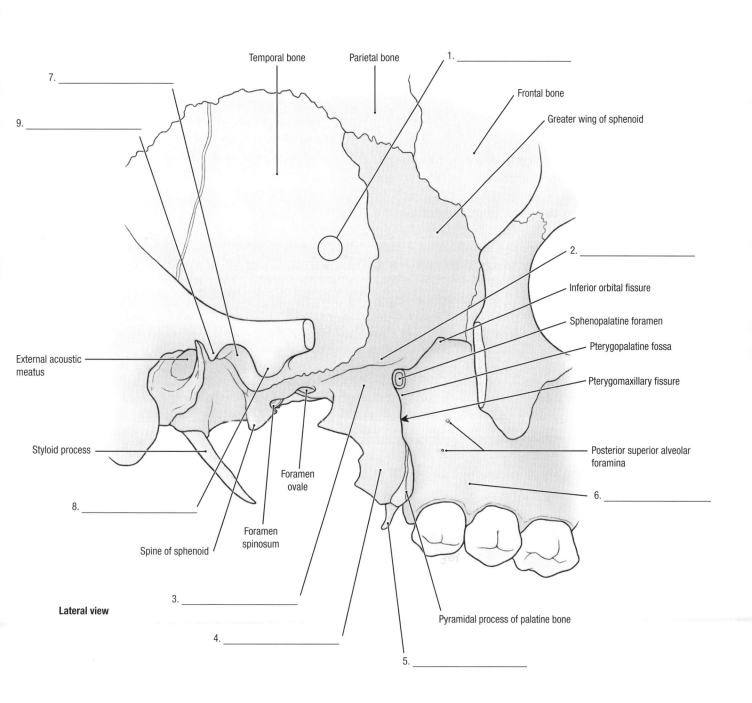

Temporal bone

Parietal bone

1. _____

7. _____

Frontal bone

9. _____

Greater wing of sphenoid

2. _____

Inferior orbital fissure

Sphenopalatine foramen

Pterygopalatine fossa

Pterygomaxillary fissure

External acoustic meatus

Posterior superior alveolar foramina

Styloid process

Foramen ovale

8. _____

6. _____

Spine of sphenoid

Foramen spinosum

Lateral view

3. _____

Pyramidal process of palatine bone

4. _____

5. _____

7.15 TEMPORALIS AND MASSETER MUSCLES

The temporalis and masseter are muscles of mastication innervated by the mandibular division of the trigeminal nerve (CN V₃). Neither of them lie within the infratemporal fossa except for the tendon of the temporalis muscle.

In this image, the skin and subcutaneous tissue over the lateral face, scalp, and upper aspect of the **sternocleidomastoid muscle** have been removed. The external ear has been removed, leaving the **external acoustic meatus** exposed. The parotid gland has also been removed from the **parotid bed** and from the lateral aspect of the mandible, leaving a remnant of the **parotid duct** as it pierces the buccinator muscle.

COLOR each of the following structures using a different color for each:

Temporalis and Masseter

○ 1. **Temporalis muscle:** Fan-shaped muscle that fills the temporal fossa. Passes deep to **zygomatic arch** to attach to the medial aspect of the coronoid process and anteromedial ramus of the mandible

○ 2. **Temporalis fascia:** Covers the superficial aspect of the temporalis muscle

○ 3. **Masseter muscle:** Covers the lateral aspect of the mandible. Courses from the zygomatic arch anterior to the TMJ posteroinferiorly to the angle of the mandible. The parotid duct, parotid gland, transverse facial artery, and branches of facial nerve travel along the superficial aspect of the masseter. The **facial artery** and **vein** pass over the inferior border of the **body of the mandible** anterior to the attachment of the masseter.

○ 4. **Buccinator muscle:** Lies medial to the masseter and is not a muscle of mastication. The buccinator keeps food between the teeth during chewing, but does not act on the mandible.

CLINICAL NOTE: BOTULINUM TOXIN TREATMENT FOR TEMPOROMANDIBULAR DISORDERS

A treatment for temporomandibular disorders involves injection of botulinum toxin into the temporalis and/or masseter muscles, which are easily accessed owing to their superficial location. The toxin acts on the neuromuscular junctions and causes the muscle(s) to relax, remitting their force on the TMJ.

Muscle	Proximal Attachment	Distal Attachment	Action
Temporalis	Floor of the temporal fossa	Medial aspect of the coronoid process and anteromedial ramus	Anterior fibers: elevation (bilateral) Posterior fibers: retraction (bilateral)
Masseter	Inferior border of the zygomatic arch	Lateral surface and angle of the mandible	Elevation and protrusion (bilateral)

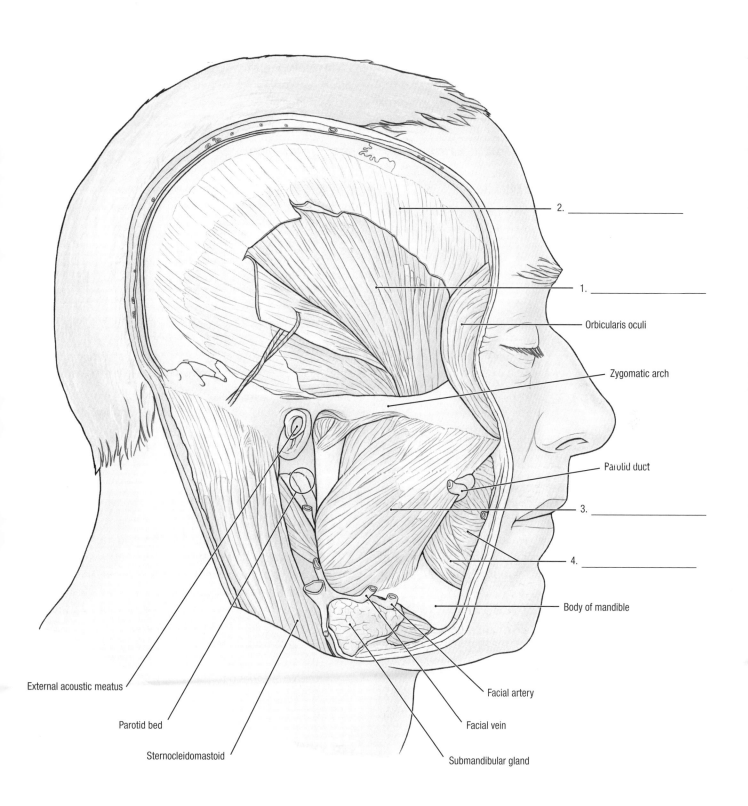

2. _____

Orbicularis oculi

Zygomatic arch

1. _____

Parotid duct

3. _____

Body of mandible

4. _____

External acoustic meatus

Facial artery

Parotid bed

Facial vein

Sternocleidomastoid

Submandibular gland

7.16 INFRATEMPORAL FOSSA I

The *maxillary artery* arises as one of the two terminal branches of the *external carotid artery*. It courses deep to the neck of the mandible, whereas the *superficial temporal artery*, the other terminal branch, courses superiorly. The maxillary artery then courses horizontally superficial, deep, or within the lateral pterygoid muscle giving rise to several branches within the infratemporal fossa. Finally, the maxillary artery traverses the pterygomaxillary fissure, entering the pterygopalatine fossa.

The branches of CN V_3 arise deep within the infratemporal fossa from the foramen ovale and, along with branches from the maxillary artery, course variably in relation to the lateral and medial pterygoid muscles.

In this image, the zygomatic arch has been removed along with the coronoid process and anterior portion of the ramus of the mandible.

COLOR each of the following structures using a different color for each:

Medial and Lateral Pterygoid Muscles

The lateral pterygoid muscle is a two-headed muscle, triangular in shape, and almost horizontal in position. The medial pterygoid muscle is also a two-headed muscle and an almost mirror image to the masseter muscle medial to the ramus of the mandible.

Muscle	Proximal Attachment	Distal Attachment	Action
◯ 1. *Lateral pterygoid, inferior head*	Lateral surface of the lateral pterygoid plate	Pterygoid fovea	Protrusion and depression of the mandible (bilateral); contralateral excursion (unilateral)
◯ 2. *Lateral pterygoid, superior head*	Inferior surface of the greater wing of the sphenoid	Articular capsule, articular disc, and pterygoid fovea	Active during elevation of the mandible against resistance
◯ 3. *Medial pterygoid, deep head*	Medial surface of the lateral pterygoid plate	Medial surface of the mandible (inferior to the mylohyoid groove near angle)	Elevation of the mandible and protrusion (bilateral); contralateral excursion (unilateral)
◯ 4. *Medial pterygoid, superficial head*	Tuberosity of the maxilla		

Neurovasculature Relationships to the Pterygoid Muscles

◯ 5. *Auriculotemporal nerve:* Travels with the superficial temporal artery after coursing posterior to the neck of the mandible supplying the *temporomandibular joint (TMJ)*

◯ 6. *Inferior alveolar nerve:* Emerges inferior to lateral pterygoid muscle and then travels between the medial pterygoid muscle and ramus of the mandible, giving rise to *nerve to the mylohyoid*. Travels with the *inferior alveolar artery* as it approaches the mandibular foramen.

◯ 7. *Lingual nerve:* Emerges inferior to the lateral pterygoid muscle medial to the inferior alveolar nerve and then travels between the medial pterygoid muscle and ramus of mandible before entering the oral cavity

◯ 8. *(Long) buccal nerve:* Emerges between the two heads of the lateral pterygoid muscle and then travels inferomedially piercing the *buccinator*, but not supplying it. Travels with the *buccal artery*.

◯ 9. *Deep temporal nerves:* Emerge superior to or through the superior head of the lateral pterygoid muscle and then travel deep to the *temporalis muscle*. Travel with the *deep temporal arteries*.

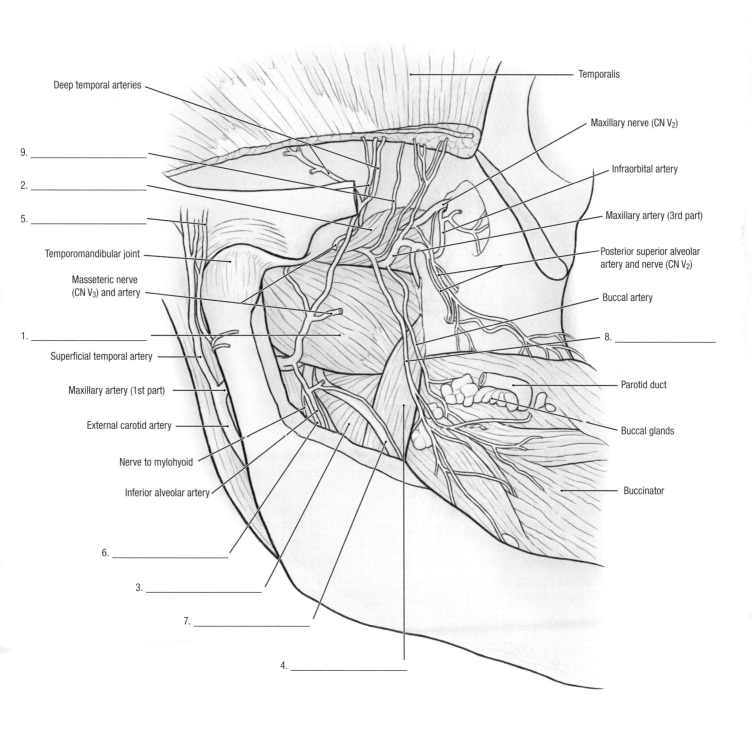

Deep temporal arteries

Temporalis

Maxillary nerve (CN V₂)

Infraorbital artery

9. _____

2. _____

5. _____

Maxillary artery (3rd part)

Temporomandibular joint

Posterior superior alveolar
artery and nerve (CN V₂)

Masseteric nerve
(CN V₃) and artery

Buccal artery

1. _____

8. _____

Superficial temporal artery

Parotid duct

Maxillary artery (1st part)

External carotid artery

Buccal glands

Nerve to mylohyoid

Inferior alveolar artery

Buccinator

6. _____

3. _____

7. _____

4. _____

Grant's

7.17   INFRATEMPORAL FOSSA II

The maxillary artery courses horizontally across the infratemporal fossa and then into the pterygopalatine fossa. The ***mandibular nerve*** emerges via the foramen ovale and immediately divides into its terminal branches.

In this image, the lateral pterygoid muscle and many of the maxillary artery branches have been removed and the ***nerve to lateral pterygoid*** and ***masseteric nerve*** have been cut.

▌ ***COLOR each of the following structures using a different color for each:***

Maxillary Artery

○ 1. ***Maxillary artery:*** Arises from the external carotid artery and can be subdivided into three portions:

First portion: passes deep to the neck of the mandible, giving rise to branches that enter bony foramina

   ○ 2. ***Middle meningeal artery:*** Courses superiorly to the foramen spinosum
Inferior alveolar artery (see figure in Section 7.16)
Second portion: gives rise to the masseteric, buccal, deep temporal, and pterygoid arteries (see figure in Section 7.16)
Third portion: passes through the pterygomaxillary fissure into the pterygopalatine fossa
   ○ 3. ***Descending palatine artery:*** Arises within the pterygopalatine fossa coursing to the palate
   ○ 4. ***Infraorbital artery:*** Travels with the ***infraorbital nerve*** through the ***inferior orbital fissure***
Posterior superior alveolar artery: travels with the posterior superior alveolar nerve (see figure in Section 7.16)

Nerves of the Infratemporal Fossa

○ 5. ***Auriculotemporal nerve:*** Courses laterally from CN V₃, crossing or encircling middle meningeal artery, passing posterior to the neck of the mandible, and then coursing superiorly anterior to the external ear. Supplies the TMJ, anterior auricle and external meatus, anterior portion of the external surface of the tympanic membrane, and the skin of the temporal region. Postsynaptic parasympathetic fibers from the lesser petrosal nerve (CN IX) via the otic ganglion "hitch a ride" to the parotid gland.

○ 6. ***Inferior alveolar nerve:*** Enters the mandibular foramen lateral to the ***sphenomandibular ligament*** and then travels within the mandibular canal, forming the inferior dental plexus. Terminates as the mental and incisive nerves. Supplies the mandibular teeth, and via the mental nerve supplies the skin and mucous membrane of the lower lip and the skin of the chin along with the vestibular gingiva of the mandibular incisors, canine, and premolars (variable).

○ 7. ***Nerve to the mylohyoid:*** Travels with the inferior alveolar nerve until the mandibular foramen where it separates to travel along the medial aspect of the mandible in the mylohyoid groove. Supplies the mylohyoid and anterior belly of the digastric muscles.

○ 8. ***Lingual nerve:*** Enters the oral cavity between the medial pterygoid muscle and ramus of the mandible to travel anteriorly in the floor of the mouth under the oral mucosa. Conducts somatic sensory (not taste) from the anterior two-thirds of tongue, mucosa of floor of the mouth, and mandibular lingual gingiva.

○ 9. ***Chorda tympani:*** Branch of CN VII that emerges from the petrotympanic fissure and "hitches a ride" on the lingual nerve. Composed of presynaptic parasympathetic fibers to the submandibular and sublingual glands that synapse in the submandibular ganglion. Also carries taste fibers from the anterior two-thirds of the tongue.

○ 10. ***(Long) buccal nerve:*** Courses inferiorly to pierce the ***buccinator***. Supplies skin over the cheek, mucous membrane lining cheek, and buccal surface of the mandibular buccal region of the molar region.

○ 11. ***Deep temporal nerves:*** Course superiorly over the infratemporal crest to the deep surface of the ***temporalis muscle***

○ 12. ***Maxillary nerve (CN V₂):*** Visible through the pterygomaxillary fissure coursing through the pterygopalatine fossa to the inferior orbital fissure where it changes name to the infraorbital nerve.

○ 13. ***Posterior superior alveolar nerves:*** Branches of CN V₂ that emerge from the pterygopalatine fossa through the pterygomaxillary fissure and then travel along the posterior aspect of the maxilla.

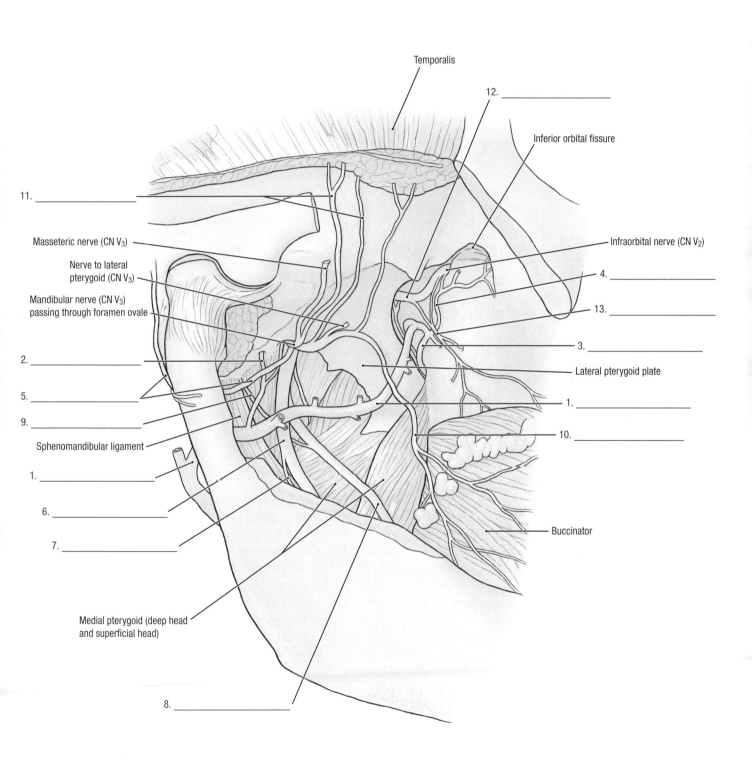

Temporalis

12. _____

Inferior orbital fissure

11. _____

Masseteric nerve (CN V₃)

Nerve to lateral
pterygoid (CN V₃)

Mandibular nerve (CN V₃)
passing through foramen ovale

Infraorbital nerve (CN V₂)

4. _____

13. _____

2. _____

3. _____

Lateral pterygoid plate

5. _____

1. _____

9. _____

10. _____

Sphenomandibular ligament

1. _____

6. _____

Buccinator

7. _____

Medial pterygoid (deep head
and superficial head)

8. _____

Grant's

7.18A and B STRUCTURES OF THE TONGUE AND FLOOR OF THE MOUTH

The oral cavity is the space between the upper and lower dental arches and is typically occupied by the tongue. The oral cavity communicates posteriorly with the oropharynx. The muscles of the tongue are innervated by the hypoglossal nerve except the palatoglossus (which is innervated by CN X).

Figure A depicts a median section of the tongue and the floor of the mouth muscles, whereas Figure B depicts the floor of the mouth structures with the tongue and mucosa removed.

COLOR each of the following structures using a different color for each:

Muscles of the Tongue

Muscle	Proximal Attachment	Distal Attachment	Action
○ 1. *Genioglossus*	Superior *mental spines*	Dorsum of the tongue; *hyoid bone*	Depresses central portion and protrudes the tongue (bilateral); deviates the tongue to the contralateral side (unilateral)
○ 2. *Hyoglossus* (B only; cut)	Body and greater horn of the hyoid bone	Inferior aspects of lateral part of the tongue	Depresses the ipsilateral side of the tongue; assists in retraction of the tongue
○ 3. *Styloglossus* (B only; cut)	Styloid process; *stylohyoid ligament*	Sides of the posterior tongue; interdigitates with the hyoglossus	Retracts the tongue and curls its sides
Palatoglossus (not shown)	Palatine aponeurosis of the soft palate	Posterolateral tongue; blends with intrinsic muscles	Elevates the posterior tongue; depresses the soft palate
○ 4. *Superior longitudinal* (A only; one of four intrinsic muscles)	Submucosal fibrous layer and median fibrous septum	Margins of the tongue and mucous membrane	Curls the tongue longitudinally upward; elevates *apex* and sides of the tongue; retracts the tongue

Floor of the Mouth Structures

○ 5. *Geniohyoid muscle:* Paired muscle lying immediately superficial to the genioglossus in the midline

○ 6. *Mylohyoid muscle:* Paired muscle lying superficial to the geniohyoid, but spans the space between the mandibular dental arch, forming a boundary between the floor of the mouth and anterior cervical region

○ 7. *Digastric muscle, anterior belly* (A only): Lies superficial to the mylohyoid muscle in the anterior cervical region

○ 8. *Platysma* (A only): Lies superficial to the anterior belly of the digastric in the anterior cervical region

○ 9. *Submandibular gland* (B only): Lies along the body of the mandible partly superficial and partly deep to the posterior edge of the mylohyoid muscle

○ 10. *Sublingual gland* (B only): Lies in the anterior aspect of the floor of the mouth between the body of the mandible and the genioglossus muscle. Multiple, small ducts open along the *sublingual fold*.

○ 11. *Submandibular duct* (B only): Arises from the deep portion of the submandibular duct, crosses anteriorly,

opens on the *sublingual caruncle* in the anterior floor of the mouth

○ 12. *Lingual nerve* (B only): Enters the oral cavity near the third mandibular molar and crosses the floor of the mouth from lateral to medial looping under the submandibular duct to reach the tongue. The submandibular ganglion is suspended by the lingual nerve superior to the deep portion of the submandibular gland.

○ 13. *Hypoglossal nerve (CN XII)* (B only): Enters the floor of the mouth lateral to the hyoglossus muscle supplying all of the intrinsic and extrinsic muscles of the tongue except the palatoglossus

○ 14. *Glossopharyngeal nerve (CN IX)* (B only): Enters the oral cavity with styloglossus and then pierces the tongue to supply somatic sensory and taste to posterior one-third of the tongue

○ 15. *Lingual artery* (B only): Enters the oral cavity medial to the hyoglossus muscle to supply the tongue and floor of the mouth structures

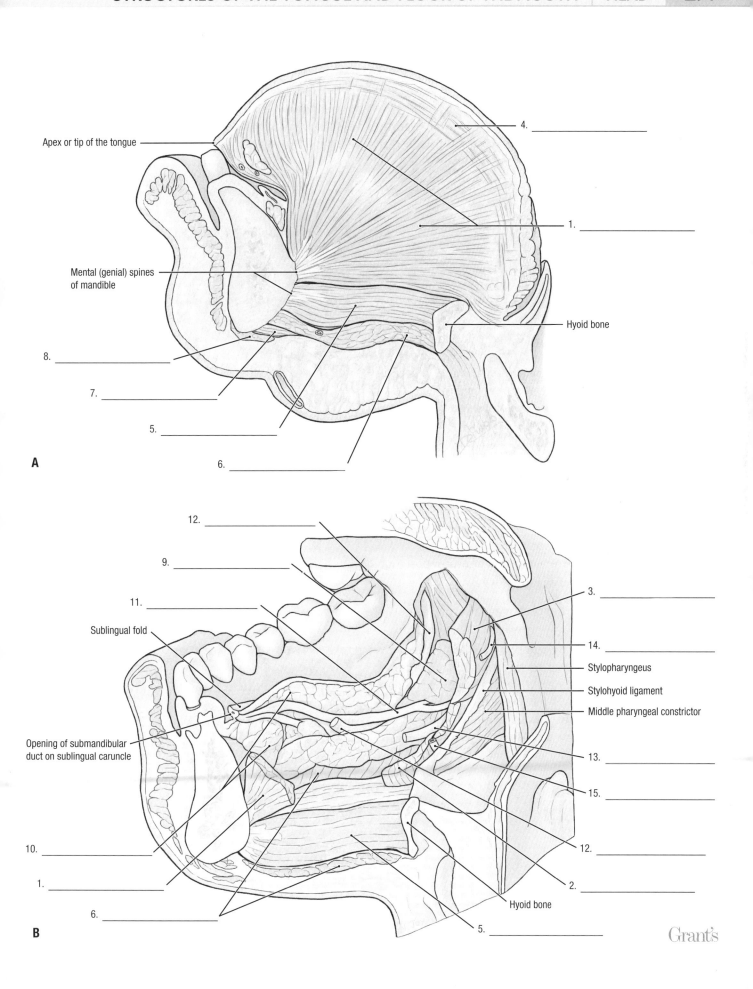

Apex or tip of the tongue

4. _____

1. _____

Mental (genial) spines
of mandible

Hyoid bone

8. _____

7. _____

5. _____

6. _____

A

12. _____

9. _____

11. _____

Sublingual fold

3. _____

14. _____

Stylopharyngeus

Stylohyoid ligament

Middle pharyngeal constrictor

Opening of submandibular
duct on sublingual caruncle

13. _____

15. _____

10. _____

12. _____

1. _____

2. _____

6. _____

Hyoid bone

5. _____

B

Grant's

7.19A and B PALATE

The palate forms the superior boundary (roof) of the oral cavity and the inferior boundary (floor) of the nasal cavity and nasopharynx. The palate consists of two regions: the **hard palate** anteriorly and the **soft palate** posteriorly. The soft palate ends posteriorly as a midline extension, the **uvula**.

Figure A depicts the bones of the hard palate, whereas Figure B depicts the structures of the soft palate and neurovasculature with the oral mucosa removed.

COLOR each of the following structures using a different color for each:

Bones of the Hard Palate

○ 1. **Palatine process of the maxilla** (A only): Bilateral, horizontal projections forming the anterior two-thirds hard palate that meet in the midline at the **intermaxillary suture**

  ○ 2. **Incisive fossa:** Midline depression posterior to the central incisors into which the incisive canals open

○ 3. **Horizontal process of palatine** (A only): Bilateral, horizontal projections forming the posterior one-third hard palate that meet in the midline at the **median palatine suture**

  ○ 4. **Greater palatine foramen** (A only): Located medial to the third maxillary molar

  Posterior nasal spine: Posteriorly directed, midline extension

○ 5. **Pyramidal process of palatine bone** (A only): Small posterior projection that fills the inferior gap between the **medial** and **lateral pterygoid plates**

  ○ 6. **Lesser palatine foramen** (A only): Located posterior to the greater palatine foramen

Soft Palate and Neurovasculature

○ 7. **Tensor veli palatini muscle** (B only): Originates from the **scaphoid fossa**, changes direction 90° at the **hamulus of the medial pterygoid plate** forming the palatine aponeurosis

○ 8. **Palatine aponeurosis** (B only): Formed by the tendon of tensor veli palatini and permits the soft palate to tense during swallowing

○ 9. **Greater palatine nerves** (B only): Branches of CN V$_2$ that emerge through the greater palatine foramen and course anteriorly to supply the gingiva, oral mucosa, and glands of most of the hard palate

○10. **Nasopalatine nerve** (B only): Branch of CN V$_2$ that emerges through the incisive canal into the incisive fossa to supply the anterior hard palate posterior to the incisors

○11. **Lesser palatine nerve** (B only): Branch of CN V$_2$ emerges through the lesser palatine foramen and courses posteriorly to supply the structures of the soft palate

○12. **Greater palatine artery** (B only): Emerges through the greater palatine foramen and travels with the greater palatine nerve

○13. **Lesser palatine artery** (B only): Emerges either through the greater or lesser palatine foramen and travels with the lesser palatine nerve

○14. **Posterior septal branch of sphenopalatine artery** (B only): Courses along the nasal septum to emerge with nasopalatine nerve through the incisive canal into the incisive fossa

---

CLINICAL NOTE: NASOPALATINE AND GREATER PALATINE NERVE BLOCKS

The nasopalatine nerves can be anesthetized by injecting an anesthetic drug into the incisive fossa, and the greater palatine nerve can be anesthetized by injecting an anesthetic drug near the greater palatine foramen. Blanching of the surrounding palatal mucosa and/or gingiva may occur because the anesthetic results in vasoconstriction of the arteries that travel with the nerves.

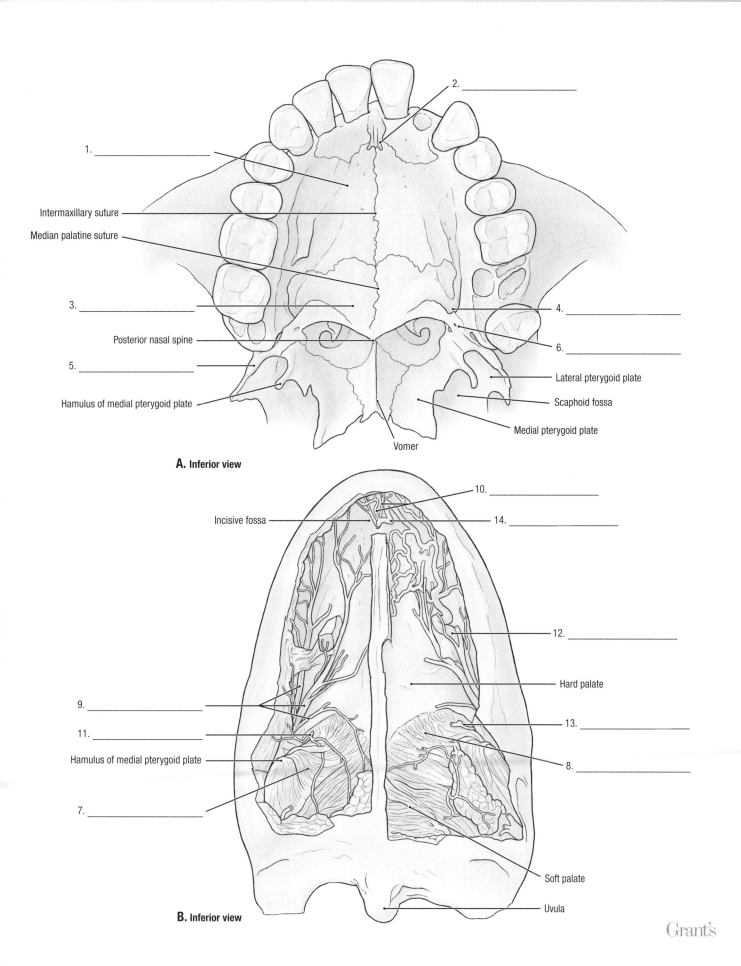

1. _____

2. _____

Intermaxillary suture

Median palatine suture

3. _____

Posterior nasal spine

4. _____

6. _____

Lateral pterygoid plate

5. _____

Scaphoid fossa

Hamulus of medial pterygoid plate

Medial pterygoid plate

Vomer

A. Inferior view

10. _____

Incisive fossa

14. _____

12. _____

Hard palate

9. _____

13. _____

11. _____

Hamulus of medial pterygoid plate

8. _____

7. _____

Soft palate

Uvula

B. Inferior view

Grant's

7.20A and B BONES OF THE NASAL WALL AND SEPTUM

The nasal cavity begins anteriorly at the nares (nostrils) and ends posteriorly at the choanae, or the open doorway through which the nasal cavity communicates with the nasopharynx.

The nasal cavity is divided by the nasal septum and communicates with paranasal sinuses and the lacrimal sac.

Figure A depicts the bones of the lateral wall, whereas Figure B depicts the bones of the nasal septum.

COLOR each of the following structures using a different color for each:

Bones of the Lateral Wall (Figure A)

○ 1. *Maxilla:* Forms most of the anterior aspect of the lateral wall
Frontal process: Articulates with the frontal bone along the lateral aspect of the nose
Palatine process: Forms the anterior portion of the floor of the nasal cavity and a portion of the *nasal crest* (see Figure B)
Anterior nasal spine: Anterior extension of the palatine process

○ 2. *Palatine:* Forms most of the posterior aspect of the lateral wall
Perpendicular plate: Vertical portion forming lateral wall of nasal cavity and medial wall of the pterygopalatine fossa and lies anterior to the *medial pterygoid plate*

　○ 3. *Sphenopalatine foramen:* Located in the superior aspect of perpendicular plate for the passage of the sphenopalatine artery and nasopalatine nerve from the pterygopalatine fossa
Horizontal plate: Forms the posterior portion of the floor of the nasal cavity and a portion of the *nasal crest* (see Figure B)
Greater palatine foramen: Opening of the greater palatine canal onto the horizontal plate

○ 4. *Ethmoid:* Forms the superior aspect of the lateral wall
Superior concha: Medial process of the ethmoid located inferior to the *cribriform plate* and anterior to the sphenoid sinus
Middle concha: Medial process of the ethmoid located inferior to the superior concha

○ 5. *Inferior concha:* Longest and broadest of the conchae inferior to the middle concha and is its own bone

Bones of the Nasal Septum (Figure B)

○ 6. *Perpendicular plate of the ethmoid:* Descends from the cribriform plate, forming the superior portion of the nasal septum. Extends superiorly into the anterior cranial fossa as the *crista galli.* Articulates with the *frontal bone* and *body of sphenoid* as well as the vomer and septal nasal cartilage.

○ 7. *Vomer:* Forms posteroinferior aspects of the nasal septum along with the nasal crest

○ 8. *Septal nasal cartilage:* Forms the anterior portion of the nasal septum

> **CLINICAL NOTE: DEVIATED NASAL SEPTUM**
> Most individuals have a slightly deviated septum without symptoms. Deviation usually occurs due to trauma, but can also occur during birth. On occasion, the deviation is severe enough that the nasal septum is in contact with one of the lateral nasal walls. Obstructed breathing and snoring often occur with severe septal deviation that can be surgically corrected.

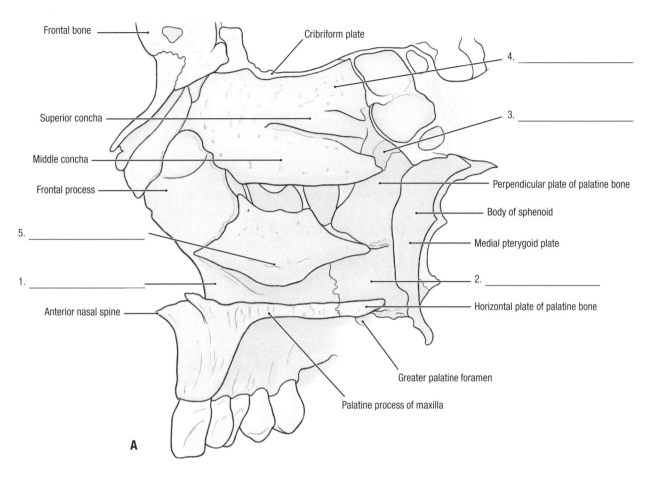

Frontal bone

Cribriform plate

4. _____

3. _____

Superior concha

Middle concha

Frontal process

Perpendicular plate of palatine bone

Body of sphenoid

Medial pterygoid plate

5. _____

1. _____

2. _____

Anterior nasal spine

Horizontal plate of palatine bone

Greater palatine foramen

Palatine process of maxilla

A

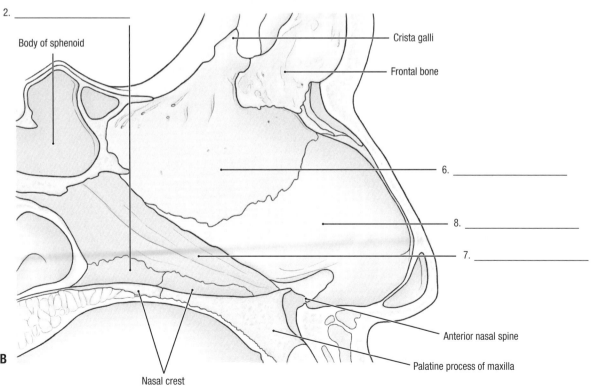

2. _____

Body of sphenoid

Crista galli

Frontal bone

6. _____

8. _____

7. _____

Anterior nasal spine

Palatine process of maxilla

Nasal crest

B

Grant's

7.21 NASAL CONCHAE AND MEATUSES

The lateral wall is marked by the formation of conchae, scroll-like convoluted structures that increase the surface area of the respiratory mucosa. Inferior to each of the conchae lies a nasal meatus (space). The paranasal sinuses and the lacrimal sac empty their contents into these meatuses.

This image depicts the medial view of the right half of the head.

COLOR each of the following structures using a different color for each:

○ 1. *Nasal vestibule:* Area immediately internal to the nares where a variable number of stiff hairs are located

○ 2. *Atrium:* Space located superior to the vestibule and anterior to the middle meatus

○ 3. *Superior concha:* Small and variable medial projection located anterior to the *sphenoid sinus*

○ 4. *Middle concha:* Medial projection locater inferior to the superior concha

○ 5. *Inferior concha:* Medial projection located inferior to the middle concha posterior to the nasal vestibule

○ 6. *Sphenoethmoidal recess:* Located posterosuperior to the superior concha

○ 7. *Superior nasal meatus:* Narrow space between the superior and middle concha

○ 8. *Middle nasal meatus:* Longer and wider space located between the middle and inferior concha

○ 9. *Inferior nasal meatus:* Horizontal space located inferior to the inferior concha and superior to the hard palate

---

CLINICAL NOTE: VISUALIZATION OF ADENOIDS THROUGH THE INFERIOR NASAL MEATUS

Inflammation of the pharyngeal tonsils, or adenoids, located in the nasopharynx posterosuperior to the *opening of the pharyngotympanic tube* can obstruct air from the nasal cavities through the choanae into the nasopharynx. Enlarged adenoids are the primary cause of snoring in children. Endoscopy through the nares into the inferior nasal meatus is noninvasive and provides direct visualization of the adenoids.

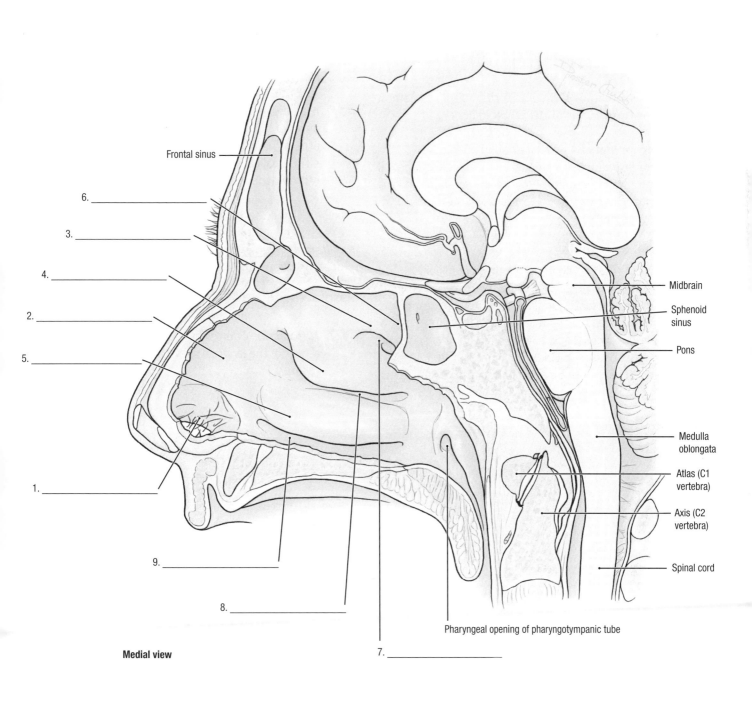

Frontal sinus

6. _____

3. _____

4. _____

2. _____

5. _____

1. _____

Midbrain

Sphenoid sinus

Pons

Medulla oblongata

Atlas (C1 vertebra)

Axis (C2 vertebra)

Spinal cord

9. _____

8. _____

Pharyngeal opening of pharyngotympanic tube

Medial view

7. _____

7.22 OPENINGS OF THE PARANASAL SINUSES AND NASOLACRIMAL DUCT

The paranasal sinuses are air-filled extensions of the nasal cavity into the frontal, sphenoid, ethmoid, and maxilla. Each paranasal sinus is named for the bone in which it resides. Paranasal sinuses continue to expand throughout life.

In this image, portions of the nasal concha have been cut away to view the openings of the paranasal sinuses. Rods represent the pathway from the sinuses to their respective openings. A small rod has also been forced through the lateral wall of the inferior meatus.

COLOR each of the following structures using a different color for each:

Middle Meatus

The middle nasal meatus is unique in that within its lateral wall are further formations of the ethmoid bone:

○ 1. **Semilunar hiatus:** Crescent-shaped opening
○ 2. **Ethmoidal bulla:** Bulge created by the middle ethmoidal cells along the superior border of the semilunar hiatus
○ 3. **Uncinate process:** Curved projection anteroinferior to semilunar hiatus

Paranasal Sinus Openings

○ 4. **Frontal sinus:** Lies posterior to the superciliary arches and root of the nose. Drains via the **frontonasal duct** into the ethmoidal infundibulum, which opens into the semilunar hiatus of the middle nasal meatus.
○ 5. **Sphenoidal sinus:** Located within the body of sphenoid bone and unevenly divided by a thin septum into right and left sinuses. Drains into the **sphenoethmoidal recess**.

○ 6. **Posterior ethmoidal air cells:** Open directly into the superior meatus. The ethmoid sinuses are multiple and are subdivided into anterior, middle, and posterior. The anterior ethmoidal cells drain to the middle nasal meatus through the ethmoidal infundibulum. The middle ethmoidal cells drain by mutliple small openings on the ethmoidal bulla into the middle nasal meatus.

Maxillary sinus: Largest of the paranasal sinuses and its medial wall is the lateral wall of the nasal cavity. Drains via the **maxillary orifice (ostium) into the semilunar hiatus** of the middle meatus.

Nasolacrimal Duct

○ 7. **Nasolacrimal duct:** Courses inferiorly from the inferior aspect of the lacrimal sac to open into the inferior nasal meatus

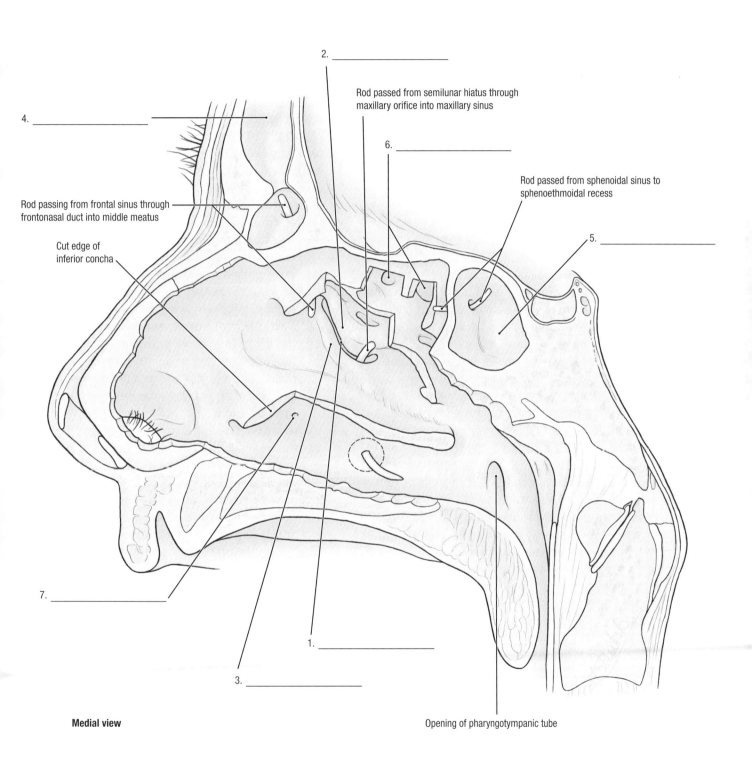

2. _____

Rod passed from semilunar hiatus through
maxillary orifice into maxillary sinus

4. _____

6. _____

Rod passed from sphenoidal sinus to
sphenoethmoidal recess

Rod passing from frontal sinus through
frontonasal duct into middle meatus

5. _____

Cut edge of
inferior concha

7. _____

1. _____

3. _____

Medial view

Opening of pharyngotympanic tube

Grant's

The pterygopalatine fossa is a small pyramidal space inferior to the apex of the orbit and medial to the infratemporal fossa. The terminal portion of the maxillary artery and its branches along with the maxillary nerve (CN V$_2$) course through the pterygopalatine fossa.

In this schematic, the pterygopalatine fossa is viewed from the infratemporal fossa along with the pathways of the branches of CN V$_2$. The lateral wall of the orbit and middle cranial fossa have been removed. A portion of the lateral wall of the *maxillary sinus* has also been removed.

COLOR each of the following structures using a different color for each:

○ 1. **Maxillary nerve (CN V$_2$):** Runs anteriorly through the foramen rotundum into the posterior aspect of the pterygopalatine fossa. Before entering the foramen rotundum, a small **meningeal branch** arises from CN V$_2$. Supplies sensory innervation to the nasal cavity, palate, tonsils, and maxillary gingivae.

○ 2. **Pterygopalatine ganglion:** Parasympathetic ganglion suspended by CN V$_2$ in the pterygopalatine fossa. Contains postsynaptic parasympathetic cell bodies that receive information from the greater petrosal nerve from the facial nerve (CN VII). Sensory fibers from CN V$_2$ and sympathetic fibers from the deep petrosal nerve pass through the pterygopalatine ganglion without synapsing.

○ 3. **Greater palatine nerve:** Courses inferiorly through the pterygopalatine fossa and exits via the palatine canal. Emerges onto the hard palate via the greater palatine foramen to innervate the palatal oral mucosa and palatal gingiva posterior to the maxillary canines.

○ 4. **Lesser palatine nerve:** Courses inferiorly through the pterygopalatine fossa exiting via the palatine canal. Emerges onto the soft palate via the lesser palatine foramen to supply the oral mucosa and glands of soft palate, uvula, and palatine tonsil.

○ 5. **Posterior superior alveolar nerve:** Exits the pterygopalatine fossa via the pterygomaxillary fissure into the infratemporal fossa. Courses along the posterior aspect of the maxilla, with some branches entering the posterior superior alveolar foramina, joining the **superior dental plexus**, and supplying most of the maxillary molars and maxillary sinus. The remaining branches do not enter

foramina and supply the vestibular (buccal) maxillary gingiva.

○ 6. **Infraorbital nerve:** Terminal branch of CN V$_2$ that enters the inferior orbital fissure and passes into the infraorbital canal. Gives rise to the middle and anterior superior alveolar nerves.

○ 7. **Middle superior alveolar nerve:** When present, arises from the infraorbital nerve, courses through the lateral wall of the maxillary sinus, joining the superior dental plexus and supplying the maxillary premolars, maxillary sinus, and maxillary vestibular (buccal) gingiva

○ 8. **Anterior superior alveolar nerve:** Arises from the infraorbital nerve proximal to the infraorbital foramen, courses through the anterior wall of the maxillary sinus joining the superior dental plexus and supplying maxillary canines and incisors and maxillary sinus.

○ 9. **Zygomatic nerve:** arises from CN V$_2$ within the pterygopalatine fossa. The zygomatic nerve divides into the zygomaticofacial and zygomaticotemporal nerves.

○10. **Communicating branch:** Arises from the zygomaticotemporal nerve and courses superiorly through bone to the lateral aspect of the orbit where it "hitches a ride" onto the lacrimal nerve. Postsynaptic parasympathetic fibers from the pterygopalatine ganglion travel on the zygomatic nerve, to the zygomaticotemporal nerve and then the communicating branch, to reach the **lacrimal nerve** (CN V$_1$ branch) to innervate the **lacrimal gland**.

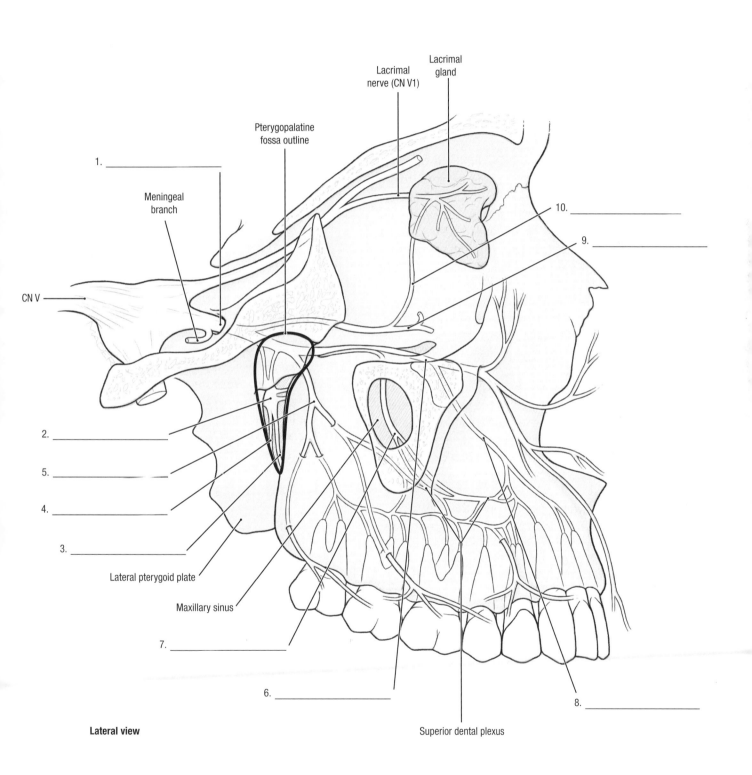

Lacrimal
nerve (CN V1)

Lacrimal
gland

Pterygopalatine
fossa outline

1. _____

Meningeal
branch

10. _____

9. _____

CN V

2. _____

5. _____

4. _____

3. _____

Lateral pterygoid plate

Maxillary sinus

7. _____

6. _____

8. _____

Lateral view

Superior dental plexus

Grant's

7.24 EXTERNAL, MIDDLE, AND INTERNAL EAR: CORONALLY SECTIONED

The ear is divided into the external, middle, and internal portions. The external and middle ear are mostly involved with hearing (transmitting sound), whereas the internal ear is involved with both hearing and balance (equilibrium).

This image depicts a coronal section through the right ear.

COLOR each of the following structures using a different color for each:

External Ear

The external ear is composed of the auricle and external acoustic meatus.

○ 1. *Auricle:* Irregular-shaped cartilage composed of several depressions and elevations located external to the external acoustic meatus

○ 2. *Concha:* Deepest of the depressions of the auricle that leads to the opening of the external acoustic meatus

○ 3. *External acoustic meatus:* Canal that leads through the tympanic part of the temporal bone from the auricle to the tympanic membrane

○ 4. *Tympanic membrane:* Thin, oval membrane at the end of the external acoustic meatus that forms the boundary between the external and middle portions of the ear

Middle Ear

The middle ear lies between the tympanic membrane and labyrinthine (medial) wall and contains the ossicles (malleus, incus, and stapes). The space of the middle ear is divided into two parts: the ***tympanic cavity*** that lies immediately internal to the tympanic membrane and the ***epitympanic recess*** that lies superior to the tympanic membrane.

○ 5. *Head of the malleus:* Extends into the epitympanic recess. The neck and handle of the malleus are attached to the tympanic membrane. The head of the malleus articulates with the incus and the incus articulates with the stapes.

○ 6. *Tensor tympani muscle:* Short muscle that attaches to the handle of the malleus. Pulls the tympanic membrane medially, tensing it, and reducing the amplitude of its oscillations. Innervated by CN V_3.

○ 7. *Pharyngotympanic (auditory) tube:* Connects the middle ear to the nasopharynx and equalizes pressure in the middle ear with atmospheric pressure allowing the tympanic membrane to move freely

Internal Ear

The inner ear is housed within the petrous portion of the temporal bone and contains the vestibulocochlear organ.

○ 8. *Cochlea:* Shell-shaped part of the bony labyrinth

○ 9. *Vestibulocochlear nerve (CN VIII):* Enters the internal ear via the ***internal acoustic meatus*** and remains within the internal ear

○10. *Facial nerve (CN VII):* Enters the internal ear via the internal acoustic meatus and then travels through the facial canal within the temporal bone

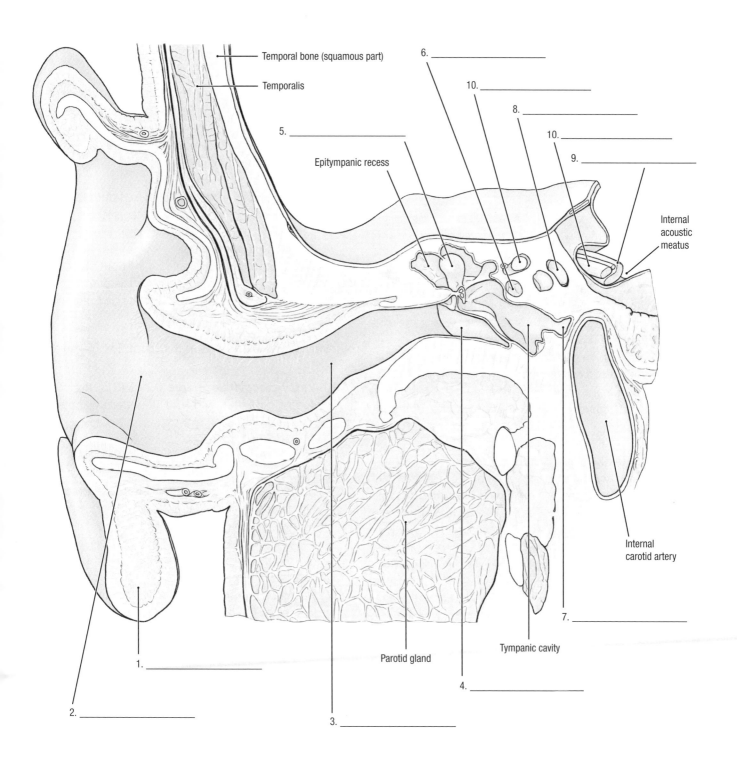

Temporal bone (squamous part)

Temporalis

6. _____

10. _____

8. _____

5. _____

10. _____

Epitympanic recess

9. _____

Internal acoustic meatus

Internal carotid artery

1. _____

2. _____

Parotid gland

3. _____

Tympanic cavity

4. _____

7. _____

Grant's

In Figure A, the tegmen tympani (roof) has been removed to expose the epitympanic recess of the middle ear. The arcuate eminence has been removed to reveal the inner ear and the course of CN VII and VIII. In Figure B, the membranous labyrinth (within a transparent otic capsule) has been isolated. The otic capsule is composed of bone that is denser than the surrounding petrous temporal bone.

COLOR each of the following structures using a different color for each:

Middle Ear

○ 1. *Malleus* (A only): The superior, rounded head extends into the epitympanic recess
○ 2. *Incus* (A only): Articulates with the malleus at the *incudomalleolar joint*

Stapes (not shown): smallest of the ossicles. The base (footplate) fits into the *oval window* of the medial wall of the tympanic cavity.

Internal Ear

The internal ear is composed of bony and membranous labyrinths. The bony labyrinth is a series of cavities within the otic capsule including the cochlea, vestibule, and semicircular canals and is filled with perilymph (similar to extracellular fluid). The membranous labyrinth consists of a series of communicating sacs and ducts that are suspended within the bony labyrinth. The membranous labyrinth contains endolymph (similar to intracellular fluid).

○ 3. *Cochlea* (A only): Portion of bony labyrinth for hearing. The *cochlear (spiral) canal* begins at the vestibule and makes 2.5 turns around a bony core, the *modiolus*. The cochlear canal also features the *round window,* which is closed off by *secondary tympanic membrane*.
○ 4. *Cochlear duct* (B only): Portion of the membranous labyrinth within the cochlear canal. Spiral tube that is closed at one end and suspended with the cochlear canal by the spiral ligament on the external wall of the canal and the *spiral lamina* of the modiolus along the internal wall.
○ 5. *Anterior (superior) semicircular canal* (A only): One of three semicircular canals that communicate with the vestibule of the bony labyrinth.
○ 6. *Semicircular duct* (B only): Component of the membranous labyrinth occupying the semicircular canals. Each semicircular duct has an *ampulla*, or swelling at one end.

The vestibule of the bony labyrinth is a small, oval chamber that features the oval window on its lateral wall. The vestibule is continuous with the cochlea anteriorly and the semicircular canals posteriorly. Two membranous labyrinth structures occupy the vestibule:

○ 7. *Utricle* (B only): Receives openings of the semicircular ducts and communicates with the saccule
○ 8. *Saccule* (B only): Continuous with the cochlear duct via the *ductus reuniens*
○ 9. *Endolymphatic sac* (B only): Blind pouch located under dura on the posterior surface of the petrous temporal bone and communicates with the utricle and saccule via the endolymphatic duct

Nerves of the Middle and Internal Ear (Figure A)

○10. *Vestibulocochlear nerve* (*CN VIII*): Enters internal acoustic meatus with CN VII where it immediately divides into the following:
 ○11. *Cochlear nerve*
 ○12. *Vestibular nerve*
○13. *Facial nerve* (*CN VII*): Enters the internal acoustic meatus, travels through the internal and middle ear within the facial canal, making a sharp bend (genu) shortly after entering the internal acoustic meatus. While traveling within the facial canal, the facial nerve gives rise to greater petrosal, stapedial, and chorda tympani nerves.
○14. *Geniculate ganglion:* Composed of sensory cell bodies located at the bend of the facial nerve
○15. *Greater petrosal nerve* (CN VII): Arises at the genu and is composed of presynaptic parasympathetic fibers to the pterygopalatine ganglion
○16. *Lesser petrosal nerve* (CN IX): Branches from the anterior aspect of the tympanic plexus formed by CN IX and is composed of presynaptic parasympathetic fibers to the otic ganglion

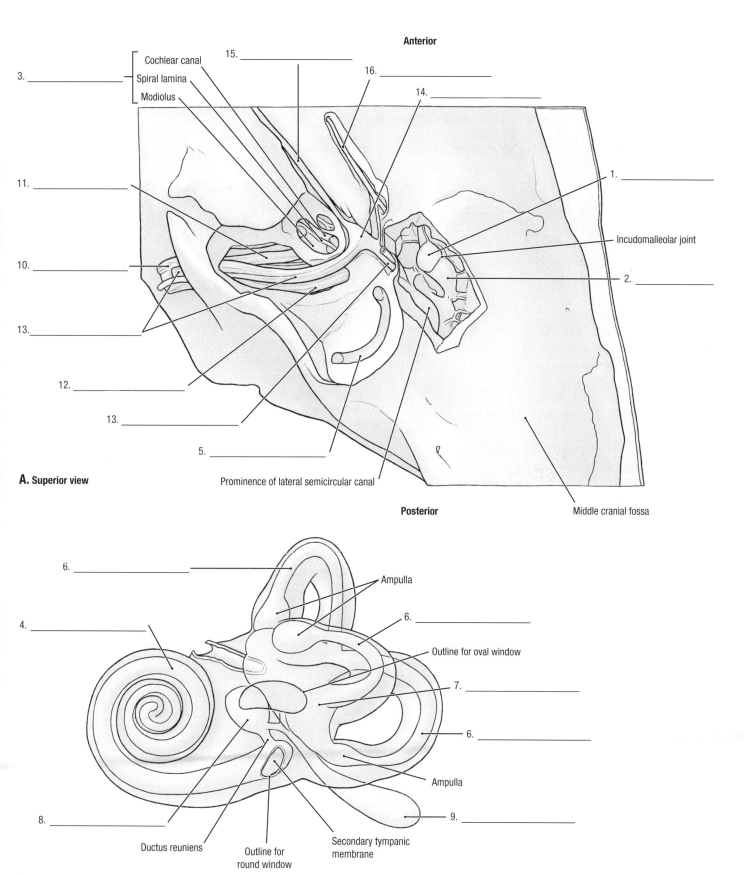

Anterior

Cochlear canal
Spiral lamina
Modiolus

3. _____

15. _____

16. _____

14. _____

1. _____

Incudomalleolar joint

2. _____

11. _____

10. _____

13. _____

12. _____

13. _____

5. _____

A. Superior view

Prominence of lateral semicircular canal

Posterior

Middle cranial fossa

6. _____

Ampulla

4. _____

6. _____

Outline for oval window

7. _____

6. _____

Ampulla

8. _____

9. _____

Ductus reuniens

Outline for round window

Secondary tympanic membrane

B. Anterolateral view of left membranous labyrinth (through transparent otic capsule)

Grant's

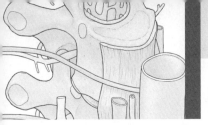

CHAPTER 8

Neck

8.1A, B, and C   BONES OF THE NECK

The bones of the neck are formed mainly by the cervical vertebrae and hyoid bone. Inferiorly, the manubrium of the sternum and the clavicles provide attachments for muscles and protection for cervical structures.

COLOR each of the following structures using a different color for each:

Hyoid Bone (Figure A)

The hyoid bone does not articulate with any other bones, which is a unique feature among the bones of the body. The hyoid lies in the anterior neck at the level of the C3 vertebra and is attached via muscles and/or ligaments to the mandible, thyroid cartilage, styloid process, manubrium, and scapulae.

○ 1. *Body:* Faces anteriorly lying in the middle of the hyoid
○ 2. *Greater horn:* Extends posterosuperiorly from each lateral end of the body
   Fibrocartilage: In younger individuals unites the greater horns to the body
○ 3. *Lesser horn:* Small projection from the superior aspect of the body near the union with the greater horn

Cervical Vertebrae (Figures B and C)

The cervical region of the vertebral column is composed of seven vertebrae. The region has the greatest range and variety of movement of all the vertebral regions due to their nearly horizontal orientation of the articular facets, small bodies, and thicker *intervertebral discs* relative to the vertebral bodies. Unique features of cervical vertebrae are described below:

○ 4. *Transverse foramen (foramen transversarium):* Oval shaped and located in each of the *transverse processes*. The vertebral part of the vertebral artery ascends from the subclavian artery through the transverse foramina from C6 to C1. Typically, only small accessory veins course through the C7 transverse foramen.
○ 5. *Groove for vertebral artery:* Located on the posterior arch of the atlas where the suboccipital portion of the vertebral artery travels after ascending through the transverse foramina and prior to entering the foramen magnum
○ 6. *Anterior tubercle of transverse process:* Anterior lateral end of the transverse process
○ 7. *Carotid tubercle:* Anterior tubercles of C6 named so due to the ability to compress the common carotid artery between them and the body to control bleeding
○ 8. *Posterior tubercle of transverse process:* Posterior lateral end of the transverse process
○ 9. *Anterior tubercle of C1:* Located in the center of the anterior aspect of the *anterior arch*
○10. *Posterior tubercle of C1:* Located in the center of the posterior aspect of the posterior arch
○11. *Dens (odontoid process) of C2:* Projects superiorly from the body and is encircled by C1

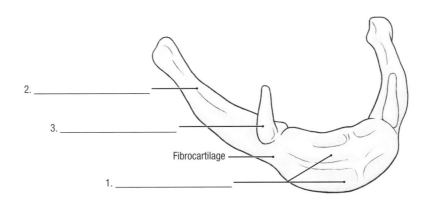

2. _____

3. _____

Fibrocartilage _____

1. _____

A. Right anterolateral view of hyoid bone

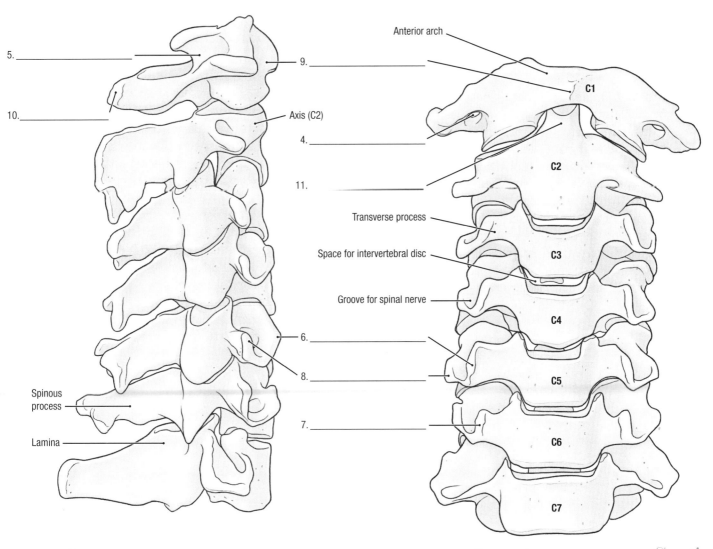

5. _____

10. _____

9. _____

Axis (C2)

4. _____

11. _____

Anterior arch

C1

C2

Transverse process

Space for intervertebral disc

C3

Groove for spinal nerve

C4

6. _____

8. _____

C5

Spinous process

7. _____

C6

Lamina

C7

B. Lateral view

C. Anterior view

Grant's

8.2 LATERAL CERVICAL REGION, SUPERFICIAL

The lateral cervical region, or posterior triangle, is located posterior to the sternocleidomastoid (SCM) muscle and anterior to the trapezius. Branches of the cervical plexus and subclavian artery pass through this region along with the external jugular vein and spinal accessory nerve (CN XI).

The overlying skin and subcutaneous tissue have been removed in this image along with the investing layer of the deep cervical fascia, which forms the roof of the lateral cervical region. Portions of the platysma have been cut to reveal the deeper structures.

COLOR each of the following structures using a different color for each:

Boundaries of the Lateral Cervical Region

○ 1. *Sternocleidomastoid:* Posterior edge forms the anterior boundary
○ 2. *Trapezius:* Anterior edge forms the posterior boundary
○ 3. *Clavicle:* Middle third forms the inferior boundary
○ 4. *Prevertebral layer of deep cervical fascia:* Forms the floor

Superior nuchal line: Located on the occipital bone where the SCM and trapezius muscles meet, forming the apex

Neurovasculature of the Lateral Cervical Region

○ 5. *External jugular vein:* Begins near the angle of the mandible and crosses SCM obliquely deep to *platysma* to enter the anteroinferior portion of the lateral cervical region and terminate into the subclavian vein
○ 6. *Spinal accessory nerve (CN XI):* Courses deep to SCM and supplies it before emerging into the lateral cervical region. Then passes posteroinferiorly deep to the investing layer of the deep cervical fascia to pass deep to the anterior border of the trapezius to supply it.
○ 7. *Occipital artery:* Courses through the apex of the lateral cervical region with the greater occipital nerve, which arises near the suboccipital triangle (posterior neck)

Cutaneous branches of the cervical plexus emerge from one location about midway along the posterior border of the SCM referred to as the nerve point of the neck. These branches supply sensory innervation to the skin of the neck, superolateral thoracic wall, and scalp between the auricle and external occipital protuberance. Additionally, the *nerve to trapezius* forms from C3 to C4 and supplies pain and proprioceptive innervation.

○ 8. *Great auricular nerve:* Arises from C2 to C3, emerges from the posterior border of SCM, and courses superiorly along the superficial aspect of SCM with the external jugular vein to the inferior aspect of the *parotid gland.* Supplies the skin over the angle of the mandible, auricle, and mastoid process along with the parotid sheath surrounding the parotid gland.
○ 9. *Transverse cervical nerve:* Arises from C2 to C3 and emerges from the posterior border of SCM inferior to the great auricular nerve. Courses along the superficial aspect of SCM deep to the external jugular vein and *platysma*. Supplies the skin covering the anterior cervical region.
○ 10. *Supraclavicular nerves:* Arise from C3 to C4 as a common trunk deep to SCM; divide into *medial*, *intermediate*, and *lateral* branches that pass over the clavicle and toward the shoulder, supplying the skin of those areas
○ 11. *Lesser occipital nerve:* Arises from C2 and emerges from the posterior border of SCM superior to the great auricular nerve. Courses superiorly along the posterior border of SCM to supply the skin posterosuperior to the auricle.

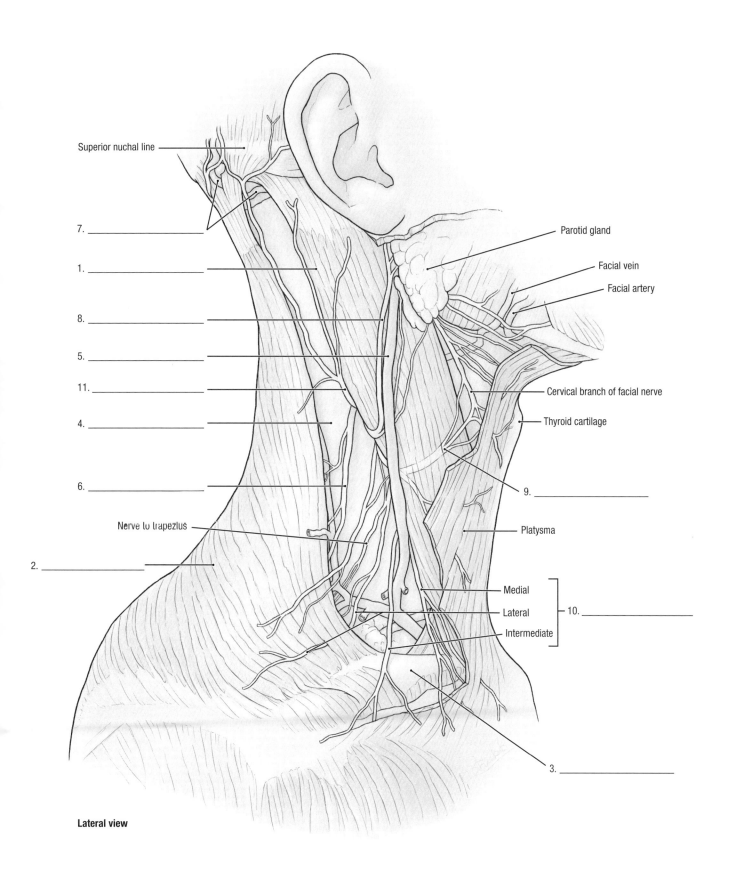

Superior nuchal line

7. _____

1. _____

8. _____

5. _____

11. _____

4. _____

6. _____

Nerve to trapezius

2. _____

Parotid gland

Facial vein

Facial artery

Cervical branch of facial nerve

Thyroid cartilage

9. _____

Platysma

Medial

Lateral   10. _____

Intermediate

3. _____

Lateral view

Grant's

The prevertebral layer of the deep cervcial fascia has been removed to reveal the underlying muscles. The middle third of the **clavicle** has been cut away along with the clavipectoral fascia covering the deltopectoral triangle between the **deltoid** and the **pectoralis major**. The **supraclavicular nerves** and **external jugular vein** have been cut as they cross the lateral cervical region.

COLOR each of the following structures using a different color for each:

Muscles of the Lateral Cervical Region

◯ 1. *Inferior belly of omohyoid*: Divides the lateral cervical region into the occipital triangle (superior) and the omo-clavicular or subclavian triangle (inferiorly). **Omohyoid fascia** covers the omoclavicular triangle. The inferior belly is separated from **the superior belly of omohyoid** by an intermediate tendon.

Four to five muscles typically form the floor of the lateral cervical region:

◯ 2. *Splenius capitis:* Located near the apex of the lateral cervical region between the **trapezius** and the **SCM**

◯ 3. *Levator scapulae:* Located anteroinferior to the splenius capitus

◯ 4. *Posterior scalene:* Located anteroinferior to the levator scapulae

◯ 5. *Middle scalene:* Located anterior to the levator scapulae and posterior scalene

◯ 6. *Anterior scalene:* Located anterior to the middle scalene

Neurovasculature of the Lateral Cervical Region

◯ 7. *Spinal accessory nerve (CN XI):* Lies superficial to the levator scapulae muscle

◯ 8. *Brachial plexus:* The roots separate the anterior and middle scalene muscles

◯ 9. *Phrenic nerve:* Arises from C3 to C5 and travels along the superficial surface of the anterior scalene

◯10. *Cervicodorsal trunk:* Branch of the subclavian artery that crosses the lateral cervical region. Also known as the transverse cervical artery.

CLINICAL NOTE: CERVICAL PLEXUS BLOCKS

A superficial cervical plexus block is indicated for superficial neck procedures such as cervical lymph node removal or carotid endarterectomy. The injection site is determined by locating the nerve point of the neck at the midpoint of the posterior border of SCM by first palpating the mastoid process and clavicular attachment of SCM. The sensory branches of the cervical plexus are typically affected, resulting in anesthesia of the anterolateral neck and periauricular area. Since ansa cervicalis and phrenic nerves course deep to SCM, they are typically not affected by a superficial cervical block. A deep cervical block administered at the C2-C4 intervertebral foramina and directly affecting the spinal roots would block the sensory and motor components of the cervical plexus.

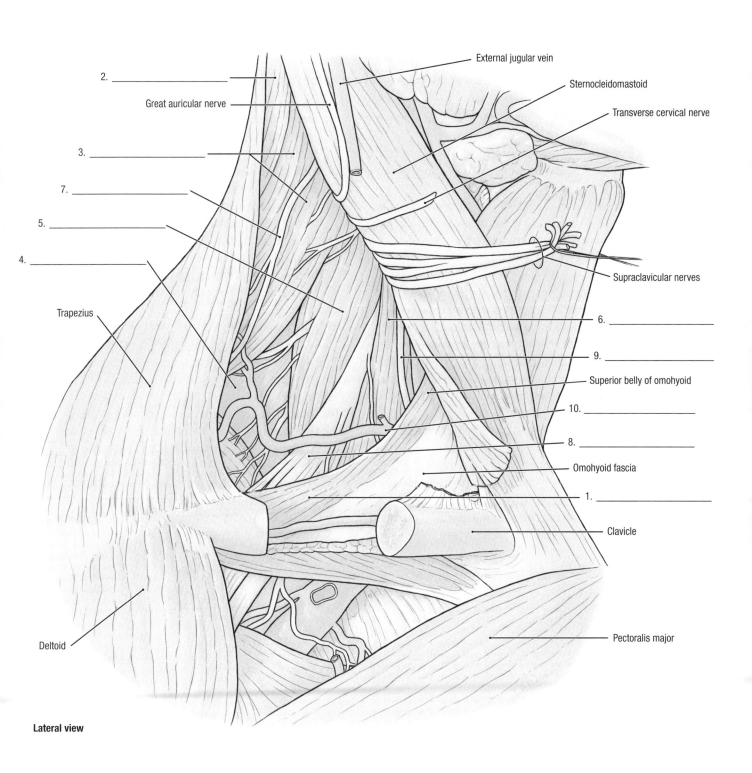

2. _____

Great auricular nerve _____

3. _____

7. _____

5. _____

4. _____

Trapezius

Deltoid

External jugular vein

Sternocleidomastoid

Transverse cervical nerve

Supraclavicular nerves

6. _____

9. _____

Superior belly of omohyoid

10. _____

8. _____

Omohyoid fascia

1. _____

Clavicle

Pectoralis major

Lateral view

Grant's

The omohyoid and omohyoid fascia have been removed to demonstrate the structures coursing through the omoclavicular (subclavian) triangle.

COLOR each of the following structures using a different color for each:

○ 1. **Anterior scalene:** Lies between the subclavian artery and the vein

○ 2. **Middle scalene:** Lies posterior to roots of the brachial plexus and pierced by **branches of anterior ramus of C5**

○ 3. **Brachial plexus:** Formed by the **anterior rami** of **C5**, **C6**, **C7**, **C8**, and **T1**. The roots of the brachial plexus course between the anterior and middle scalenes and then form the superior, middle, and inferior trunks superior to the **clavicle**.

○ 4. **Subclavian artery:** Courses between the anterior and middle scalenes with the roots of the brachial plexus. Can be subdivided into three parts based on the anterior scalene: first part located medial, second part located posterior, and third part located lateral. The third portion passes through the omoclavicular triangle and then changes names to **axillary artery** as it passes the first rib.

○ 5. **Cervicodorsal artery:** Crosses the phrenic nerve superficially and then crosses or passes through the trunks of the brachial plexus. When present, terminates as the superficial cervical artery and dorsal scapular artery.

○ 6. **Dorsal scapular artery:** Arises either as a branch of the cervicodorsal artery or as an independent branch from the third part of the subclavian artery. When it is an independent branch, courses through the trunks of the brachial plexus. Regardless of its origin, runs deep to the levator scapulae and rhomboids, supplying them.

○ 7. **Suprascapular artery:** Crosses the phrenic nerve superficially inferior to the cervicodorsal artery. Passes laterally deep to the clavicle with the suprascapular vein crossing the cords of the brachial plexus to reach the supraspinatus and infraspinatus muscles.

○ 8. **Suprascapular nerve:** Arises from the superior trunk of the brachial plexus; runs laterally across the lateral cervical region to supply supraspinatus and infraspinatus muscles.

○ 9. **Subclavian vein:** Courses through the inferior portion of the lateral cervical region, passing superficially to the anterior scalene muscle. Receives venous drainage from the **axillary vein** and typically from the external jugular vein.

○10. **Internal jugular vein:** Structure of the anterior cervical region, which joins the subclavian vein at the medial border of the anterior scalene to form the **brachiocephalic vein**

○11. **Phrenic nerve:** Lies anterior to the anterior scalene passing deep to the subclavian vein into the thoracic cavity. Crossed superficially by the suprascapular and cervicodorsal artery.

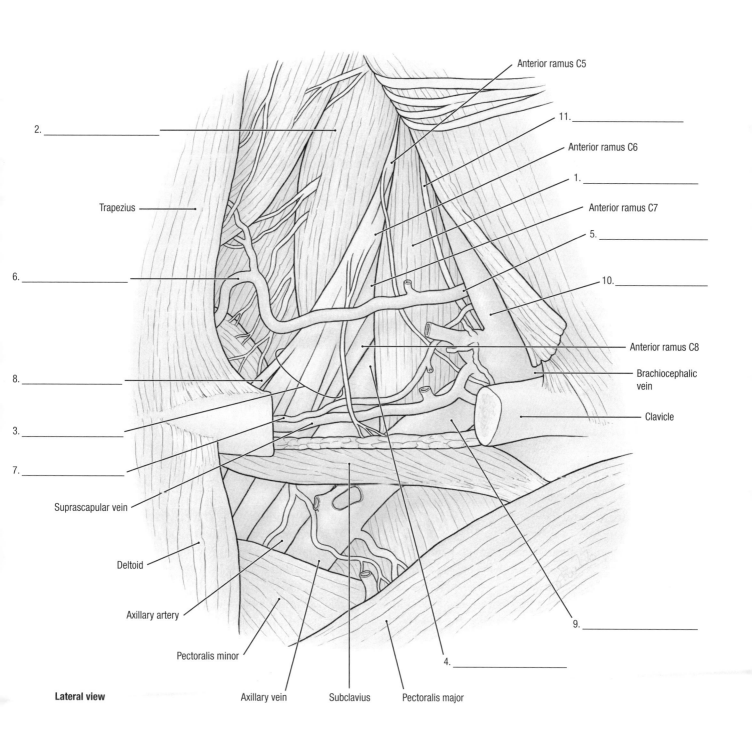

Anterior ramus C5

2. _____

11. _____

Anterior ramus C6

Trapezius ───

1. _____

Anterior ramus C7

5. _____

6. _____

10. _____

Anterior ramus C8

Brachiocephalic vein

8. _____

3. _____

Clavicle

7. _____

Suprascapular vein

Deltoid

Axillary artery

9. _____

Pectoralis minor

4. _____

Lateral view

Axillary vein   Subclavius   Pectoralis major

8.5 ANTERIOR CERVICAL REGION

The anterior cervical region (triangle) lies between the midline of the neck, the mandible, and the anterior border of the SCM. The digastric and omohyoid muscles subdivide the anterior cervical region into four triangles: submental, submandibular, muscular, and carotid.

In this image, the submental and muscular triangles are highlighted. The submental triangle is unpaired and lies inferior to the chin. The muscular triangle lies between the superior belly of the omohyoid, the anterior border of the SCM, and the median plane of the neck. The remaining two triangles are highlighted in figures in Sections 8.6, 8.10, and 8.11. The paired submandibular triangles lie between anterior and posterior bellies of the digastric and the mandible. The carotid triangle lies between the posterior belly of the digastric, superior belly of the omohyoid, and anterior border of SCM.

COLOR each of the following structures using a different color for each:

Boundaries of the Anterior Cervical Region

○ 1. *Sternocleidomastoid:* Anterior edge forms the posterior border
○ 2. *Mandible:* Inferior aspect forms the superior border
○ 3. *Manubrium:* Jugular notch forms the apex
○ 4. *Investing layer of deep cervical fascia:* Forms the roof
○ 5. *Visceral layer of pretracheal fascia:* Forms the floor

Submental and Submandibular Triangles

○ 6. *Anterior belly of digastric:* Paired muscle forming the lateral boundaries of the submental triangle and separates the submental and submandibular triangles
○ 7. *Mylohyoid muscle:* Paired muscle uniting in the midline by a fibrous ***median raphe***. Forms the boundary between the oral cavity and the submental and submandibular triangles.
○ 8. *Hyoid bone:* Forms the inferior boundary of the submental triangle
○ 9. *Submental lymph nodes:* Primary structures found within the submental triangle and receiving drainage from the mandibular incisors and gingivae, chin, middle of lower lip, and tip of the tongue. Drain to the submandibular and deep cervical nodes.
○ 10. *Submandibular gland (covered in fascia):* Almost fills the submandibular triangle and covered by the investing layer of the deep cervical fascia

Muscular Triangle

The muscular triangle contains the infrahyoid muscles along with thyroid and parathyroid glands. The infrahyoid muscles stabilize and depress the hyoid and larynx during swallowing and speaking. The infrahyoid muscles are arranged into superficial and deep layers. The superior belly of the omohyoid and sternohyoid lies in the superficial plane, whereas the sternohyoid and thyrohyoid (see figure in Section 8.6) lie in the deep plane.

○ 11. *Superior belly of omohyoid:* Paired muscle forming the superolateral boundary of the muscular triangle and separating the muscular and carotid triangles. Attaches to the inferior border of the hyoid and to the intermediate tendon of the omohyoid, which is connected to the clavicle via a fascial thickening.
○ 12. *Sternohyoid:* Paired muscle attaching to the body of the hyoid bone, the manubrium of the sternum, and the medial end of the clavicle
○ 13. *Sternothyroid:* Paired muscle lying deep to the sternohyoid. Attaches to the oblique line of the ***thyroid cartilage*** and the posterior surface of the manubrium of the sternum.
○ 14. *Anterior jugular vein:* Paired veins coursing through the subcutaneous tissue of the anterior neck and typically uniting the superior and the manubrium to form the ***jugular venous arch***

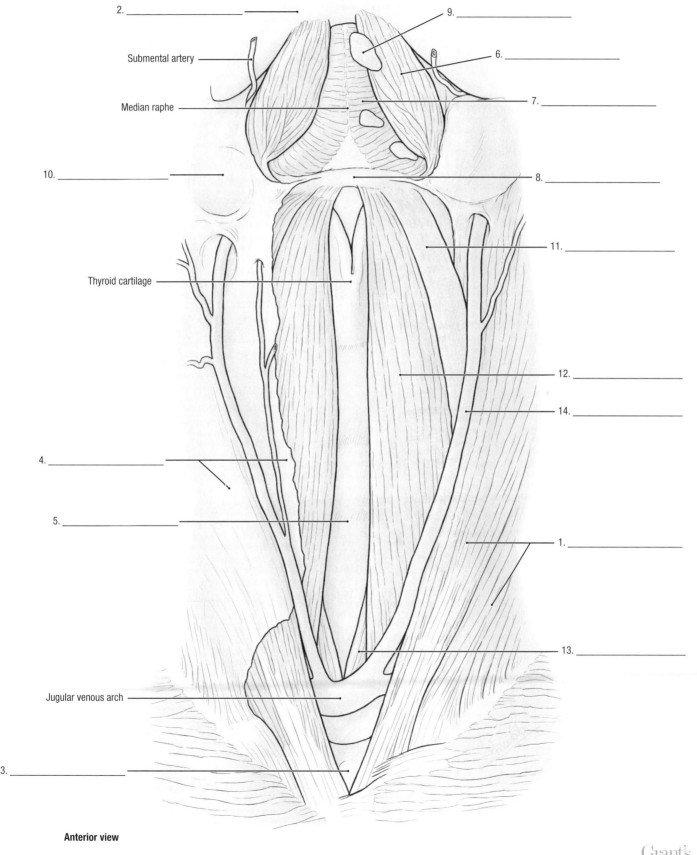

2. _____

Submental artery _____

Median raphe _____

10. _____

Thyroid cartilage _____

4. _____

5. _____

Jugular venous arch _____

3. _____

9. _____

6. _____

7. _____

8. _____

11. _____

12. _____

14. _____

1. _____

13. _____

Anterior view

8.6 ANTERIOR CERVICAL REGION, SUBMANDIBULAR TRIANGLE

The suprahyoid muscles include the mylohyoid, digastrics, stylohyoid, and geniohyoid muscles. The suprahyoid muscles elevate the *hyoid* and larynx during swallowing and speaking and also form the floor of the mouth, providing support for movements of the tongue.

In this image, a majority of the submandibular gland and a portion of the *body of the mandible* have been removed. The segment of the facial artery related to the submandibular gland has also been removed.

COLOR each of the following structures using a different color for each:

Boundaries of the Submandibular Triangle

○ 1. *Digastric, anterior belly:* Forms the medial boundary of the submandibular triangle and separates it from the submental triangle. Attaches to the digastric fossa of the mandible and the *intermediate tendon of digastric*, which is attached to the body and greater horn of the hyoid.

○ 2. *Mylohyoid:* Forms the floor of the submental and submandibular triangles and separates them from the oral cavity. Attaches to the mylohyoid line of the mandible and to the median raphe and the middle of the body of the hyoid.

○ 3. *Hyoglossus:* Forms the posteromedial aspect of the floor of the submandibular triangle. Attaches to the greater horn of the hyoid and inserts into intrinsic muscles of the tongue.

Body of mandible forms the superior boundary of the submandibular triangle; the posterior belly of the digastric (not shown) forms the posterolateral boundary as it attaches the intermediate tendon to the digastric (mastoid) notch of the temporal bone.

Contents of the Submandibular Triangle

○ 4. *Submandibular gland:* Superficial lobe of the gland almost completely fills the submandibular triangle. The deep lobe extends into the oral cavity superior to the posterior edge of the mylohyoid muscle. The *submandibular duct* is associated with the deep aspect of the gland.

○ 5. *Facial artery:* Branch of the external carotid artery that passes superiorly deep to the posterior belly of digastric and stylohyoid muscles. It then travels within the deep aspect of the superficial lobe of the submandibular gland supplying it. The facial artery then passes over the inferior border of the mandible to the face.

○ 6. *Submental artery:* Arises from the facial artery as it courses through the submandibular gland. Supplies structures of the floor of the mouth.

○ 7. *Hypoglossal nerve (CN XII):* Passes through the submandibular triangle and then enters the gap between hyoglossus and mylohyoid to enter the oral cavity

○ 8. *Nerve to thyrohyoid:* Branch of the anterior ramus of C1, which becomes bound to CN XII as it passes through the neck. Branches away from CN XII to innervate the *thyrohyoid* prior to CN XII entering the oral cavity.

○ 9. *Nerve to mylohyoid:* Branch of CN V_3 that arises from the inferior alveolar nerve prior to the mandibular foramen. Innervates the mylohyoid and anterior belly of the digastric.

○ 10. *Stylohyoid muscle:* Attaches to the styloid process and the body of the hyoid. Closely associated with the posterior belly of the digastric and often splits around the intermediate tendon of the digastric to attach to the hyoid.

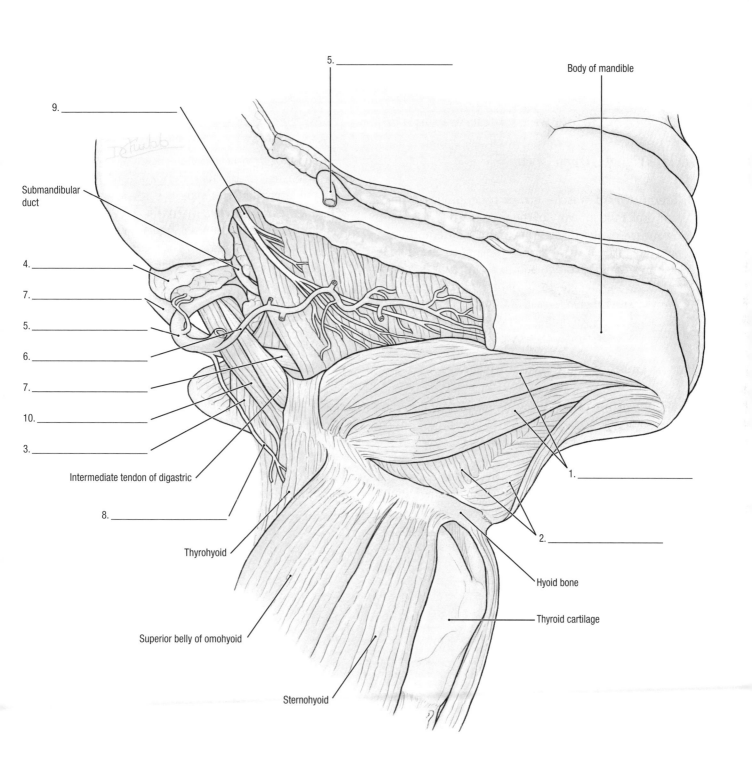

5. _____

Body of mandible

9. _____

Submandibular
duct

4. _____

7. _____

5. _____

6. _____

7. _____

10. _____

3. _____

Intermediate tendon of digastric

8. _____

Thyrohyoid

Superior belly of omohyoid

Sternohyoid

1. _____

2. _____

Hyoid bone

Thyroid cartilage

8.7 ANTERIOR CERVICAL REGION, MUSCULAR TRIANGLE, AND CERVICAL VISCERA

The cervical viscera of the neck are arranged in three layers from superficial to deep: endocrine, respiratory, and alimentary. The endocrine layer includes the thyroid and parathyroid glands, the respiratory layer includes the larynx and trachea, and the alimentary layer includes the pharynx and esophagus.

In this image, the **sternohyoid** muscle has been reflected superiorly and inferiorly on the left side. On the right, the middle portion of the sternothyroid has been cut away to reveal the right lobe of the thyroid gland.

COLOR each of the following structures using a different color for each:

Muscular Triangle, Deep Layer

1. **Sternothyroid muscle:** Covers the superficial aspect and limits the mobility of the thyroid gland
2. **Thyrohyoid muscle:** Lies superior to the sternothyroid and deep to the sternohyoid. Attaches to the oblique line of **thyroid cartilage** and to the inferior border of the body and the greater horn of the **hyoid bone**.
3. **Nerve to thyrohyoid:** Branch of C1 anterior ramus, which is bound to CN XII during part of its course. Descends from CN XII to supply the thyrohyoid muscle.

Endocrine Layer of the Cervical Viscera

4. **Thyroid gland:** Lies deep to sternothyroid and sternohyoid muscles at the level of C5-T1 vertebrae. Consists of right and left lobes with an **isthmus** that unites the two lobes.
5. **Accessory thyroid gland:** May develop lateral to the thyroid cartilage typically superficial to the thyrohyoid muscle (not usually present)
6. **Superior thyroid artery:** Arises from the **external carotid artery** and descends to supply the anterosuperior aspect of the thyroid gland

7. **Superior thyroid vein:** Accompanies the superior thyroid artery and drains the **superior pole of thyroid gland** to the internal jugular vein
8. **Middle thyroid vein:** Drains the middle of the right and left lobes to the internal jugular vein
9. **Inferior thyroid vein:** Drains the **inferior pole of thyroid gland** to the brachiocephalic veins

Structures Lateral to the Cervical Viscera

10. **Common carotid artery:** Ascends in the carotid sheath with the internal jugular vein and vagus nerve (CN X)
11. **Subclavian artery:** Courses horizontally through the root of the neck
12. **Brachiocephalic trunk:** Bifurcates into the right subclavian and common carotid arteries
13. **Internal jugular vein:** Lies laterally within the carotid sheath
14. **Vagus nerve (CN X):** Lies posteriorly within the carotid sheath between the internal jugular vein and the common carotid artery

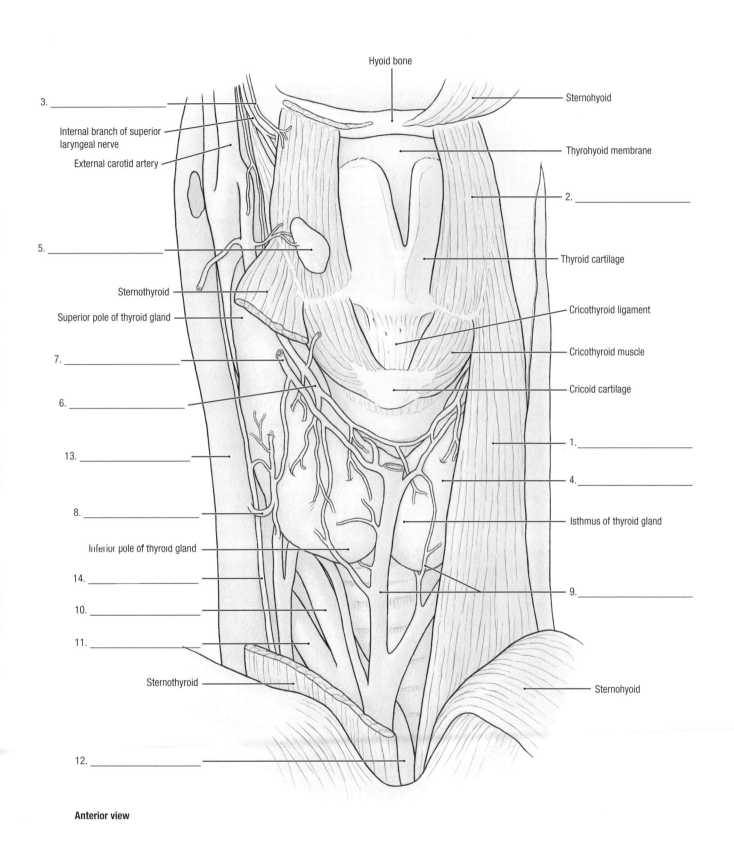

Hyoid bone

Sternohyoid

3. _____

Internal branch of superior
laryngeal nerve

External carotid artery

Thyrohyoid membrane

2. _____

5. _____

Thyroid cartilage

Sternothyroid

Superior pole of thyroid gland

Cricothyroid ligament

Cricothyroid muscle

7. _____

6. _____

Cricoid cartilage

1. _____

13. _____

4. _____

8. _____

Isthmus of thyroid gland

Inferior pole of thyroid gland

14. _____

10. _____

9. _____

11. _____

Sternothyroid

Sternohyoid

12. _____

Anterior view

Grant's

The larynx and trachea comprise the respiratory viscera of the neck. The larynx is a complex of cartilages described in detail in figures in Sections 8.20 and 8.21. The trachea extends from the larynx into the thorax.

In this image, the middle portion of the ***sternothyroid muscle*** has been removed and the isthmus of the thyroid gland cut and the left lobe reflected laterally.

COLOR each of the following structures using a different color for each:

Endocrine Layer of the Cervical Viscera

○ 1. *Thyroid gland:* The isthmus usually lies anterior to the second and third tracheal rings. A dense ***fascial band*** attaches the capsule that surrounds the thyroid gland to the cricoid cartilage and superior tracheal rings.

○ 2. *Inferior parathyroid gland:* One of four parathyroid glands that lie on the posterior surface of each lobe of the thyroid gland

○ 3. *Superior thyroid artery:* First branch of the external carotid artery; gives rise to the superior laryngeal artery and then descends to the thyroid gland traveling part of its path with the external laryngeal nerve

○ 4. *Superior thyroid vein:* Travels with the superior thyroid artery to the internal jugular vein

○ 5. *Inferior thyroid vein:* Travels along the anterior aspect of the trachea to the brachiocephalic vein

Respiratory Layer of the Cervical Viscera

○ 6. *Thyroid cartilage:* Largest and most superiorly placed of the laryngeal cartilages

○ 7. *Thyrohyoid membrane:* Connects the superior border of the thyroid cartilage to the hyoid bone

○ 8. *Internal branch of superior laryngeal nerve:* Branch of the vagus nerve (CN X) that pierces the thyrohyoid membrane

○ 9. *Superior laryngeal artery:* Branch of the superior thyroid artery that travels with the internal branch of the superior laryngeal nerve through the thyrohyoid membrane

○10. *Cricoid cartilage:* Only complete ring of the airway located inferior to the thyroid cartilage

○11. *Cricothyroid ligament:* Connects the cricoid cartilage to the inferior border of the thyroid cartilage

○12. *Cricothyroid muscle:* Paired muscle attaching to the anterolateral cricoid cartilage and inferior border and horn of the thyroid cartilage

○13. *External branch of superior laryngeal nerve:* Branch of the vagus nerve (CN X) that innervates the cricothyroid muscle

○14. *Cricotracheal ligament:* Connects the inferior margin of the cricoid cartilage to the first tracheal ring

○15. *Trachea:* Fibrocartilaginous tube composed of incomplete C-shaped cartilages that face anteriorly

Structures Lateral to the Cervical Viscera

○16. *Common carotid artery:* The right common carotid artery begins at the bifurcation of the brachiocephalic trunk, whereas the left common carotid branches directly off the arch of the aorta

○17. *Subclavian artery:* Other terminal branch of the brachiocephalic trunk on the right side. The left subclavian artery arises directly from the arch of the aorta.

○18. *Internal jugular vein:* Receives superior and middle thyroid veins and lies within carotid sheath

○19. *Vagus nerve (CN X):* Courses vertically in the neck within the carotid sheath giving rise to the superior laryngeal nerve, which branches into internal and external laryngeal nerves

○20. *Left recurrent laryngeal nerve:* Branch of CN X that loops under the arch of the aorta and then travels lateral to the trachea. The right recurrent laryngeal nerve loops under the right subclavian artery.

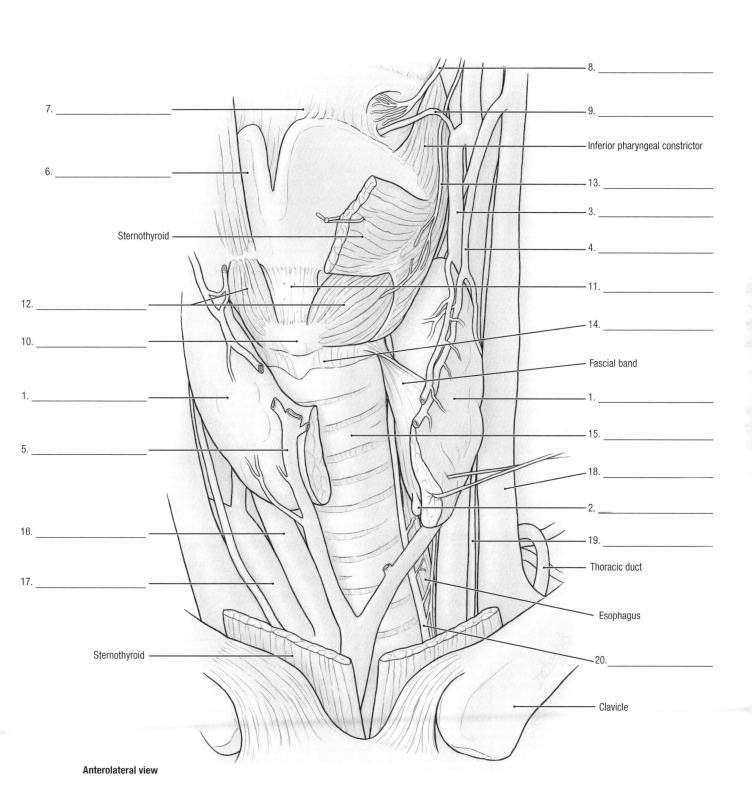

7. _____

6. _____

Sternothyroid _____

12. _____

10. _____

1. _____

5. _____

16. _____

17. _____

Sternothyroid _____

8. _____

9. _____

Inferior pharyngeal constrictor

13. _____

3. _____

4. _____

11. _____

14. _____

Fascial band

1. _____

15. _____

18. _____

2. _____

19. _____

Thoracic duct

Esophagus

20. _____

Clavicle

Anterolateral view

Grant's

The pharynx and esophagus comprise the alimentary viscera of the neck. The pharynx directs food into the esophagus and also directs air into the larynx. The esophagus marks the beginning of the alimentary canal or digestive tract.

In this image, the **sternothyroid** muscles are cut. On the left side, the **internal jugular vein**, **common carotid artery**, and **vagus nerve (CN X)** are retracted laterally by a string.

COLOR each of the following structures using a different color for each:

Endocrine and Respiratory Layers of Cervical Viscera

○ 1. **Thyroid gland:** Lobes lie anterolateral to the trachea and lateral to the esophagus

○ 2. **Parathyroid glands:** The two superior parathyroid glands lie near the inferior border of the cricoid cartilage, whereas the two inferior glands are more variable in their position

○ 3. **Inferior thyroid vein:** May be confused with the thyroid ima artery when present. The thyroid ima artery branches from the brachiocephalic trunk and travels on the anterior aspect of the trachea to the isthmus of the thyroid gland.

○ 4. **Superior thyroid vein:** Drains to the internal jugular vein typically at the level of the thyroid cartilage

○ 5. **Superior thyroid artery:** Typically arises from the external carotid artery near the bifurcation of the common carotid artery

○ 6. **Thyroid cartilage:** Composed of two plates, or laminae, which form an anterior-facing shield

○ 7. **Cricoid cartilage:** Marks the transition point of the pharyngoesophageal junction

○ 8. **Trachea:** Composed of C-shaped cartilages that are closed posteriorly by the trachealis muscle, allowing the esophagus to expand during swallowing

Alimentary Layer of the Cervical Viscera

○ 9. **Esophagus:** Muscular tube that connects the pharynx to the stomach. Lies posterior to the trachea.

○10. **Inferior pharyngeal constrictor:** Inferiormost of the three pharyngeal constrictors that attach to the oblique line of the thyroid cartilage and cricoid cartilage

Structures Lateral to the Cervical Viscera

○11. **Left recurrent laryngeal nerve:** Travels in the tracheoesophageal groove prior to passing deep to the inferior pharyngeal constrictor to reach structures of the larynx

○12. **Inferior thyroid artery:** Branches from the thyrocervical trunk (branch of the subclavian artery) and passes medially to supply the posterior aspect of the thyroid gland and all four of the parathyroid glands. Typically, gives rise to the **ascending cervical artery**.

○13. **Thoracic duct:** Major lymphatic duct of the body draining to the left venous angle between the left internal jugular and subclavian veins

○14. **Sympathetic trunk:** Travels posterior to the carotid sheath embedded or superficial to the **prevertebral fascia**. In the cervical region, composed of ascending presynaptic sympathetic fibers, which synapse within one of three paravertebral cervical ganglia.

○15. **Middle cervical ganglion:** Typically located anterior to or near the inferior thyroid artery at the level of the cricoid cartilage

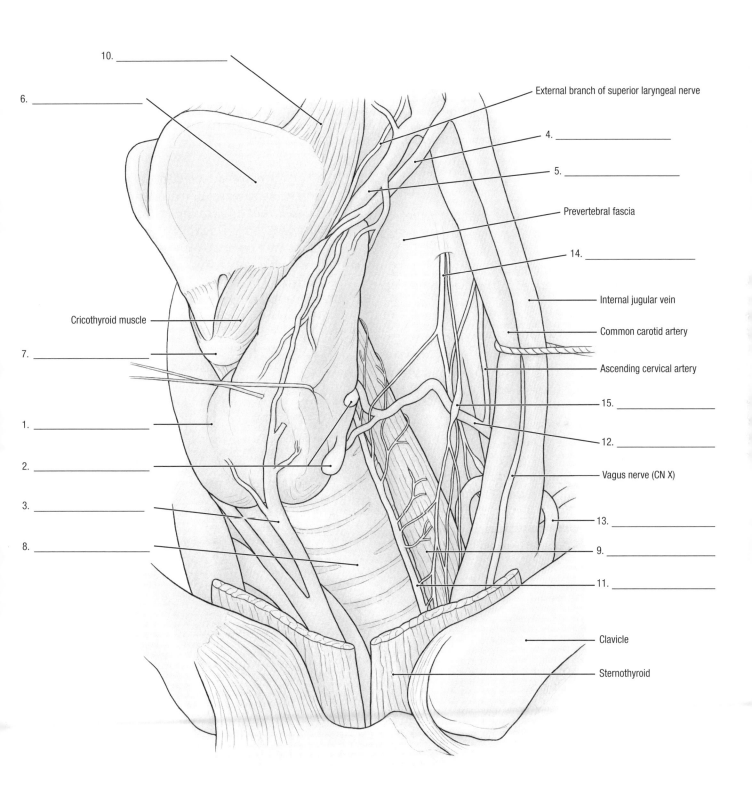

10. _____

6. _____

External branch of superior laryngeal nerve

4. _____

5. _____

Prevertebral fascia

14. _____

Internal jugular vein

Common carotid artery

Cricothyroid muscle

Ascending cervical artery

7. _____

15. _____

1. _____

12. _____

2. _____

Vagus nerve (CN X)

3. _____

13. _____

8. _____

9. _____

11. _____

Clavicle

Sternothyroid

Grant's

8.10 CAROTID TRIANGLE, SUPERFICIAL

The carotid triangle lies between the superior belly of the omohyoid, the posterior belly of the digastric, and the anterior border of the SCM. The carotid arterial and internal jugular venous systems lie within the depths of the triangle.

In this image, the skin, subcutaneous tissue, and investing layer of the deep cervical fascia have been removed. Two pins hold the anterior border of the SCM laterally. Structures of the submandibular triangle and lower mandibular region are also visible.

COLOR each of the following structures using a different color for each:

Boundaries of the Carotid Triangle

○ 1. *Sternocleidomastoid:* Forms the posterior boundary
○ 2. *Superior belly of omohyoid:* Forms the anterior boundary

The posterior belly of the digastric forms the superior boundary and the roof is formed by the investing layer of the deep cervical fascia.

Contents of the Carotid Triangle

○ 3. *Internal jugular vein:* Lies within the carotid sheath. Receives the venous drainage from:
  ○ 4. *Superior thyroid vein*
  ○ 5. *Common facial vein:* Typically a short vein that forms in the superior neck
    ○ 6. *Facial vein:* Travels superficially over the **sub-mandibular gland** in the submandibular triangle
    ○ 7. *Anterior branch of retromandibular vein:* Travels inferiorly through **parotid gland**
○ 8. *Superior root of ansa cervicalis:* Composed of C1 fibers, which are bound to CN XII during its course. Exits

CN XII to descend superficial or embedded within the anterolateral aspect of the carotid sheath
○ 9. *Inferior root of ansa cervicalis:* Composed of C2-C3 fibers and forms a loop by uniting with the superior root of the ansa cervicalis along the anterolateral aspect of the carotid sheath. Ansa cervicalis innervates all of the infrahyoid muscles except for the **thyrohyoid**.
○ 10. *Spinal accessory nerve* **(CN XI):** After exiting the jugular foramen courses through the carotid triangle to reach SCM

CLINICAL NOTE: SUBMANDIBULAR GLAND RESECTION

The submandibular gland is most often removed due to a tumor, but it may also be excised due to chronic infection caused by the presence of salivary stones. The incision is often superficially placed to the submandibular gland parallel to the inferior border of the mandible. If the incision is placed too deeply, the facial vein or the gland itself may be incised. The **marginal mandibular branch of the facial nerve** (CN VII) is also at risk during the incision through the skin and platysma muscle. The **facial artery** and vein are isolated and ligated (along with the submandibular duct within the oral cavity) prior to removal of the gland.

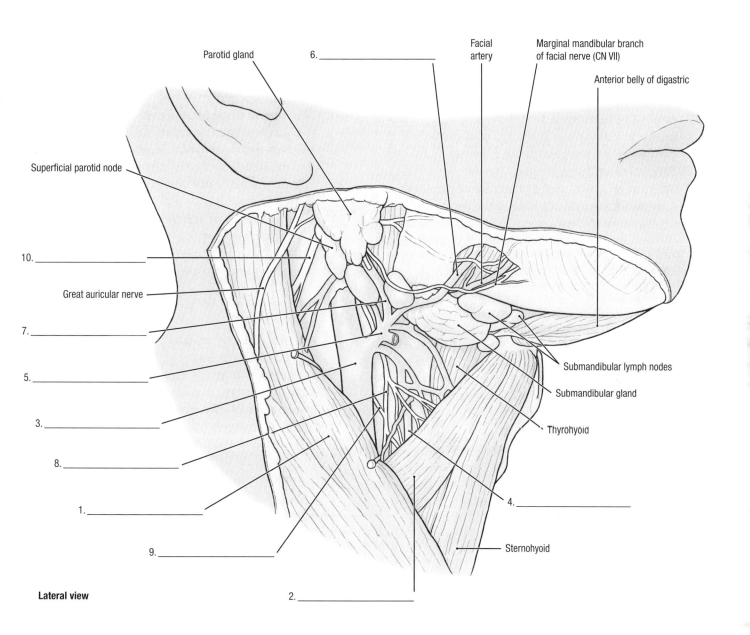

Parotid gland

6. _____

Facial
artery

Marginal mandibular branch
of facial nerve (CN VII)

Anterior belly of digastric

Superficial parotid node

10. _____

Great auricular nerve

7. _____

5. _____

3. _____

8. _____

1. _____

9. _____

Submandibular lymph nodes

Submandibular gland

Thyrohyoid

4. _____

Sternohyoid

2. _____

Lateral view

Grant's

8.11 CAROTID TRIANGLE, DEEP DISSECTION

The external carotid artery gives rise to several branches within the carotid triangle.

In this image, the SCM has been cut and reflected and the investing layer of deep cervical and pretracheal fascia removed.

The submandibular gland has also been removed within the submandibular triangle.

COLOR each of the following structures using a different color for each:

Contents of the Carotid Triangle

○ 1. *Internal carotid artery:* Arises from the **common carotid artery** at the level of the superior border of thyroid cartilage. Does not give off any branches in the neck.

○ 2. *External carotid artery:* Arises from the common carotid artery at the same level as the internal carotid artery. Gives rise to several branches in the neck:

  ○ 3. *Superior thyroid artery:* First anterior branch and descends to the thyroid gland supplying it as well as SCM and infrahyoid muscles

  ○ 4. *Common trunk for facial and lingual arteries:* The lingual and facial arteries are the second and third anterior branches and at times may arise from a common trunk. The lingual artery passes deep to CN XII, **stylohyoid**, and posterior belly digastric to enter the oral cavity medial to the hyoglossus.

  ○ 5. *Facial artery:* Passes superiorly deep to the posterior belly of the digastric and stylohyoid muscles and submandibular gland to pass over the inferior border of the mandible and onto the face. Gives rise to the **submental artery**.

  ○ 6. *Occipital artery:* Posterior branch that arises at the same level as or superior to the facial artery and then crosses CN XII as it passes superiorly

○ 7. *Internal jugular vein*

○ 8. *Spinal accessory nerve (CN XI):* Enters the deep aspect of SCM

○ 9. *Hypoglossal nerve (CN XII):* Descends from the hypoglossal canal lateral to the carotids and then turns anteriorly at the level of the oral cavity. C1 fibers become bound to it and then exit as:

○ 10. *Superior root of ansa cervicalis:* First C1 branch off CN XII and descends

○ 11. *Nerve to thyrohyoid:* Second C1 branch off CN XII and travels to the thyrohyoid muscle

○ 12. *Inferior root of ansa cervicalis:* C2-C3 fibers, which unite with the superior root

○ 13. *Internal branch of superior laryngeal nerve:* Pierces the thyrohyoid membrane

○ 14. *External branch of superior laryngeal nerve:* Innervates the cricothyroid muscle

Review of Cervical Triangles

○ 15. *Anterior belly of digastric:* Separates submental and submandibular triangles

○ 16. *Mylohyoid:* Forms the roof of submental and submandibular triangles

○ 17. *Superior belly of omohyoid:* Separates carotid and muscular triangles

○ 18. *Sternohyoid:* Located medial to the superior belly of the omohyoid with the muscular triangle

○ 19. *Sternothyroid:* Located deep to the sternohyoid within the muscular triangle

○ 20. *Thyrohyoid:* Located superior to the sternothyroid within the muscular triangle

○ 21. *Inferior belly of omohyoid:* Divides the lateral cervical region into omoclavicular and occipital triangles

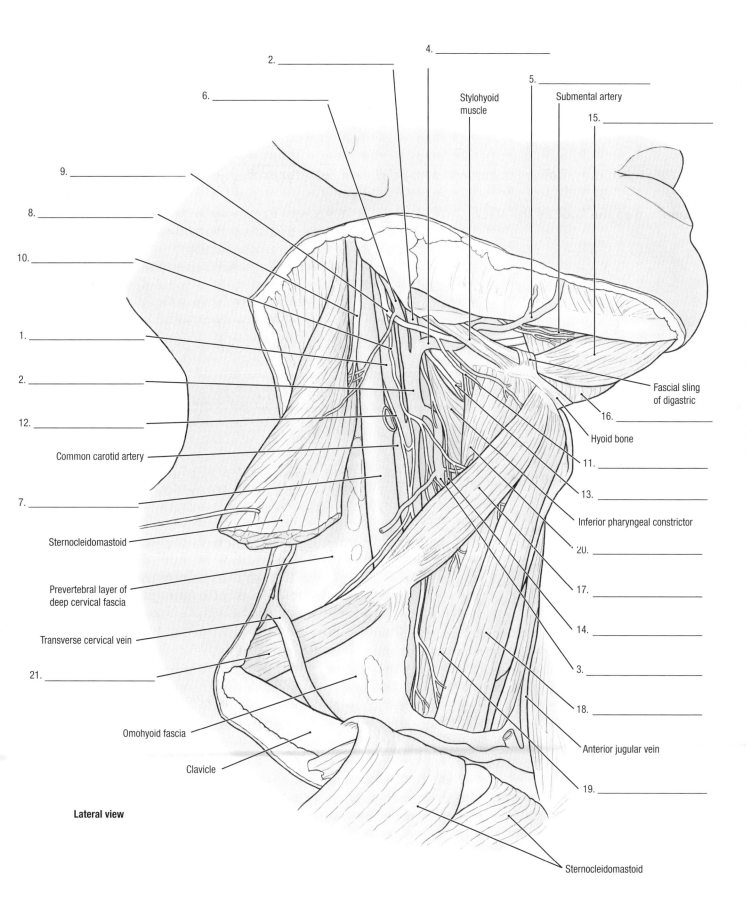

2. _____

6. _____

4. _____

Stylohyoid
muscle

5. _____
Submental artery

15. _____

9. _____

8. _____

10. _____

1. _____

2. _____

12. _____

Common carotid artery

7. _____

Sternocleidomastoid

Prevertebral layer of
deep cervical fascia

Transverse cervical vein

21. _____

Omohyoid fascia

Clavicle

Fascial sling
of digastric

16. _____

Hyoid bone

11. _____

13. _____
Inferior pharyngeal constrictor

20. _____

17. _____

14. _____

3. _____

18. _____

Anterior jugular vein

19. _____

Sternocleidomastoid

Lateral view

Grant's

8.12 ROOT OF THE NECK

The root of the neck is the area between the neck and the thorax. All structures from the head and neck to the thorax and vice versa pass through the superior thoracic aperture, which is formed by the first pair of ribs and their costal cartilages, manubrium of sternum, and body of T1 vertebra.

In this image, the middle portions of the right common carotid artery and *internal jugular vein* have been removed. The *clavicle* has been cut and the *right lobe of the thyroid gland* is retracted anteriorly by a string.

▎*COLOR each of the following structures using a different color for each:*

Vasculature of the Root of the Neck

○ 1. *Brachiocephalic trunk:* Arises in the midline posterior to the manubrium and divides into the right common carotid and subclavian arteries posterior to the *sterno-clavicular joint*

○ 2. *Common carotid artery:* Ascends in the neck within the carotid sheath with the internal jugular vein lateral to the cervical viscera

○ 3. *Subclavian artery:* Passes superolaterally from the brachiocephalic trunk posterior to the anterior scalene muscle. Divided into three segments relative to the anterior scalene: medial, posterior, and lateral to it.

○ 4. *Inferior thyroid artery:* Branches from the thyrocervical trunk coursing medially toward the thyroid gland

○ 5. *Ascending cervical artery:* Typically arises from the inferior thyroid artery and ascends on the superficial aspect of the anterior scalene

○ 6. *Cervicodorsal trunk:* Passes laterally from the thyrocervical trunk. Also known as the transverse cervical artery.

○ 7. *Superficial cervical artery:* Passes laterally from the cervicodorsal trunk crossing the phrenic nerve and the anterior scalene muscle anteriorly

○ 8. *Suprascapular artery:* Can arise independently from the thyrocervical trunk or from a common trunk with the other branches. Passes laterally inferior to the superficial cervical artery, crossing the phrenic nerve and anterior scalene anteriorly.

○ 9. *Dorsal scapular artery:* Arises either independently from the third part of the subclavian artery or as a branch of the cervicodorsal trunk

○ 10. *Subclavian vein:* Passes anterior to the anterior scalene muscle

○ 11. *Vertebral vein:* Drains to the subclavian vein medial to the anterior scalene muscle

Nerves of the Root of the Neck

○ 12. *Phrenic nerve:* Arises from C3 to C5, descends along the anterior surface of the anterior scalene muscle passing deep to the superficial cervical artery, suprascapular artery, and subclavian vein to continue into the thorax to supply the diaphragm

○ 13. *Vagus nerve (CN X):* Passes vertically posterior to the internal jugular vein and common carotid artery. Passes anterior to the subclavian artery to descend into the thorax.

○ 14. *Right recurrent laryngeal nerve:* Branches from CN X and loops under the right subclavian artery to then travel in the tracheoesophageal groove between the lateral aspects of the *trachea* and esophagus

○ 15. *Sympathetic trunk:* Lies anterolateral to the vertebral column embedded in or superficial to the *prevertebral fascia* covering the prevertebral muscles. The paravertebral ganglia of the cervical sympathetic trunk coalesce to form three ganglia: superior, middle, and inferior.

○ 16. *Middle cervical ganglion:* Smallest of the three ganglia and typically located near the inferior thyroid artery

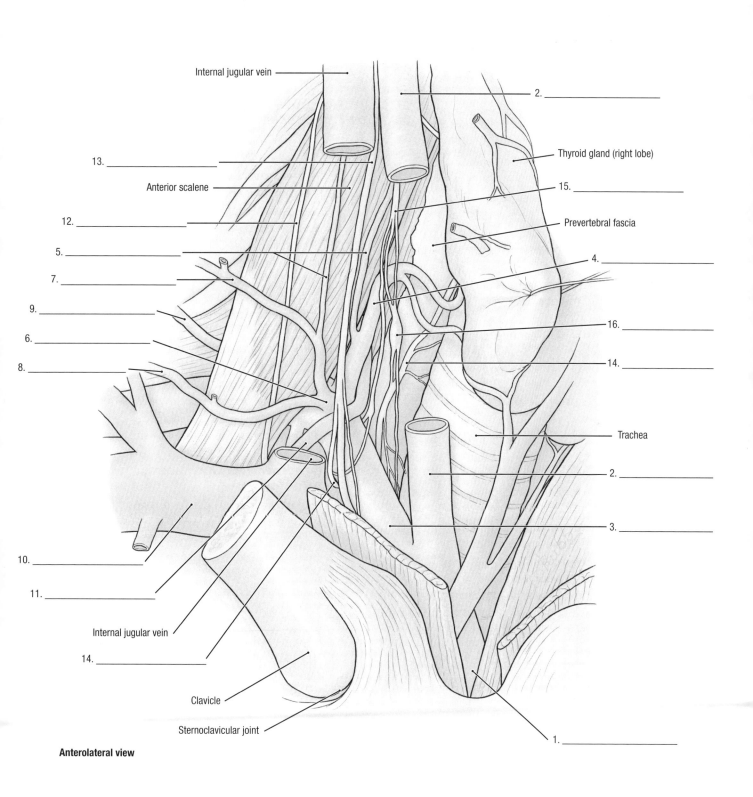

Internal jugular vein

2. _____

Thyroid gland (right lobe)

13. _____

Anterior scalene

15. _____

Prevertebral fascia

12. _____

5. _____

4. _____

7. _____

9. _____

16. _____

6. _____

8. _____

14. _____

Trachea

2. _____

3. _____

10. _____

11. _____

Internal jugular vein

14. _____

Clavicle

Sternoclavicular joint

1. _____

Anterolateral view

Grant's

8.13   ROOT OF THE NECK, DEEP

In this image, the superior components of the ***thyroid gland***, ***trachea***, and ***esophagus*** have been cut away. The ***common carotid arteries*** and vagus nerves have been cut inferiorly. On the left the ***internal jugular vein*** has been cut and reflected inferiorly with a string. On the right side, the ***right brachiocephalic vein*** has been cut with the internal jugular and subclavian veins removed.

COLOR each of the following structures using a different color for each:

Muscles of the Root of the Neck

○ 1. ***Anterior scalene:*** Attaches to the first rib and the transverse processes of C3-C6 vertebrae
○ 2. ***Middle scalene:*** Attaches to the first rib posterior to the groove of the subclavian artery and the posterior tubercles of transverse processes of C5-C7 vertebrae
○ 3. ***Longus capitis:*** Attaches to the basilar part of the occipital bone and the anterior tubercles of C3-C6 transverse processes
○ 4. ***Longus colli:*** Attaches to bodies of C1-C3 and transverse processes of C3-C6 vertebrae and then to bodies of C5-T3 vertebrae and transverse processes of C3-C5

Root of the Neck Neurovasculature

○ 5. ***Subclavian artery:*** Passes superolaterally, reaching its apex posterior to the anterior scalene. The first part (medial to anterior scalene) gives rise to:
   ○ 6. ***Vertebral artery:*** Ascends between the anterior scalene and prevertebral muscles
   ○ 7. ***Thyrocervical trunk:*** Short trunk arising lateral to the vertebral artery and giving rise to:
     ○ 8. ***Inferior thyroid artery***
     ○ 9. ***Ascending cervical artery***
     ○ 10. ***Suprascapular artery***

Cervicodorsal (transverse cervical) trunk

○ 11. ***Internal thoracic artery:*** Descends into the thorax superficial to the ***cervical parietal pleura***
○ 12. ***Dorsal scapular artery:*** Can arise either as a branch from the cervicodorsal trunk or independently from the third part of the subclavian artery
○ 13. ***Vertebral vein:*** Courses anterior to vertebral and subclavian arteries to drain into the ***subclavian vein***
○ 14. ***Internal thoracic vein:*** Travels with the internal thoracic artery to typically drain into the brachiocephalic vein
○ 15. ***Inferior thyroid vein:*** Drains to the brachiocephalic veins
○ 16. ***Thoracic duct:*** Enters the left venous angle from a posteromedial approach
○ 17. ***Anterior rami of C5, C6, C7, C8, T1:*** Form the roots of the brachial plexus between the anterior and the middle scalene muscle
○ 18. ***Phrenic nerve:*** Descends into the thorax superficial to the cervical parietal pleura
○ 19. ***Vagus nerve (CN X):*** Descends into the thorax medial to the phrenic nerve
○ 20. ***Sympathetic trunk:*** Passes posteriorly with the vertebral column through the superior thoracic aperture

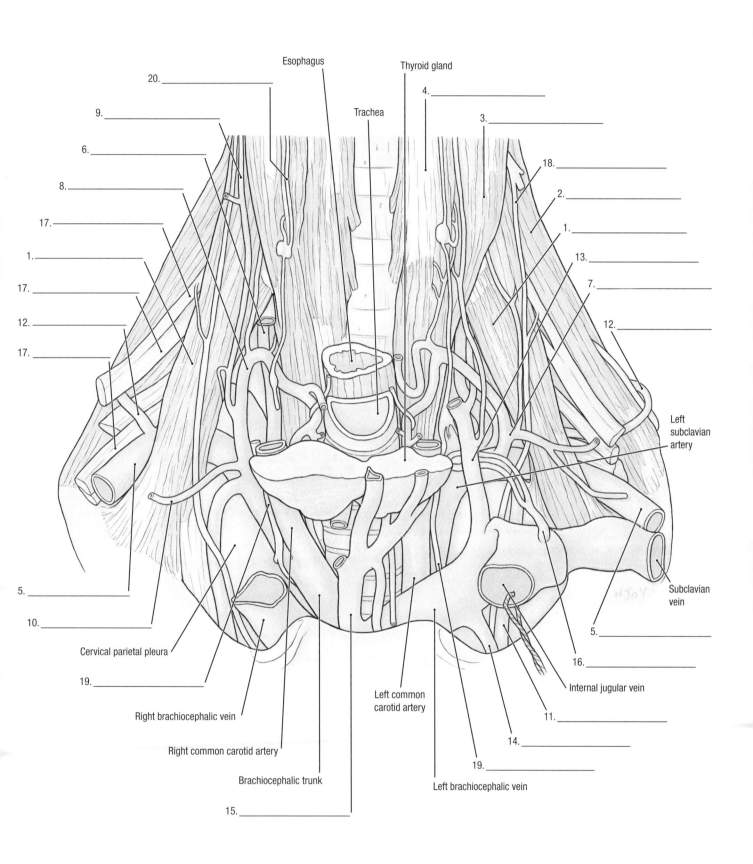

Esophagus

Thyroid gland

Trachea

20. _____

9. _____

6. _____

8. _____

17. _____

1. _____

17. _____

12. _____

17. _____

4. _____

3. _____

18. _____

2. _____

1. _____

13. _____

7. _____

12. _____

Left
subclavian
artery

Subclavian
vein

5. _____

10. _____

Cervical parietal pleura

19. _____

Right brachiocephalic vein

Right common carotid artery

Brachiocephalic trunk

15. _____

Left common
carotid artery

Left brachiocephalic vein

Internal jugular vein

5. _____

16. _____

11. _____

14. _____

19. _____

8.14 EXTERNAL PHARYNX, POSTERIOR VIEW

The pharynx is unique compared with the remainder of the alimentary tract in that the circular (constrictor) muscles lie external to the longitudinal muscles.

In this image, the cervical vertebrae and a wedge of the occipital bone have been removed, along with the buccopharyngeal fascia that lines the pharynx posteriorly. The internal jugular veins have been removed except at the jugular foramen. On the specimen's right, **common carotid**, **external carotid**, and **internal carotid arteries** have been removed along with most of the nerves that lie lateral to pharynx.

COLOR *each of the following structures using a different color for each:*

Pharyngeal Muscles and Esophagus

Constrictor muscles meet in the midline at the pharyngeal raphe and are stacked within one another.

○ 1. **Superior pharyngeal constrictor:** Paired muscle attaching in the midline to the **pharyngeal tubercle** of the occipital bone

○ 2. **Middle pharyngeal constrictor:** Paired muscle that superficially overlaps the inferior aspect of the superior constrictor

○ 3. **Inferior pharyngeal constrictor:** Paired muscle that superficially covers the inferior aspect of the middle constrictor

○ 4. **Esophagus:** Extends inferiorly from the pharyngoesophageal junction, which is the narrowest portion of the esophagus

○ 5. **Pharyngobasilar fascia:** Strong, internal fascial lining between the muscles and the mucosa of the pharynx

○ 6. **Stylopharyngeus:** One of the longitudinal muscles that courses from the styloid process through the gap between the superior and middle constrictors to the internal pharynx

Structures Lateral to the Pharynx

○ 7. **Sympathetic trunk:** Lies at or medial to the carotids and gives rise to the **sympathetic plexus**, which travels on the carotid arterial system

○ 8. **Superior cervical ganglion:** Bulge of the sympathetic trunk located at C1-C2 vertebral levels and is a useful landmark for differentiating the sympathetic trunk from CN X

○ 9. **Middle cervical ganglion:** Located at C6 vertebral level

○ 10. **Inferior cervical ganglion:** Lies anterior to the transverse process of C7 vertebra

○ 11. **Vagus nerve (CN X):** Lies immediately lateral to the sympathetic trunk and gives rise to the **superior laryngeal** and recurrent laryngeal nerves and to the **pharyngeal plexus**

○ 12. **Hypoglossal nerve (CN XII):** Lies immediately lateral to CN X but descends only to the level of the angle of the mandible and then courses anteriorly to enter the oral cavity

○ 13. **Spinal accessory nerve (CN XI):** Lies lateral to CN XII and enters the deep surface of the **sternocleidomastoid (SCM)**

○ 14. **Glossopharyngeal nerve (CN IX):** Lies on the stylopharyngeus muscle supplying it and participating in the pharyngeal plexus

○ 15. **Recurrent laryngeal nerve:** Dives deep to the inferior pharyngeal constrictor

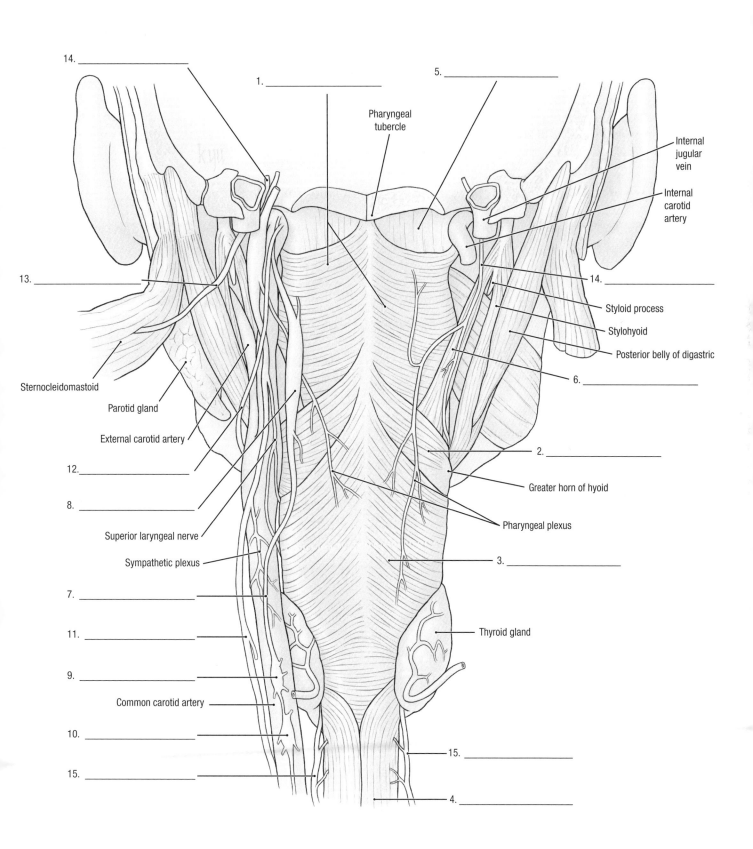

14. _____

1. _____

Pharyngeal tubercle

5. _____

Internal jugular vein

Internal carotid artery

13. _____

14. _____

Styloid process

Stylohyoid

Posterior belly of digastric

Sternocleidomastoid

6. _____

Parotid gland

External carotid artery

2. _____

12. _____

Greater horn of hyoid

8. _____

Superior laryngeal nerve

Pharyngeal plexus

Sympathetic plexus

3. _____

7. _____

11. _____

Thyroid gland

9. _____

Common carotid artery

10. _____

15. _____

15. _____

4. _____

Grant's

8.15   EXTERNAL PHARYNX, LATERAL VIEW

The overlapping nature and lateral attachments of the pharyngeal constrictors leave four gaps for structures to enter or exit the pharynx. The lateral boundaries of the oral cavity and oropharynx are continuous due to the attachment of the *buccinator* and superior pharyngeal constrictor to the *pterygomandibular raphe*.

In this image, the rami of the mandible and zygomatic arch have been removed along with the buccopharyngeal fascia covering the buccinator and the posterior aspect of the pharynx. The *stylohyoid muscle* and the *digastric tendon* have been cut. *CN X* and *XII* are retracted posteriorly by a hook.

COLOR *each of the following structures using a different color for each:*

Pharyngeal Muscles

Muscle	Proximal Attachment	Distal Attachment	Innervation
○ 1. *Superior pharyngeal constrictor*	Pterygoid hamulus, pterygomandibular raphe	Pharyngeal tubercle	Pharyngeal nerve (CN X) and pharyngeal plexus
○ 2. *Middle pharyngeal constrictor*	Stylohyoid ligament and *greater horn of hyoid*	Pharyngeal raphe	
○ 3. *Inferior pharyngeal constrictor*	Oblique line of *thyroid cartilage* and lateral *cricoid cartilage*	Pharyngeal raphe and inferior portion encircles pharyngoesophageal junction	

Gaps Between the Pharyngeal Constrictors

○ 4. *Levator veli palatini:* Passes through the gap between the superior pharyngeal constrictor and the base of the cranium

○ 5. *Stylopharyngeus:* Passes through the gap between the superior and middle pharyngeal constrictors

○ 6. *Glossopharyngeal nerve (CN IX):* Travels with the stylopharyngeus muscle

○ 7. *Internal branch of superior laryngeal nerve:* Passes through the gap between middle and inferior pharyngeal constrictors with the superior laryngeal artery to pierce through the *thyrohyoid membrane*

○ 8. *Recurrent laryngeal nerve:* Passes through a gap inferior to the inferior pharyngeal constrictor

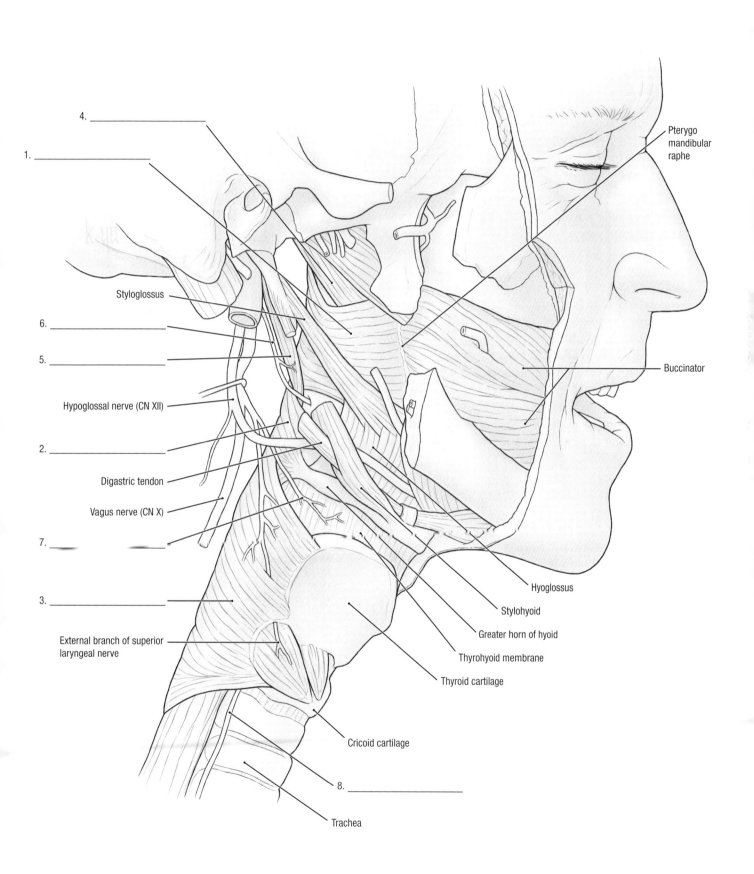

4. _____

1. _____

Pterygo mandibular raphe

Styloglossus

6. _____

5. _____

Buccinator

Hypoglossal nerve (CN XII)

2. _____

Digastric tendon

Vagus nerve (CN X)

7. _____

Hyoglossus

Stylohyoid

3. _____

Greater horn of hyoid

External branch of superior laryngeal nerve

Thyrohyoid membrane

Thyroid cartilage

Cricoid cartilage

8. _____

Trachea

Grant's

8.16   INTERNAL PHARYNX

The pharynx extends from the cranial base to the inferior border of the cricoid cartilage anteriorly and the inferior border of C6 vertebra posteriorly. The pharynx is the widest at the level of the hyoid and narrowest as it becomes continuous with the esophagus. The pharynx is divided into three parts: nasopharynx, oropharynx, and laryngopharynx.

In this image, the ***posterior wall of the pharynx*** has been cut in the midline and each side retracted laterally to reveal the internal aspect of the pharynx.

COLOR *each of the following structures using a different color for each:*

Nasopharynx

The ***nasopharynx*** lies posterior to the nasal cavity and has a respiratory function only.

○ 1. ***Choanae:*** Paired openings or doorways between the nasal cavity and the nasopharynx. The choanae are separated by the posterior aspect of the ***nasal septum***.

○ 2. ***Salpingopharyngeal fold:*** Vertical fold of the mucosa that extends inferiorly from the ***posterior lip of the opening of the pharyngotympanic tube***

○ 3. ***Pharyngeal recess:*** Slit-like depression that lies posterior to the salpingopharyngeal fold

○ 4. ***Soft palate:*** Separates the nasopharynx from the oropharynx. The ***uvula*** is a midline posterior extension of the soft palate.

Oropharynx

The ***oropharynx*** lies posterior to the oral cavity and has a digestive function.

○ 5. ***Posterior (base) of tongue:*** Separated by the isthmus of the fauces from the oropharynx. The posterior tongue is marked by the ***foramen cecum*** and ***terminal sulcus***.

○ 6. ***Lateral glossoepiglottic fold:*** Paired mucosal fold connecting the posterior tongue to the lateral aspect of the epiglottis

○ 7. ***Epiglottis:*** Superior border separates the oropharynx from the laryngopharynx

Laryngopharynx

The ***laryngopharynx*** lies posterior to the larynx and serves a digestive function.

○ 8. ***Ary-epiglottic fold:*** Mucosal fold that surrounds the lateral and posterior aspects of the ***inlet of the larynx (aditus to larynx)***

○ 9. ***Piriform recess*** (fossa)***:*** Small depression on either side of the laryngeal inlet

○ 10. ***Cricoid cartilage:*** Inferior border separates the laryngopharynx from the ***esophagus***

CLINICAL NOTE: FOREIGN OBJECTS IN THE PIRIFORM RECESS

Ingestion of a foreign object may occur at any age, but occurs most often in infants and children. In adults, bones (chicken or fish) or metal objects (pins/wires) are more commonly reported. Objects may become lodged near the base of the tongue and the vallecula, tonsillar bed, piriform recess, or esophagus or within the lower respiratory tract. The piriform recess is narrow at its superior and inferior margins as the thyroid and cricoid cartilages form its boundaries, permitting objects to become lodged within it. Deep to the mucosa of the recess lies the internal branch of the superior laryngeal nerve. This nerve may become damaged by a sharp object that pierces the mucosa or during removal of the object. A lesion to the nerve may result in anesthesia of the laryngeal mucosa superior to the vocal fold.

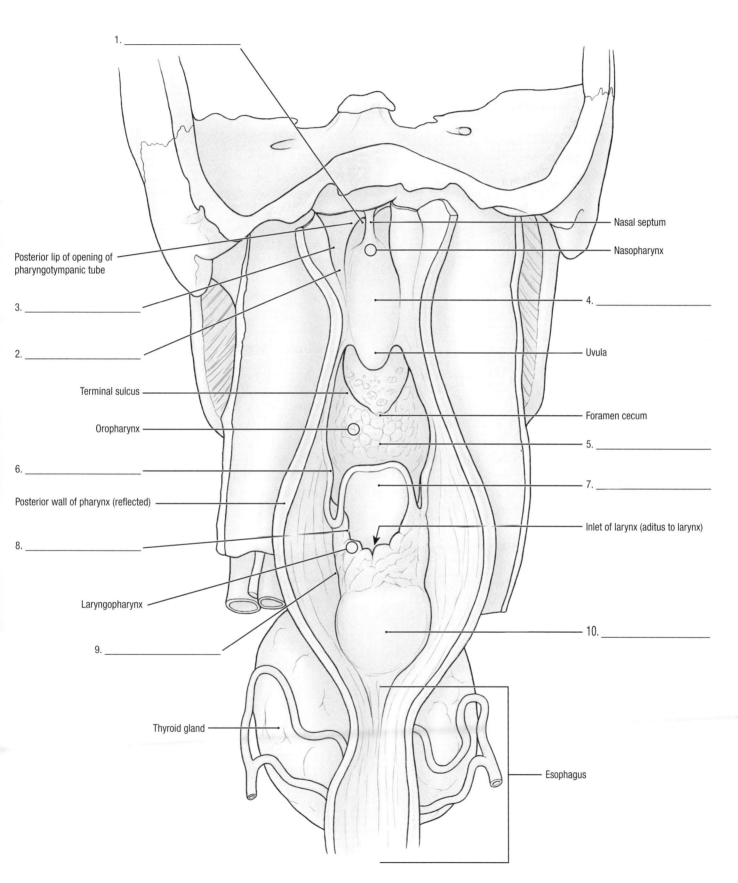

1. _____

Posterior lip of opening of
pharyngotympanic tube

3. _____

2. _____

Terminal sulcus

Oropharynx

6. _____

Posterior wall of pharynx (reflected)

8. _____

Laryngopharynx

9. _____

Thyroid gland

Nasal septum

Nasopharynx

4. _____

Uvula

Foramen cecum

5. _____

7. _____

Inlet of larynx (aditus to larynx)

10. _____

Esophagus

Grant's

8.17 INTERNAL PHARYNX, MUCOSA REMOVED

The posterior wall of the pharynx has been cut in the midline and each side reflected laterally as in figure in Section 8.16; the mucosa has then been removed to expose the underlying musculature.

COLOR *each of the following structures using a different color for each:*

Longitudinal Muscles of the Pharynx

Muscle	Proximal Attachment	Distal Attachment	Innervation
○ 1. *Salpingopharyngeus*	*Cartilaginous part of the pharyngotympanic tube*	Blends with the palatopharyngeus	Pharyngeal nerve (CN X) and pharyngeal plexus
○ 2. *Palatopharyngeus*	Hard palate and palatine aponeurosis	Posterior border of the lamina of the thyroid cartilage and blends into sides of the pharynx and esophagus	
Stylopharyngeus (see figure in Section 8.15)	Styloid process	Posterior and superior borders of the thyroid cartilage with palatopharyngeus	Glossopharyngeal nerve (CN IX)

Nasopharynx

○ 3. *Levator veli palatini:* Attaches to the pharyngotympanic tube and palatine aponeurosis

○ 4. *Pharyngobasilar fascia:* Forms the superior aspect of the posterior wall of the nasopharynx

○ 5. *Superior pharyngeal constrictor:* Forms the inferior aspect of the posterior wall of the nasopharynx and the superior aspect of the posterior wall of the oropharynx

○ 6. *Musculus uvulae:* Muscular portion of the *uvula*

Oropharynx

○ 7. *Middle pharyngeal constrictor:* Forms the inferior aspect of the posterior wall of the oropharynx

○ 8. *Palatine tonsil:* Lies within the fauces, the space between the oropharynx and the oral cavity

Laryngopharynx

○ 9. *Arytenoid muscle:* Laryngeal muscle on the posterior aspect of the arytenoid cartilages

○10. *Ary-epiglottic muscle:* Lies within the ary-epiglottic fold

○11. *Posterior crico-arytenoid muscle:* Laryngeal muscle on the posterior aspect of the cricoid cartilage

○12. *Inferior pharyngeal constrictor:* Forms the posterior wall of the laryngopharynx

Esophagus

○13. *Circular muscle:* Internal

○14. *Longitudinal muscle:* External

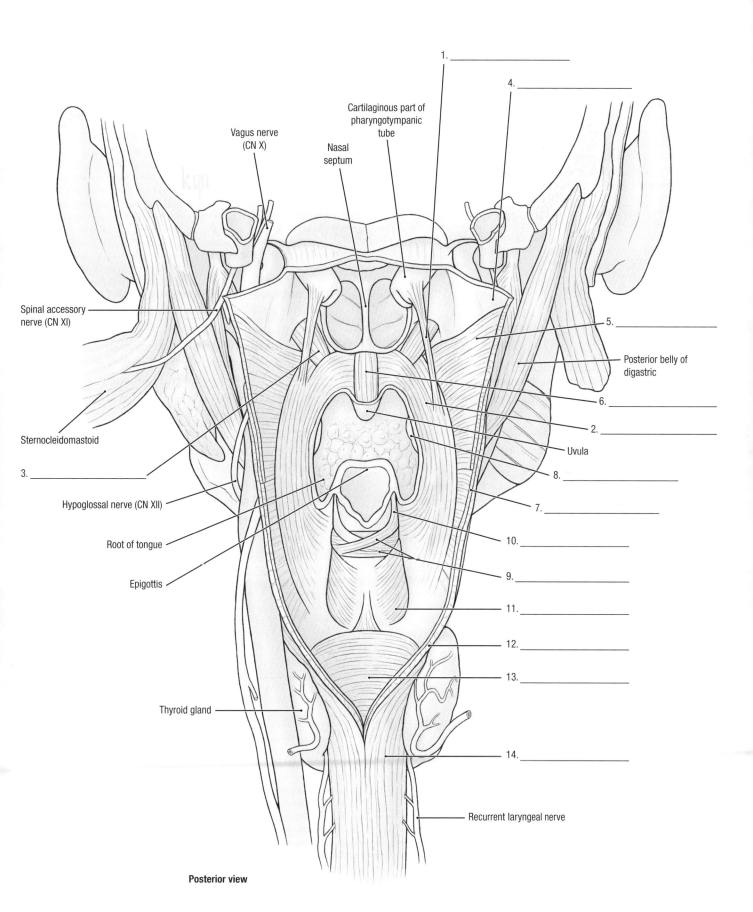

1. _____

4. _____

Cartilaginous part of
pharyngotympanic
tube

Vagus nerve
(CN X)

Nasal
septum

Spinal accessory
nerve (CN XI)

5. _____

Posterior belly of
digastric

6. _____

2. _____

Uvula

Sternocleidomastoid

8. _____

3. _____

7. _____

Hypoglossal nerve (CN XII)

10. _____

9. _____

Root of tongue

Epigottis

11. _____

12. _____

13. _____

Thyroid gland

14. _____

Recurrent laryngeal nerve

Posterior view

Grant's

8.18A and B   ISTHMUS OF FAUCES AND LATERAL WALL OF THE NASOPHARYNX

The fauces is the space between the oral cavity and the oropharynx. It is bounded by the soft palate superiorly, ***dorsum of the tongue*** inferiorly, and palatoglossal and palatopharyngeal arches laterally. The isthmus of the fauces refers to the space between the palatoglossal and palatopharyngeal folds. The nasopharynx lies superior to the fauces, with the soft palate as its inferior boundary.

Figure A depicts the oral cavity and isthmus of fauces from an anterior view. On the specimen's right the mucosa has been removed to reveal the underlying neurovasculature and muscles. Figure B depicts a medial view of the right isthmus of fauces and the nasopharynx.

COLOR *each of the following structures using a different color for each:*

Fauces

○ 1. *Hard palate:* Forms anterior portion of the palate separating the oral and nasal cavities
○ 2. *Soft palate:* Forms posterior portion of the palate separating the nasopharynx and fauces, ending posteriorly as the ***uvula***. ***Palatine glands*** lie deep to the mucosa covering the hard and soft palate.
○ 3. *Palatoglossal arch:* Mucosal fold covering the palatoglossus muscle that courses from the soft palate to the lateral aspect of the tongue
○ 4. *Palatopharyngeal arch:* Mucosal fold covering the palatopharyngeus muscle that courses from the soft palate and blends with the muscles of the pharynx
○ 5. *Tonsillar fossa* (B only): Located between the palatoglossal and palatopharyngeal arches
○ 6. *Palatine tonsil* (A only): Lymphoid tissue occupying the tonsillar fossa

Nasopharynx (B only)

○ 7. *Opening of pharyngotympanic tube:* Located posterior to the ***inferior nasal concha*** of the nasal cavity and permits communication to the middle ear
○ 8. *Torus tubarius:* Medial, blunt end of the cartilage that forms the pharyngotympanic tube covered by mucosa. Located posterosuperior to the opening of the pharyngotympanic tube.
○ 9. *Salpingopharyngeal fold:* Fold of mucosa extending inferiorly from the torus tubarius covering the salpingopharyngeus muscle. Blends into the wall of the pharynx.
○ 10. *Pharyngeal recess:* Depression located posterosuperior to the torus tubarius and salpingopharyngeal fold
○ 11. *Pharyngeal tonsil:* Lymphoid tissue located within the roof and posterior wall of the nasopharynx posterosuperior to the pharyngeal recess
○ 12. *Torus levatorius:* Ridge of the mucosa located inferior to the opening of the pharyngotympanic tube that covers the levator veli palatini muscle

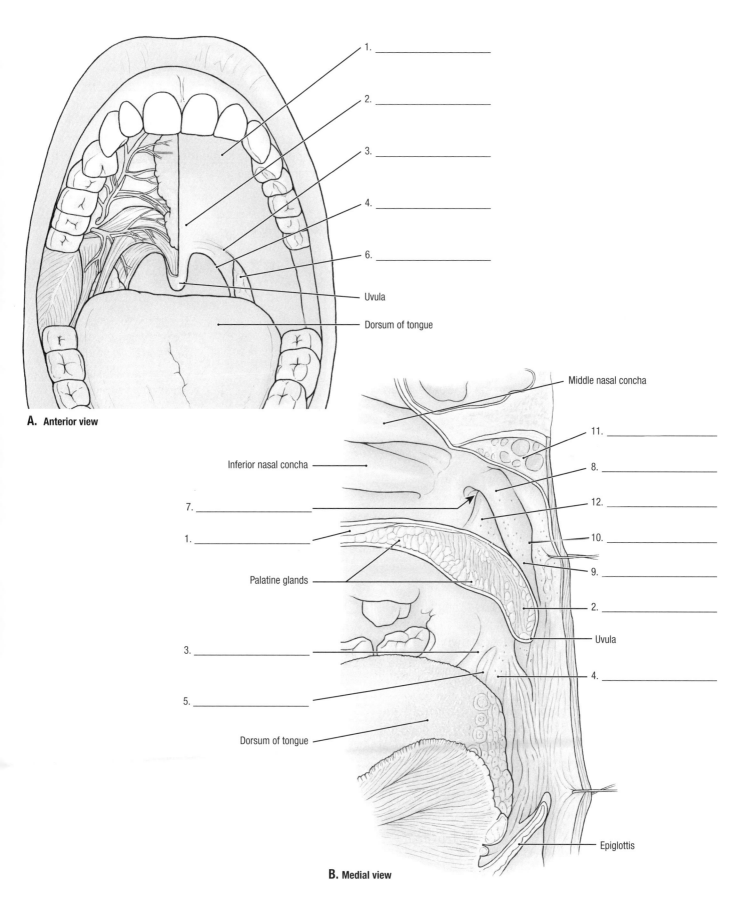

A. Anterior view

1. _____
2. _____
3. _____
4. _____
6. _____
Uvula
Dorsum of tongue

Middle nasal concha
11. _____
8. _____
12. _____
10. _____
9. _____
2. _____
Uvula
4. _____

Inferior nasal concha
7. _____
1. _____
Palatine glands
3. _____
5. _____
Dorsum of tongue
Epiglottis

B. Medial view

Grant's

8.19A and B   ISTHMUS OF FAUCES AND LATERAL WALL OF NASOPHARYNX, MUCOSA REMOVED

The muscles of the soft palate are innervated by the pharyngeal branch of the vagus nerve (CN X) except for the tensor veli palatini, which is innervated by the mandibular division of the trigeminal nerve (CN V$_3$).

In Figure A, the mucosa has been removed along with the palatine and pharyngeal tonsils. The pharyngobasilar fascia has also been removed except the portion superior to the superior pharyngeal constrictor. The *tongue* has been pulled anteriorly with a string. In Figure B, the inferior portion of the superior pharyngeal constrictor has also been removed, revealing the medial aspect of the *submandibular gland* within the submandibular triangle.

COLOR *each of the following structures using a different color for each:*

Muscles of the Soft Palate

Muscle	Proximal Attachment	Distal Attachment	Main Action
○ 1. *Tensor veli palatini* (A only)	Scaphoid fossa and *cartilage of the pharyngotympanic tube*	Palatine aponeurosis	Tenses the soft palate and opens the pharyngotympanic tube during swallowing and yawning
○ 2. *Levator veli palatini* (A only)	Cartilage of the pharyngotympanic tube and the petrous part of the temporal bone		Elevates the soft palate during swallowing and yawning
○ 3. *Palatoglossus*	Palatine aponeurosis	Side of the tongue	Elevates the posterior part of the tongue and draws the soft palate inferiorly
○ 4. *Palatopharyngeus*	Hard palate and palatine aponeurosis	Lateral wall of the pharynx	Tenses the soft palate and pulls the pharyngeal walls superiorly, anteriorly, and medially during swallowing
○ 5. *Musculus uvulae* (A only)	Posterior nasal spine and palatine aponeurosis	Mucosa of the uvula	Shortens the uvula and pulls it superiorly

○ 6. *Salpingopharyngeus* (A only): Longitudinal muscle of the pharynx extending from the cartilage of the pharyngotympanic tube and blending with the other longitudinal muscles of the pharynx

○ 7. *Superior pharyngeal constrictor:* Forms the lateral wall of the tonsillar fossa

○ 8. *Pharyngobasilar fascia* (A only): Attaches to the pharyngeal tubercle of the *basilar part of the occipital bone* and courses between the mucosa and pharyngeal muscles. Also contributes to the formation of the tonsillar fossa.

○ 9. *Middle pharyngeal constrictor:* Forms the lateral and posterior walls of the oropharynx

○ 10. *Styloglossus* (B only): Muscle of the tongue passing anteromedially from the styloid process to blend with the *hyoglossus* as it inserts into the intrinsic muscles of the tongue

○ 11. *Stylopharyngeus* (B only): Courses medially from the styloid process to blend with the other longitudinal muscles of the pharynx

○ 12. *Stylohyoid ligament* (B only): Courses from the tip of the styloid process to the lesser horn of the *hyoid bone*

○ 13. *Glossopharyngeal nerve* (CN IX): Follows the styloglossus muscle to the posterior third of the tongue supplying both taste and general sensory

○ 14. *Tonsillar branch of facial artery:* Arises from the facial artery within the submandibular triangle supplying the palatine tonsil

○ 15. *Ascending palatine branch of facial artery* (A only): Arises from the facial artery within the submandibular triangle supplying muscles and glands of the soft palate and the palatine tonsil

○ 16. *External palatine (paratonsillar) vein:* Drains to the facial vein within the submandibular triangle

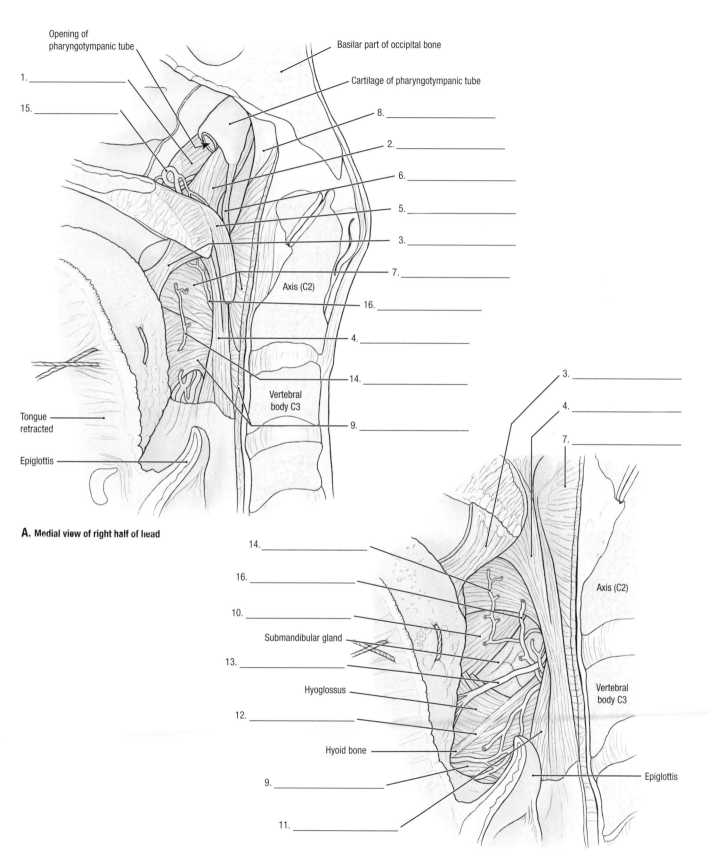

Opening of
pharyngotympanic tube

Basilar part of occipital bone

Cartilage of pharyngotympanic tube

1. _____

15. _____

8. _____

2. _____

6. _____

5. _____

3. _____

7. _____

Axis (C2)

16. _____

4. _____

14. _____

Vertebral
body C3

9. _____

Tongue
retracted

Epiglottis

A. Medial view of right half of head

3. _____

4. _____

7. _____

Axis (C2)

14. _____

16. _____

10. _____

Submandibular gland

13. _____

Hyoglossus

12. _____

Hyoid bone

9. _____

11. _____

Vertebral
body C3

Epiglottis

B. Medial view of right half of head

Grant's

8.20A and B LARYNGEAL SKELETON, ANTERIOR AND LATERAL VIEWS

The larynx lies anterior to the vertebral bodies of C3-C6 connecting the laryngopharynx to the **_trachea_**. The laryngeal skeleton is composed of nine cartilages (three single and three paired) joined by ligaments and membranes.

Figure A depicts an anterior view of the laryngeal skeleton, whereas Figure B depicts a lateral view.

COLOR each of the following structures using a different color for each:

○ 1. **_Thyroid cartilage:_** Largest of the laryngeal cartilages composed of two **_laminae_**.

   ○ 2. **_Laryngeal prominence:_** Formed by the fusion of the inferior two-thirds of the lamina in the midline. Commonly referred to as the "Adam's apple" and is more pronounced at approximately 90° in males.

   ○ 3. **_Superior horn_** (B only)**_:_** Superior projection from the posterior border

   ○ 4. **_Inferior horn_** (B only)**_:_** Inferior projection from the posterior border

   ○ 5. **_Oblique line_** (B only)**_:_** Located on the lateral aspect of each lamina

○ 6. **_Cricoid cartilage:_** Located inferior to the thyroid cartilage at the level of C6 vertebral body. Smaller, but thicker and stronger, than the thyroid cartilage. Only complete ring of cartilage of the airway.

   ○ 7. **_Arch_** (B only)**_:_** Anterior portion

   ○ 8. **_Lamina_** (B only)**_:_** Posterior portion

○ 9. **_Epiglottis:_** Located posterior to the hyoid bone

○ 10. **_Thyrohyoid membrane:_** Connects the **_greater horns_** and the **_body of the hyoid bone_** to the superior horns and superior border of the thyroid cartilage. By connecting the hyoid bone to the trachea, muscles that attach to the hyoid also move the larynx as a whole.

○ 11. **_Median cricothyroid ligament:_** Attaches the inferior border of the thyroid cartilage to the arch of the cricoid cartilage

○ 12. **_Capsule of the cricothyroid joint_** (B only)**_:_** Articulation of the inferior horns of the thyroid cartilage to the cricoid cartilage

○ 13. **_Cricotracheal ligament_** (B only)**_:_** Attaches the inferior border of the cricoid cartilage to the superior border of the **_1st trachea cartilage_**

CLINICAL NOTE: LARYNGEAL FRACTURES

Laryngeal cartilage fractures can occur following direct trauma to the neck region from a motor vehicle accident or direct blows during assaults or sports. Common symptoms with laryngeal trauma include hoarseness, neck pain, dyspnea (difficult breathing), odynophonia (pain when using voice), or odynophagia (pain when swallowing). Laryngeal fractures produce submucosal hemorrhage and edema and possible respiratory obstruction. Dislocation of cartilages may also occur, which can affect the crico-arytenoid and cricothyroid joints, altering voice production. Crushing or compression injuries may also damage the laryngeal nerves.

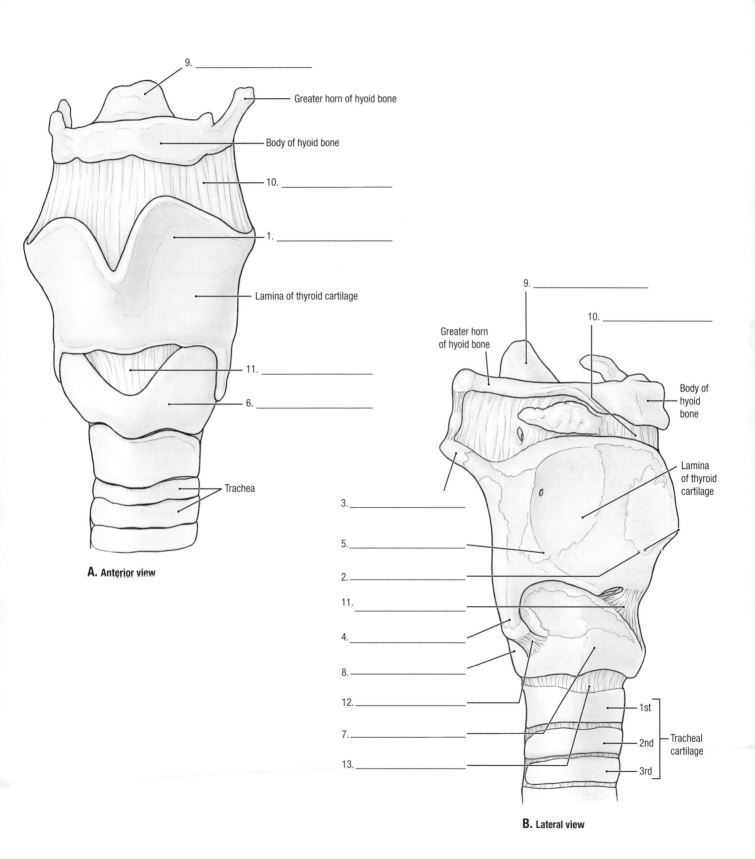

9. _____

Greater horn of hyoid bone

Body of hyoid bone

10. _____

1. _____

Lamina of thyroid cartilage

11. _____

6. _____

Trachea

A. Anterior view

9. _____

10. _____

Greater horn
of hyoid bone

Body of
hyoid
bone

Lamina
of thyroid
cartilage

3. _____

5. _____

2. _____

11. _____

4. _____

8. _____

12. _____

7. _____

13. _____

1st

2nd   Tracheal
cartilage

3rd

B. Lateral view

Grant's

8.21A and B   LARYNGEAL SKELETON, POSTERIOR AND INTERNAL VIEWS

Figure A depicts the posterior view of the articulated laryngeal skeleton. In Figure B, the posterior wall of the larynx has been split and two sides held apart by a **surgical needle spreading** *cricoid cartilage*. On the right side of the specimen, the mucosa has been removed to reveal the underlying cartilages, membranes, and ligaments.

▌ COLOR *each of the following structures using a different color for each:*

○ 1. **Epiglottic cartilage:** The broader superior end is free, whereas the narrow inferior end is attached to the posterior aspect of the thyroid cartilage. The anterior aspect is attached to the hyoid and to the tongue.

○ 2. **Lamina of thyroid cartilage:** The posterior border extends lateral to the arytenoid cartilages, with the prominent **superior horns** projecting superoposteriorly. The **inferior horns** articulate with the cricoid cartilage, forming the cricothyroid joints.

○ 3. **Lamina of cricoid cartilage:** Faces posteriorly and is taller than the anteriorly facing arch

○ 4. **Cricothyroid joint ligaments** (A only)*:* Permit rotation and gliding of the thyroid cartilage at the cricothyroid joint that changes the length of the vocal folds

○ 5. **Arytenoid cartilage:** Paired, three-sided pyramidal cartilages that articulate with the superior border of the lamina of the cricoid cartilage. The **vocal process** extends anteriorly and provides the attachment of the vocal ligament. The **muscular process** extends laterally and provides attachment for the muscles that move the **crico-arytenoid joint**. The apex projects superiorly.

○ 6. **Corniculate cartilage:** Attaches to the apex of the arytenoid cartilage and appears as a small **tubercle** in the **ary-epiglottic fold**

○ 7. **Cuneiform cartilage:** Does not directly attach to any of the laryngeal cartilages and appears as a small **tubercle** in the ary-epiglottic fold

○ 8. **Thyrohyoid membrane** (A only)*:* Lies anterior to the epiglottis

○ 9. **Quadrangular membrane:** Thin connective tissue sheet that extends between the lateral aspects of the arytenoid cartilages and epiglottis

○ 10. **Vestibular ligament** (B only)*:* Inferior free margin of the quadrangular membrane. When covered by the mucosa, forms the **vestibular fold** or false vocal fold

○ 11. **Conus elasticus** (B only)*:* Fills the triangular area superior to the cricoid cartilage to the arytenoid cartilages anteriorly to the interior angle of the thyroid cartilage

○ 12. **Vocal ligament** (B only)*:* Superior free margin of the conus elasticus. When covered by mucosa, forms the **vocal fold** or true vocal fold.

○ 13. **Ventricle** (B only)*:* Space between the vestibular and vocal folds

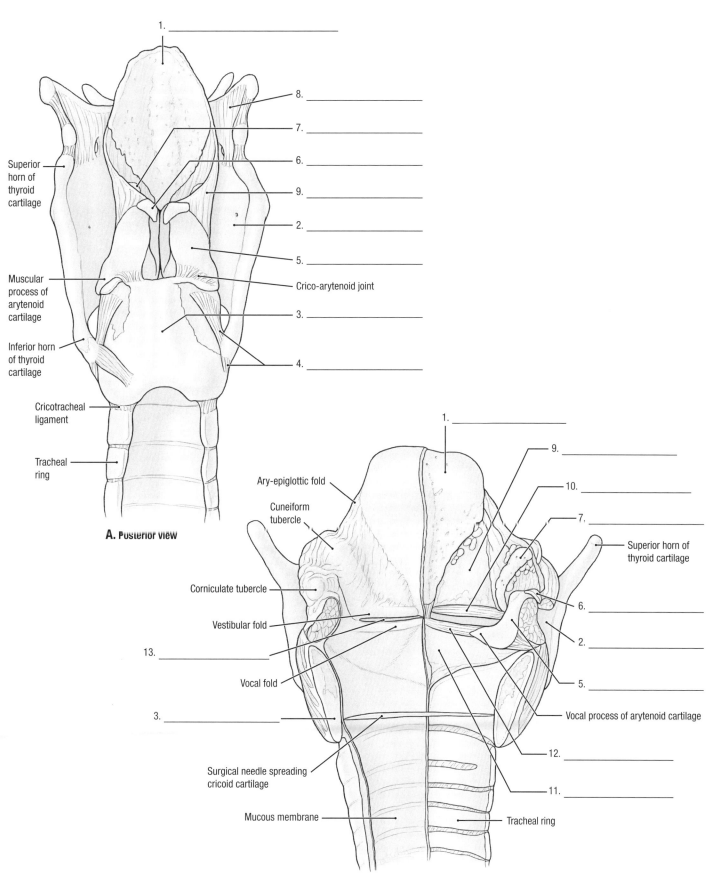

1. _____

8. _____

7. _____

6. _____

9. _____

2. _____

Superior horn of thyroid cartilage

Crico-arytenoid joint

5. _____

Muscular process of arytenoid cartilage

3. _____

Inferior horn of thyroid cartilage

4. _____

Cricotracheal ligament

Tracheal ring

A. Posterior view

1. _____

9. _____

Ary-epiglottic fold

10. _____

Cuneiform tubercle

7. _____

Superior horn of thyroid cartilage

Corniculate tubercle

6. _____

Vestibular fold

2. _____

13. _____

5. _____

Vocal fold

Vocal process of arytenoid cartilage

3. _____

12. _____

Surgical needle spreading cricoid cartilage

11. _____

Mucous membrane

Tracheal ring

B. Posterior view (after incision and spreading of posterior wall of larynx and trachea)

Grant's

8.22A and B MUSCLES OF THE LARYNX, LATERAL VIEWS

Extrinsic muscles of the larynx (infrahyoid and suprahyoid muscles along with the stylopharyngeus) move the larynx as a whole during speaking and swallowing. Intrinsic muscles move one laryngeal cartilage in relation to another. These movements either change the shape of the rima glottidis (space between the vocal folds) for phonation or alterations in breathing (forced respiration) or change the length (tension) of the vocal fold resulting in pitch changes.

Figure A depicts the lateral view of an intact larynx. In Figure B, the right ***thyroid lamina*** has been cut and reflected anteriorly with the right cricothyroid joint separated between the ***thyroid articular surface*** and the ***facet for the cricoid cartilage***.

▌COLOR *each of the following structures using a different color for each:*

Intrinsic Muscles of the Larynx

Muscle	Proximal Attachment	Distal Attachment	Main Action
○ 1. *Cricothyroid* (A only)	Anterolateral ***cricoid cartilage***	Inferior margin and ***inferior horn*** of the ***thyroid cartilage***	Tenses vocal fold
○ 2. *Lateral crico-arytenoid* (B only)	Arch of the cricoid cartilage	Muscular process of the arytenoid cartilage	Adducts vocal fold
○ 3. *Posterior crico-arytenoid* (B only)	Posterior surface of the cricoid lamina		Abducts vocal fold
○ 4. *Arytenoid* (B only)	Arytenoid cartilage	Opposite arytenoid cartilage	Brings arytenoid cartilages closer together (closing laryngeal inlet)
○ 5. *Thyro-arytenoid* (B only)	Posterior surface of the thyroid cartilage	Muscular process of the arytenoid cartilage	Relaxes the vocal fold

○ 6. *Ary-epiglottic muscle* (B only): Acts as a sphincter bringing the ary-epiglottic folds together and pulling the arytenoid cartilages toward the esophagus to close the laryngeal inlet during swallowing

○ 7. *Thyro-epiglottic muscle* (B only): Works with the ary-epiglottic muscle to close the laryngeal inlet during swallowing

Nerves of the Larynx

○ 8. *Recurrent laryngeal nerve:* Supplies sensory innervation to the mucosa of the larynx inferior to the vocal fold and supplies all of the intrinsic muscles of the larynx except the cricothyroid muscle, which is innervated by the external branch of the superior laryngeal nerve

○ 9. *Internal branch of superior laryngeal nerve* (B only): Supplies the sensory innervation to the mucosa of the larynx superior to the vocal fold

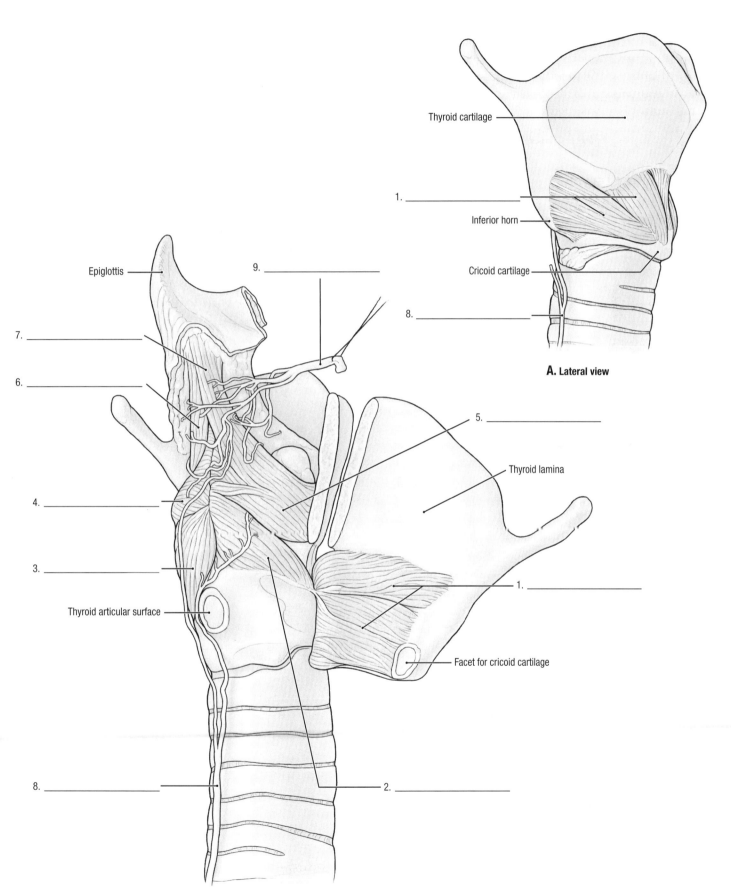

Thyroid cartilage

1. _____

Inferior horn

Cricoid cartilage

8. _____

A. Lateral view

Epiglottis

9. _____

7. _____

6. _____

5. _____

Thyroid lamina

4. _____

3. _____

Thyroid articular surface

1. _____

Facet for cricoid cartilage

8. _____

2. _____

B. Lateral view

Grant's

8.23 MUSCLES OF THE LARYNX, POSTERIOR VIEW

The posterior wall of the pharynx has been cut and each side reflected laterally. The *longitudinal muscles of the pharynx* and the *pharyngobasilar fascia* are intact on the right side of the image. The longitudinal muscles have been removed on the left side to reveal the *middle* and *inferior pharyngeal constrictors*. The posterior wall of the *esophagus* has been cut and the sides held open by two pins.

COLOR *each of the following structures using a different color for each:*

Muscles of the Larynx

○ 1. *Posterior crico-arytenoid:* Paired muscle covering the posterior aspect of the cricoid lamina and the only abductor of the vocal folds. Pulls the muscular processes of the arytenoids posteriorly, which rotates the vocal processes laterally and widens/opens the rima glottidis.

○ 2. *Arytenoid muscle:* Composed of both transverse and oblique fibers connecting one arytenoid cartilage to the opposite one. Along with the lateral crico-arytenoid muscle, adducts the vocal folds or narrows the rima glottidis.

Nerves of the Larynx

○ 3. *Internal branch of superior laryngeal nerve:* Pierces the thyrohyoid membrane and passes through the piriform recess of the laryngopharynx to supply the sensory innervation to the mucosa of the larynx superior to the vocal fold

○ 4. *Recurrent laryngeal nerve:* Courses deep to the inferior pharyngeal constrictor passing superiorly toward the piriform recess and changing its name at this point to *inferior laryngeal nerve*. Travels posterior to the lateral aspect of the posterior crico-arytenoid muscle, supplying it and the other intrinsic muscles of the larynx except cricothyroid. Supplies sensory innervation to the mucosa inferior to the vocal fold.

CLINICAL NOTE: INJURIES TO LARYNGEAL NERVES

Damage to the recurrent laryngeal or inferior laryngeal nerve results in paralysis of the vocal fold on the ipsilateral (same) side because it innervates all the intrinsic laryngeal muscles except the cricothyroid. Typically, the patient initially presents with hoarseness because the paralyzed vocal fold cannot adduct to meet the other vocal fold. With time, the intact vocal fold crosses midline to meet the paralyzed vocal fold, and vocal production improves. Damage to the superior laryngeal nerve affects both internal and external branches. Anesthesia of the superior laryngeal mucosa occurs due to loss of the internal branch. A monotone voice occurs because of the loss of innervation of the external branch to the cricothyroid muscle, which alters tension and length of the vocal fold.

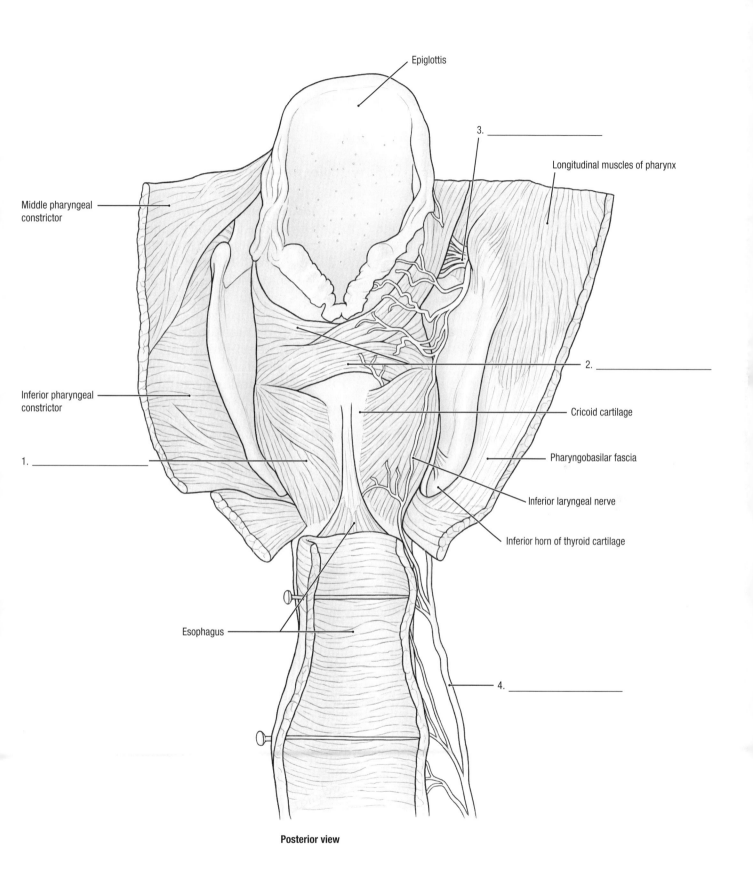

Epiglottis

3. _____

Longitudinal muscles of pharynx

Middle pharyngeal
constrictor

Inferior pharyngeal
constrictor

2. _____

Cricoid cartilage

1. _____

Pharyngobasilar fascia

Inferior laryngeal nerve

Inferior horn of thyroid cartilage

Esophagus

4. _____

Posterior view

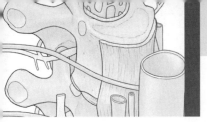

CHAPTER 9

Cranial Nerves

9.1 CRANIAL NERVES IN RELATION TO THE BASE OF THE BRAIN

Cranial nerves are numbered in a rostrocaudal direction as they exit the cranial cavity but can also be identified as they emerge from the brain and spinal cord.

COLOR each of the following structures using a different color for each:

○ 1. **Olfactory bulb:** Primary olfactory neurons (CN I) lie in the olfactory epithelium of the nasal cavity and project their special sensory fibers to the olfactory bulb. The olfactory bulb lies along the inferior (orbital) surface of the **frontal lobe** of the cerebral hemisphere. The olfactory bulb is composed of mitral cells that send their fibers through the **olfactory tract**. Fibers from the olfactory tract primarily project directly to the olfactory cortex.

○ 2. **Optic nerve (CN II):** Composed of special sensory fibers of retinal ganglion cells that lie in the retina of the eyeball. Each optic nerve exits the orbit postero-medially via the optic canal forming the **optic chiasm** near the **infundibulum** of the pituitary gland. At the optic chiasm, fibers from the medial (nasal) half of the retina decussate (cross) to join uncrossed fibers from the lateral (temporal) half of the retina to form the **optic tract**. The optic tracts project primarily to the lateral geniculate bodies of the thalamus.

○ 3. **Oculomotor nerve (CN III):** Emerges from the **midbrain** and is composed of somatic motor and presynaptic parasympathetic fibers

○ 4. **Trochlear nerve (CN IV):** Only cranial nerve that emerges from the dorsal surface of the midbrain and then passes anteriorly around the brainstem. Composed of somatic motor fibers.

○ 5. **Trigeminal nerve (CN V):** Emerges from the lateral aspect of the **pons** and is composed of a large somatic **sensory root** and a small somatic **motor root**

○ 6. **Abducens nerve (CN VI):** Emerges from the brainstem between the pons and the **medulla oblongata** and is composed of somatic motor fibers

○ 7. **Facial nerve (CN VII):** Emerges from the junction of the pons and medullas as two components, the facial nerve proper and the **intermediate nerve**. The facial nerve proper is composed of somatic motor fibers, whereas the intermediate nerve is composed of special sensory (taste), presynaptic parasympathetic, and somatic sensory fibers.

○ 8. **Vestibulocochlear nerve (CN VIII):** Emerges from the junction of the pons and medulla and is composed of special sensory fibers for hearing and balance

○ 9. **Glossopharyngeal nerve (CN IX):** Emerges from the lateral aspect of the medulla and is composed of somatic motor, presynaptic parasympathetic, somatic sensory, and special sensory (taste) fibers

○10. **Vagus nerve (CN X):** Emerges as a series of rootlets along the lateral aspect of the medulla and is composed of somatic motor, somatic sensory, presynaptic parasympathetic, special sensory (taste), and visceral sensory fibers

○11. **Spinal accessory nerve (CN XI):** Emerges as a series of rootlets from the first six cervical segments of the **spinal cord** (only the superior aspect is shown). Composed of somatic motor fibers.

○12. **Hypoglossal nerve (CN XII):** Emerges as a series of rootlets from the medulla and is composed of somatic motor fibers

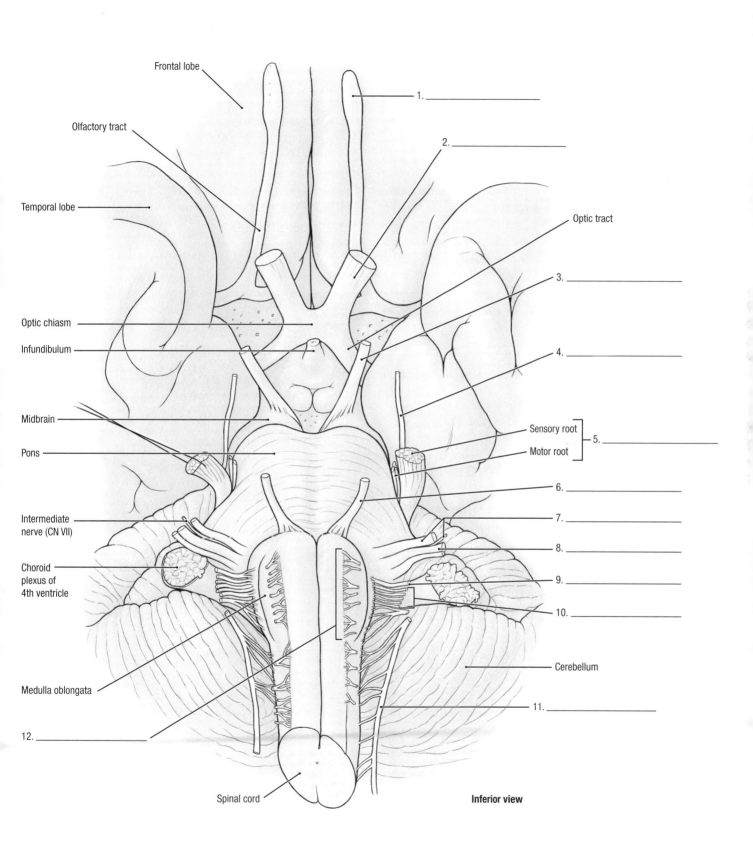

Frontal lobe

1. _____

Olfactory tract

2. _____

Temporal lobe

Optic tract

Optic chiasm

3. _____

Infundibulum

4. _____

Midbrain

Sensory root

5. _____

Pons

Motor root

6. _____

Intermediate nerve (CN VII)

7. _____

8. _____

Choroid plexus of 4th ventricle

9. _____

10. _____

Cerebellum

Medulla oblongata

11. _____

12. _____

Spinal cord

Inferior view

Grant's

9.2 CRANIAL NERVE NUCLEI

Nuclei are groups of cell bodies in the brain or spinal cord, and ganglia are groups of cell bodies located near, but outside of, the brain and spinal cord. Nuclei are composed of cell bodies of the same function (somatic motor, somatic sensory, parasympathetic, visceral sensory, and special sensory). Most sensory pathways involve three neurons (first-, second-, and third-order neurons). First-order neurons are located in a sensory ganglion and send their fibers to second-order neurons located in a nucleus. Motor pathways involve two neurons with a lower motor neuron (somatic) or presynaptic parasympathetic (visceral) located in a nucleus.

A somatic motor pathway has an upper motor neuron located in the cerebral cortex that projects to the lower motor neuron. Presynaptic parasympathetic cell bodies synapse on postsynaptic parasympathetic cell bodies located in one of the four parasympathetic ganglia in the head (ciliary, otic, pterygopalatine, and submandibular).

In this image, the cerebellum has been removed and a dorsal view of the brainstem is depicted with the location of the nuclei demarcated. The mesencephalic, principal sensory, and spinal nuclei of the trigeminal nerve collectively form the *sensory nucelus of CN V*.

COLOR each of the following structures using a different color for each:

Cranial Nerve Nuclei

Nucleus	Location	Components
◯ 1. *Nucleus of oculomotor nerve (CN III)*	Midbrain	Somatic motor
◯ 2. *Edinger-Westphal nucleus of oculomotor nerve (CN III)*	Midbrain	Presynaptic parasympathetic
◯ 3. *Nucleus of trochlear nerve (CN IV)*	Midbrain	Somatic motor
◯ 4. *Motor nucleus of trigeminal nerve (CN V)*	Pons	Somatic motor
◯ 5. *Mesencephalic nucleus of trigeminal nerve (CN V)*	Midbrain and pons	Somatic sensory
◯ 6. *Principal (chief, main, pontine) sensory nucleus of trigeminal nerve (CN V)*	Pons	Somatic sensory
◯ 7. *Spinal trigeminal nucleus of trigeminal nerve (CN V)*	Medulla, caudal pons, and rostral spinal cord	Somatic sensory
◯ 8. *Nucleus of abducens nerve (CN VI)*	Pons	Somatic motor
◯ 9. *Motor nucleus of facial nerve (CN VII)*	Pons	Somatic motor
◯ 10. *Superior salivatory nucleus (CN VII)*	Pons	Presynaptic parasympathetic
◯ 11. *Vestibular nuclei (CN VIII)*	Pons and medulla	Special sensory (balance)
◯ 12. *Cochlear nuclei (CN VIII)*	Pons	Special sensory (hearing)
◯ 13. *Inferior salivatory nucleus (CN IX)*	Medulla	Presynaptic parasympathetic
◯ 14. *Nucleus ambiguus (CNs IX, X)*	Medulla	Somatic motor
◯ 15. *Posterior (motor) nucleus of vagus nerve (CN X)*	Medulla	Presynaptic parasympathetic
◯ 16. *Nuclei of solitary tract (CNs VII, IX, X)* *Gustatory nucleus* and *cardiorespiratory nucleus*	Pons and medulla	Special sensory (taste) and visceral sensory
◯ 17. *Nucleus of hypoglossal nerve (CN XII)*	Medulla	Somatic motor
◯ 18. *Nucleus of spinal accessory nerve (CN XI)*	Upper spinal cord	Somatic motor

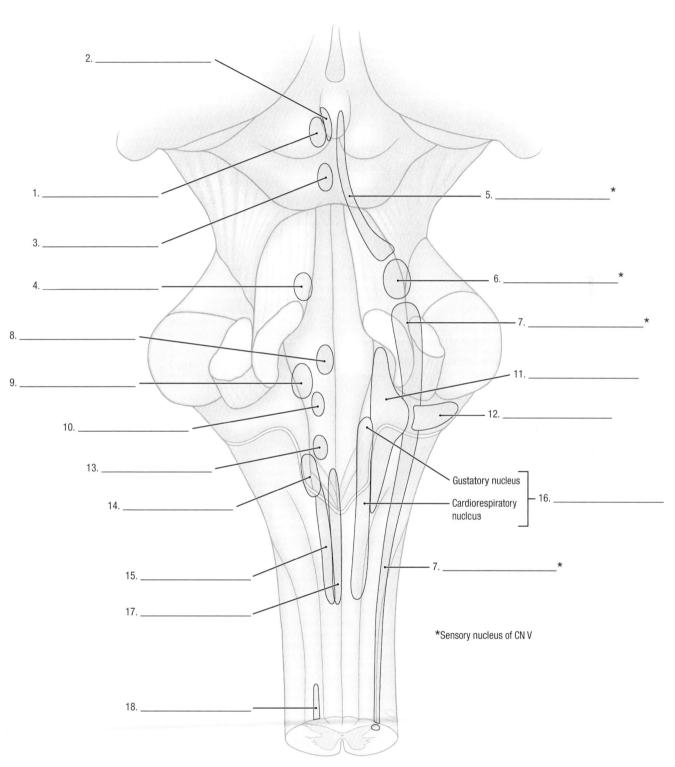

2. _____

1. _____

3. _____

4. _____

5. _____ *

6. _____ *

7. _____ *

8. _____

9. _____

11. _____

12. _____

10. _____

13. _____

Gustatory nucleus

14. _____

16. _____

Cardiorespiratory
nuclcus

15. _____

7. _____ *

17. _____

*Sensory nucleus of CN V

18. _____

Posterior (dorsal) view

Grant's

9.3 OLFACTORY NERVE (CN I)

The function of the olfactory nerve is special sensory for smell (olfaction). The sensory neurons of this pathway are bipolar neurons in that they have peripheral and central processes.

The olfactory pathway is unique among sensory pathways in that most of its fibers do not pass through the thalamus and it is only a two-neuron pathway.

COLOR the following structure:

○ 1. **Neurosensory cell:** Primary olfactory, or first-order, neurons located in the **olfactory part of nasal mucosa (olfactory epithelium)** in the roof of the nasal cavity. The **central processes of olfactory sensory neurosensory** **cells** collectively form the right and left olfactory nerve (CN I). Olfactory nerves, approximately 20 on each side, pass through the **cribriform plate of ethmoid bone** to reach the **olfactory bulb** in the anterior cranial fossa.

TRACE the lines of the following components:

○ 2. **Mitral cells:** Second-order neurons of the olfactory pathway located in the olfactory bulb. The central processes form the **olfactory tract**. Each olfactory tract (right and left) divides into lateral and medial olfactory striae at the olfactory trigone. The **medial olfactory stria** projects to contralateral olfactory structures, whereas the **lateral olfactory stria** projects to the piriform cortex of the temporal lobe and the uncus.

○ 3. **Efferent fibers:** Fibers from the contralateral medial stria

CLINICAL NOTE: CRIBRIFORM PLATE FRACTURES

Anosmia, or loss of smell, can result from damage to the olfactory nerve (CN I) after head trauma. Fractures of the cribriform plate may present with leakage of cerebrospinal fluid into the nasal cavity due to the proximity of the olfactory bulb and surrounding the **subarachnoid space**. Although rare, complications such as meningitis, encephalitis, or brain abscess can occur.

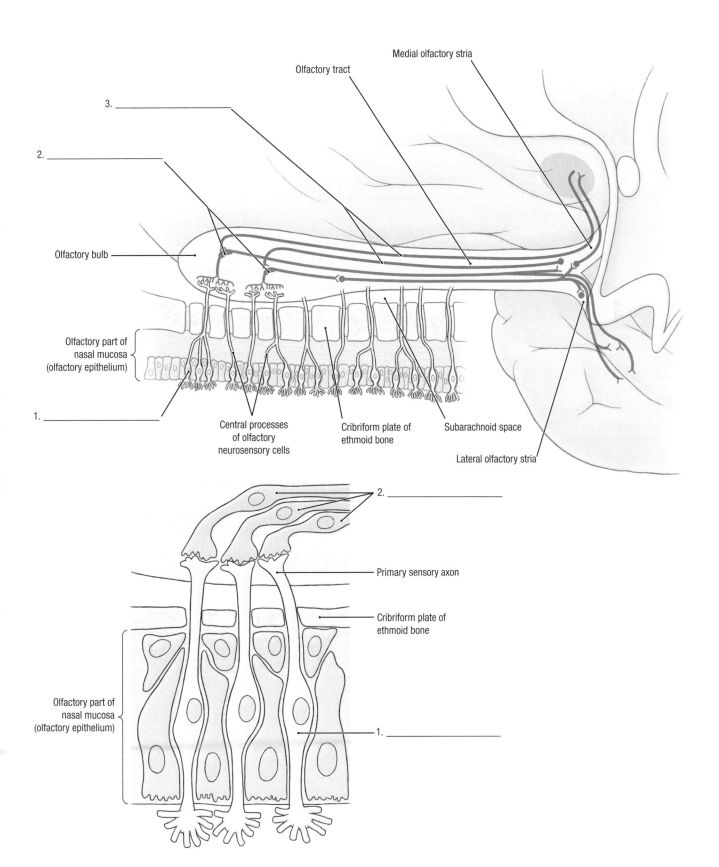

Olfactory tract

Medial olfactory stria

3. _____

2. _____

Olfactory bulb _____

Olfactory part of
nasal mucosa
(olfactory epithelium)

1. _____

Central processes
of olfactory
neurosensory cells

Cribriform plate of
ethmoid bone

Subarachnoid space

Lateral olfactory stria

2. _____

Primary sensory axon

Cribriform plate of
ethmoid bone

Olfactory part of
nasal mucosa
(olfactory epithelium)

1. _____

Medial view of sagittal section through cribriform plate of ethmoid bone

9.4 OPTIC NERVE (CN II)

The optic nerve provides the special sense of sight. The field of vision that the two eyes can observe in primary (straight-forward) gaze is *termed* the *visual field*. Each **eyeball** sees only a segment of the visual field. The visual field can be divided into right and left hemifields that project onto nasal (medial) or temporal (lateral) aspects of the **retina**. The right and left hemifields overlap extensively in the central portion, leading to the binocular field of vision.

COLOR each of the following structures using a different color for each and then trace the lines in the same colors from the visual field to the appropriate section of the retina:

○ 1. **Right visual field:** Projects its image onto the temporal left retina and nasal right retina

○ 2. **Left visual field:** Projects its image onto the nasal left retina and temporal right retina

○ 3. **Center visual field:** Projects its image onto the fovea of the retina where the cones are most concentrated.

TRACE the lines in the same colors used previously representing the visual fields as they travel through the following components:

Optic nerve (CN II): Composed of axons of retinal ganglion cells (first-order neurons of the visual pathway) passing through the posteromedial orbit and exiting through the optic canal

Optic chiasm: Fibers from the nasal half of each retina decussate (cross) in the chiasm and join uncrossed fibers from the temporal half of the retina

Optic tract: Composed of fibers from the ipsilateral (same) halves of both retinas conveying the contralateral visual field. For example, the right optic tract conveys the right halves of both retinas conveying the left visual field.

Lateral geniculate nucleus: One of many nuclei of the thalamus and composed of the second-order neurons of the visual pathway.

Optic radiations: Composed of fibers from the second-order neurons in the lateral geniculate nucleus.

The optic radiations subdivide with the fibers carrying information about the superior visual field (forming Meyer's loop through the temporal lobe) and the fibers carrying information about the inferior visual field traveling through the parietal lobe. Optic radiations terminate in the **visual cortex (occipital lobe)**.

CLINICAL NOTE: VISUAL PATHWAY LESIONS

Damage to the optic nerve can result in loss of the nasal and temporal visual fields of the ipsilateral eye or complete blindness in the eye. A lesion to the optic chiasm, most commonly from a pituitary gland tumor, can result in bitemporal hemianopia or loss of the right and left temporal visual fields. Damage to an optic tract can result in contralateral hemianopia, or a loss of the opposite side of the visual field. The optic radiations subdivide the visual field into superior and inferior fields as well as right and left. Damage to one optic radiation can result in contralateral quadrantanopia or loss of a quadrant of the opposite side of the visual field.

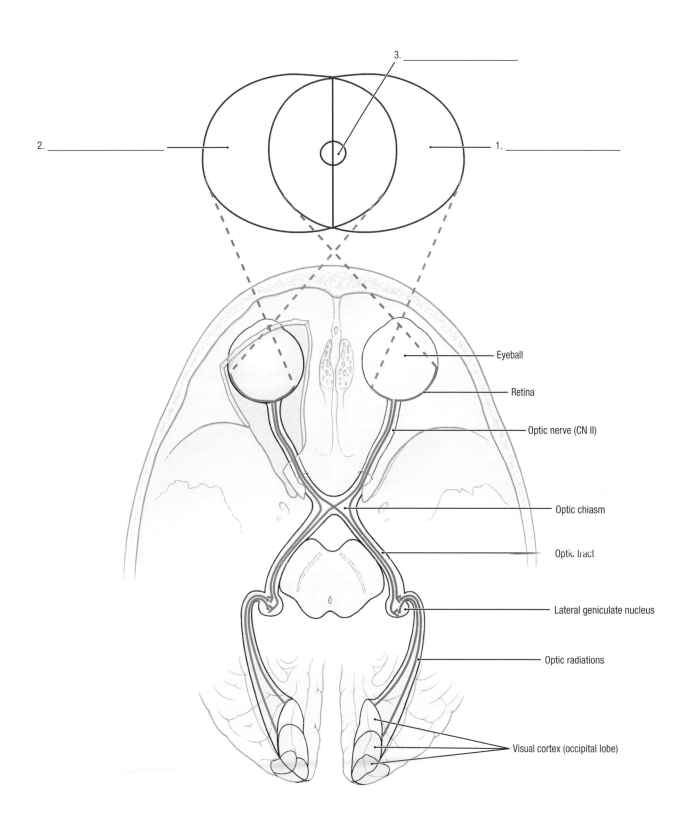

3. _____

2. _____

1. _____

Eyeball

Retina

Optic nerve (CN II)

Optic chiasm

Optic tract

Lateral geniculate nucleus

Optic radiations

Visual cortex (occipital lobe)

9.5 OCULOMOTOR, TROCHLEAR, AND ABDUCENS NERVES (CN III, IV, VI)

The oculomotor, trochlear, and abducens nerves together supply all of the extraocular muscles of the orbit. Additionally, the oculomotor nerve supplies parasympathetic innervation to the sphincter pupillae and ciliary muscles that regulate tension on the lens. In this image, the lateral rectus muscle has been cut at its insertion into the eyeball and reflected to show its medial surface.

Oculomotor Nerve (CN III)

COLOR each of the following structures using a different color for each:

○ 1. *Oculomotor nerve:* Composed of somatic motor fibers from the motor nucleus of the oculomotor nerve and presynaptic parasympathetic fibers from the Edinger-Westphal nucleus. Enters the *superior orbital fissure* and then divides into:
Superior division of CN III: Composed only of somatic motor fibers. Pierces the inferior aspect of the *superior rectus* and then sends fibers to the *levator palpebrae superioris*, supplying both muscles.
Inferior division of CN III: Composed of somatic motor and presynaptic parasympathetic fibers. Somatic motor fibers supply the *medial rectus*, *inferior rectus*, and *inferior oblique* muscles.

TRACE the lines of each of the following components (cell bodies and axons) of the parasympathetic innervation to the eyeball using a different color for presynaptic and postsynaptic:

Presynaptic parasympathetic fibers (represented by dotted line): Arise from the Edinger-Westphal nucleus and then travel as part of the oculomotor nerve. Exclusively travel through the inferior division of the oculomotor nerve and then exit via a communicating branch to the *ciliary ganglion*.

Postsynaptic parasympathetic cell bodies and fibers (represented by solid line): Ciliary ganglion is composed of postsynaptic parasympathetic cell bodies whose axons "hitch a ride" on *short ciliary nerves*, branches of CN V$_1$, to pierce the posterior aspect of the eyeball. Innervate the sphincter (constrictor) pupillae and ciliary muscles.

COLOR each of the following structures using a different color for each:

Trochlear Nerve (CN IV)

○ 2. *Trochlear nerve (CN IV):* Composed of somatic motor fibers; enters superior orbital fissure and immediately pierces the superior aspect of the *superior oblique* muscle, innervating it

Abducens Nerve (CN VI)

○ 3. *Abducens nerve (CN VI):* Composed of somatic motor fibers; enters superior orbital fissure and immediately pierces the medial aspect of the *lateral rectus* muscle, innervating it

---

CLINICAL NOTE: CN III, IV, VI LESIONS

A lesion to the oculomotor nerve (CN III) can result in a dilated pupil due to loss of parasympathetic innervation to the constrictor pupillae and a pupil that appears "down and out" due to unopposed action of the lateral rectus and superior oblique muscles. Damage to the trochlear nerve (CN IV) can result in the inability to look inferiorly when the pupil is in the medial position. Damage to the abducens nerve (CN VI) can result in the inability to look laterally.

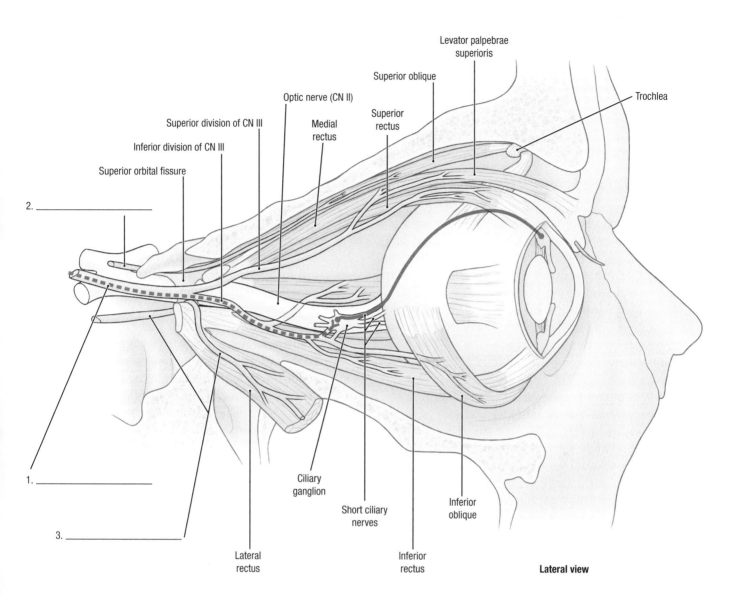

Levator palpebrae superioris

Superior oblique

Trochlea

Optic nerve (CN II)

Superior rectus

Superior division of CN III

Medial rectus

Inferior division of CN III

Superior orbital fissure

2. _____

Ciliary ganglion

1. _____

Short ciliary nerves

Inferior oblique

3. _____

Lateral rectus

Inferior rectus

Lateral view

Grant's

9.6 TRIGEMINAL NERVE (CN V)

The trigeminal nerve is the primary sensory nerve of the head. Additionally, the mandibular division supplies the somatic motor innervation to the first pharyngeal arch muscles. The *trigeminal ganglion* is composed of first-order sensory neurons for touch, pain, and temperature (somatic sensory) and lies in the trigeminal (Meckel's) cave in the middle cranial fossa. The sensory root of the *trigeminal nerve (CN V)* is composed of the central processes of the neurons composing the trigeminal ganglion. The peripheral processes form the three divisions: ophthalmic, maxillary, and mandibular nerves. Fibers of the motor root of CN V pass inferiorly to trigeminal ganglion and exclusively travel with the mandibular nerve.

COLOR each of the following structures using a different color for each:

○ 1. **Ophthalmic nerve (CN V₁):** Supplies the skin and mucous membranes of the forehead, frontal sinus, cornea, superior eyelid, ethmoid sinus, sphenoid sinus, and superior nasal cavity. Enters the superior orbital fissure and divides into:
   Nasociliary nerve: Gives rise to long ciliary, short ciliary, sensory root of ciliary ganglion, infratrochlear, anterior and posterior ethmoidal nerves
   Frontal nerve: Gives rise to supraorbital and supratrochlear nerves
   Lacrimal nerve: Receives the communicating branch of the zygomatic nerve of CN V₂

○ 2. **Maxillary nerve (CN V₂):** Supplies the skin and mucous membranes of the inferior eyelid, posteroinferior nasal cavity, maxillary sinus, palate, maxillary teeth, anterior cheek, and upper lip. Courses through foramen rotundum into pterygopalatine fossa and then gives rise to:

   Zygomatic nerve: Gives rise to zygomaticofacial and zygomaticotemporal nerves along with the communicating branch to lacrimal nerve
   Infraorbital nerve: Gives rise to *anterior* and *middle superior alveolar nerves*
   Posterior superior alveolar nerve
   Greater and lesser palatine nerves

○ 3. **Mandibular nerve (CN V₃):** Supplies sensory innervation to the skin and mucous membranes of the floor of the mouth, anterior two-thirds of the tongue, mandibular teeth, lower lip, chin, parotid region, and temporal region. Also supplies motor innervation to derivatives of the first pharyngeal arch. Courses through the foramen ovale into infratemporal fossa and then divides into *auriculotemporal*, *inferior alveolar*, *lingual*, (long) *buccal*, *deep temporal nerves*, and nerves to masseter, lateral and medial pterygoid, mylohyoid, tensor tympani, and tensor veli palatini.

Parasympathetic Ganglia Associated with Trigminal Nerve

All four of the parasympathetic ganglia of the head are associated with the division of CN V. Postsynaptic parasympathetic fibers from these ganglia "hitch a ride" on branches of CN V.

○ 4. **Ciliary ganglion:** Postsynaptic fibers join short ciliary nerves of CN V₁

○ 5. **Pterygopalatine ganglion:** Postsynaptic fibers join all branches of CN V₂

○ 6. **Otic ganglion:** Postsynaptic fibers join the auriculotemporal nerve of CN V₃

○ 7. **Submandibular ganglion:** Postsynaptic fibers join the lingual nerve of CN V₃

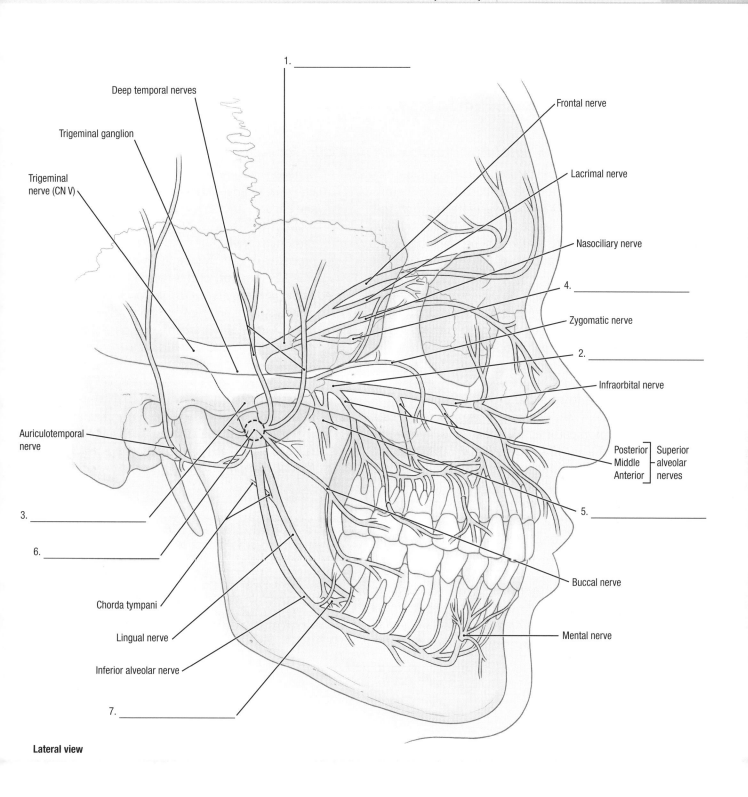

1. _____

Deep temporal nerves

Trigeminal ganglion

Trigeminal nerve (CN V)

Frontal nerve

Lacrimal nerve

Nasociliary nerve

4. _____

Zygomatic nerve

2. _____

Infraorbital nerve

Auriculotemporal nerve

Posterior ⎤ Superior
Middle ⎬ alveolar
Anterior ⎦ nerves

3. _____

5. _____

6. _____

Buccal nerve

Chorda tympani

Lingual nerve

Mental nerve

Inferior alveolar nerve

7. _____

Lateral view

Grant's

9.7 FACIAL NERVE (CN VII)

The *facial nerve (CN VII)* innervates the muscles responsible for facial expression and other second pharyngeal arch structures and supplies taste to the anterior two-thirds tongue, presynaptic parasympathetic fibers to the submandibular and pterygopalatine ganglia, and somatic sensory fibers to the external ear.

COLOR each of the following structures using a different color for each:

The facial nerve courses through the *internal acoustic meatus* and then travels anteriorly for only a short distance before making a sharp bend posteriorly. The *geniculate ganglion*, the sensory ganglion of CN VII, lies at this bend. While traveling through the facial canal of the temporal bone, the facial nerve gives rise to the following branches:

1. *Greater petrosal nerve:* Composed of presynaptic parasympathetic fibers. Arises at the bend, or genu, of the facial nerve and joins the *deep petrosal nerve* (composed of postsynaptic sympathetic fibers) near the foramen lacerum forming the *nerve of the pterygoid canal*. The nerve of the pterygoid canal enters the pterygopalatine fossa and the greater petrosal nerve fibers synapse in the *pterygopalatine ganglion*. Postsynaptic parasympathetic fibers then "hitch a ride" on branches of the *maxillary nerve (CN V₂)* to the glands of the nasal cavity and palate and to the lacrimal nerve of CN V₁ supplying the *lacrimal gland*.

2. *Nerve to stapedius:* Composed of somatic motor fibers supplying the stapedius muscle of the middle ear

3. *Chorda tympani:* Composed of taste and presynaptic parasympathetic fibers. Arises superior to the *stylomastoid foramen* and traverses the middle ear cavity medial to the handle of the malleus. Passes through the *petrotympanic fissure* entering the infratemporal fossa to hitch a ride on the *lingual nerve* from the *mandibular nerve (CN V₃)*. Fibers synapse in the *submandibular*

ganglion and postsynaptic fibers and then either directly enter the *submandibular gland* or hitch a ride back onto the lingual nerve as it travels through the floor of the mouth to reach the *sublingual gland*. Taste fibers from the anterior two-thirds of the tongue are the peripheral processes of sensory neurons in the geniculate ganglion that travel as part of the chorda tympani.

4. *Facial nerve at stylomastoid foramen:* Contains only somatic motor and sensory fibers. After emerging from the stylomastoid foramen, gives off the *posterior auricular branch* that supplies the auricular muscles and a small area of the skin of the external ear. The sensory fibers are peripheral fibers of sensory cell bodies located in the geniculate ganglion. The facial nerve then travels through the parotid gland and forms the parotid plexus that gives rise to the branches that supply the muscles responsible for facial expression: *temporal*, *zygomatic*, *buccal*, *marginal mandibular*, and *cervical*.

CLINICAL NOTE: CN VII LESIONS

Facial muscle paralysis is a common feature of Bell's palsy, which is caused by inflammation of the facial nerve. Paralysis may occur across all facial expression muscles on one side of the face; if only one motor branch is damaged, only some muscles may be affected. Dry mouth and abnormal taste may occur if the chorda tympani or the facial nerve proximal to the branching point of the chorda tympani get damaged. Dry eye may also occur if the greater petrosal nerve or facial nerve proximal to the genu is damaged.

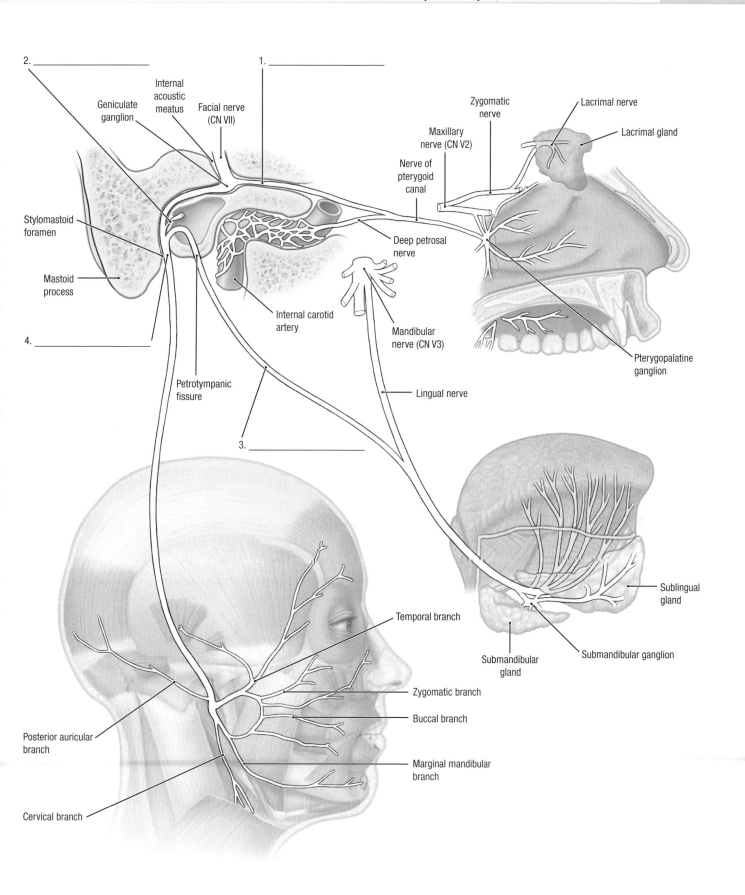

2. _____

1. _____

Internal
acoustic
meatus

Geniculate
ganglion

Facial nerve
(CN VII)

Zygomatic
nerve

Lacrimal nerve

Maxillary
nerve (CN V2)

Lacrimal gland

Nerve of
pterygoid
canal

Stylomastoid
foramen

Deep petrosal
nerve

Mastoid
process

Internal carotid
artery

Mandibular
nerve (CN V3)

Pterygopalatine
ganglion

4. _____

Petrotympanic
fissure

Lingual nerve

3. _____

Sublingual
gland

Temporal branch

Submandibular ganglion

Posterior auricular
branch

Submandibular
gland

Zygomatic branch

Buccal branch

Marginal mandibular
branch

Cervical branch

Grant's

9.8   VESTIBULOCOCHLEAR NERVE (CN VIII)

The *vestibulocochlear nerve (CN VIII)* is the nerve for hearing and balance. It traverses the *internal acoustic meatus* with CN VII.

COLOR each of the following structures using a different color for each:

○ 1. *Vestibular nerve:* Composed of the central processes of the first-order neurons located in the *vestibular ganglion*. The peripheral processes extend to the *maculae* of the *utricle* and *saccule* (sensitive to linear acceleration) and to the *ampullae of the semicircular ducts* (sensitive to rotational acceleration).

○ 2. *Cochlear nerve:* Composed of the central processes of the first-order neurons located in the cochlear *(spiral) ganglion*. The peripheral processes extend to the spiral organ of the *cochlear duct* for the sense of hearing.

CLINICAL NOTE: ACOUSTIC NEUROMA (VESTIBULAR SCHWANNOMA)

Vestibular schwannoma is a benign, slow-growing tumor of CN VIII. As the tumor grows, dizziness and loss of balance along with ipsilateral hearing loss and/or tinnitus (ringing in the ear) can occur. Due to proximity of CN VII at the internal acoustic meatus, further growth of the tumor can result in ipsilateral facial expression paralysis. CN V may also be compressed by an acoustic neuroma.

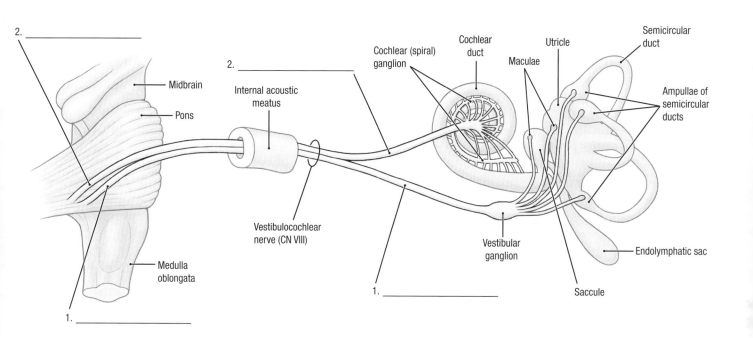

2. _____

Midbrain

Pons

Medulla
oblongata

1. _____

2. _____

Internal acoustic
meatus

Vestibulocochlear
nerve (CN VIII)

1. _____

Cochlear (spiral)
ganglion

Cochlear
duct

Maculae

Utricle

Semicircular
duct

Ampullae of
semicircular
ducts

Endolymphatic sac

Vestibular
ganglion

Saccule

9.9 GLOSSOPHARYNGEAL NERVE (CN IX)

The glossopharyngeal nerve (CN IX) supplies the stylopharyngeus muscle and provides sensory innervation to the middle ear, carotid sinus and body, oropharynx, posterior tongue, and isthmus of fauces and taste innervation to the posterior one-third of the tongue. It also provides presynaptic parasympathetic fibers to the otic ganglion. CN IX is associated with two sensory ganglia: superior and inferior.

COLOR each of the following structures using a different color for each:

○ 1. *Glossopharyngeal nerve:* Emerges from the lateral medulla and passes through the jugular foramen. The *superior* and *inferior ganglia* are located near the jugular foramen. Descends and follows the *stylopharyngeus*, innervating it. Peripheral processes of the sensory cell bodies extend to the *carotid sinus* and *carotid body*, and form *lingual branches* to the posterior one-third of the tongue and *tonsillar branches* to the isthmus of the fauces and to the *pharyngeal plexus*.

○ 2. *Tympanic nerve:* Composed of somatic sensory fibers of the middle ear and forming the *tympanic plexus* on the promontory of the middle ear. Presynaptic parasympathetic fibers "hitch a ride" on the tympanic nerve to the tympanic plexus and then exit via the *lesser petrosal nerve*. Lesser petrosal nerve exits the cranium via the foramen ovale to synapse in the otic ganglion. Postsynaptic parasympathetic fibers hitch a ride on the *auriculotemporal nerve* of CN V_3 to reach the *parotid gland*.

CLINICAL NOTE: JUGULAR FORAMEN SYNDROME

Isolated symptoms from CN IX lesions are rare since CN IX travels in proximity to CN X and CN XI. Often a tumor located near the jugular foramen results in symptoms from compression of all three nerves, resulting in jugular foramen (Vernet) syndrome. Symptoms from CN IX compression include dysphagia (difficulty in swallowing), loss of sensation and taste from posterior one-third of the tongue, decreased parotid gland secretion, and loss of the gag reflex.

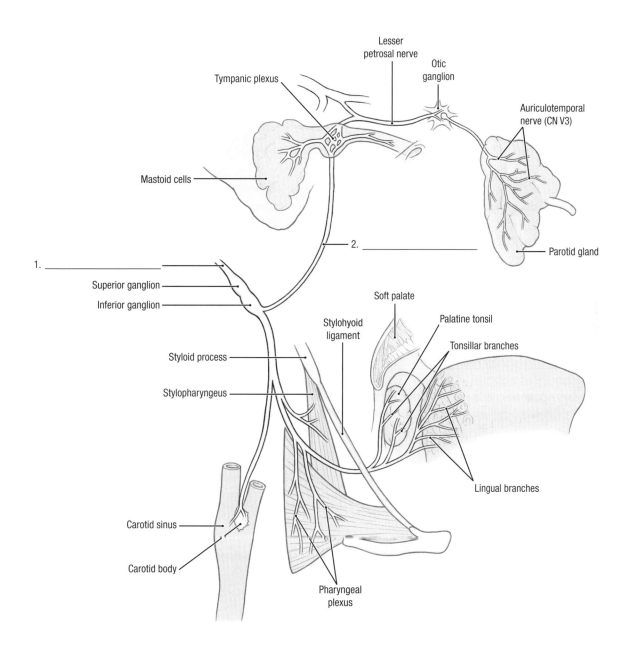

Lesser
petrosal nerve

Otic
ganglion

Tympanic plexus

Auriculotemporal
nerve (CN V3)

Mastoid cells

2. _____

Parotid gland

1. _____

Superior ganglion

Inferior ganglion

Soft palate

Palatine tonsil

Stylohyoid
ligament

Tonsillar branches

Styloid process

Stylopharyngeus

Lingual branches

Carotid sinus

Carotid body

Pharyngeal
plexus

9.10　VAGUS NERVE (CN X)

The vagus nerve (CN X) provides sensory innervation from the auricle via the **_auricular branches_**, inferior pharynx, and larynx along with thoracic and abdominal organs; taste from the root of the tongue and epiglottis, muscles of the palate, pharynx, and larynx; and presynaptic parasympathetic innervation to thoracic and abdominal organs. Two sensory **_ganglia_**, **_superior_** and **_inferior_**, are associated with the vagus nerve.

COLOR each of the following structures using a different color for each:

○ 1. **_Vagus nerve (CN X):_** Has the longest course and extensive distribution inferior to the head. CN X leaves the cranium through the jugular foramen and descends through the neck within the carotid sheath with the common carotid artery and internal jugular vein entering the thorax, providing visceral sensory and presynaptic parasympathetic innervation to the thoracic and abdominal viscera to the left colic flexure.

○ 2. **_Pharyngeal branch:_** Arises inferior to the jugular foramen and provides the motor component of the pharyngeal plexus and **_branchial motor branch to muscles of palate_** (except tensor veli palatini)

○ 3. **_Superior laryngeal nerve:_** Arises inferior to the pharyngeal branch carrying somatic motor and visceral sensory fibers

○ 4. **_Internal branch:_** Arises from the superior laryngeal nerve and supplies sensory innervation to the mucosa of the inferior pharynx and larynx superior to the vocal folds

○ 5. **_External branch:_** Arises from the superior laryngeal nerve and supplies the **_cricothyroid_** muscle

○ 6. **_Recurrent laryngeal nerve:_** Loops under the subclavian artery on the right and the arch of the aorta on the left. Supplies the intrinsic muscles of the larynx except the cricothyroid and sensory innervation to the mucosa of the larynx inferior to the vocal folds.

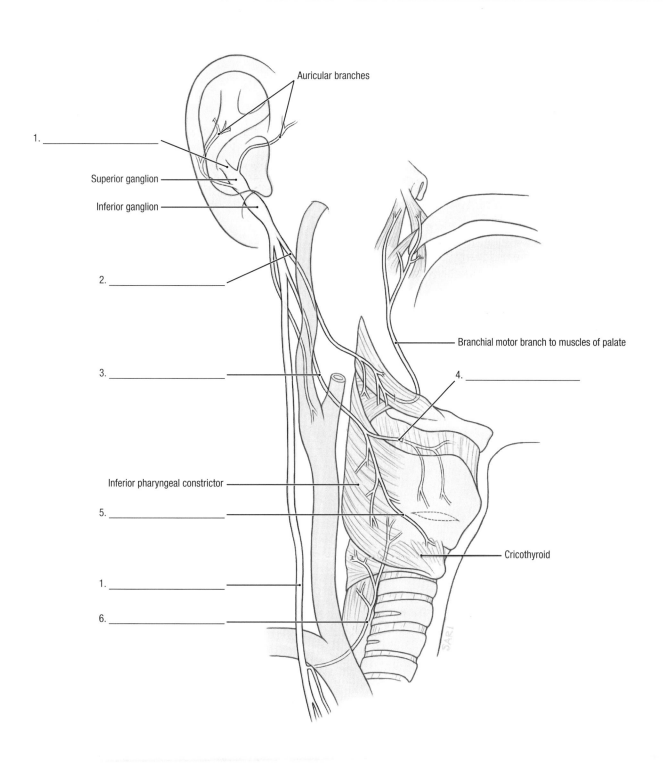

Auricular branches

1. _____

Superior ganglion

Inferior ganglion

2. _____

Branchial motor branch to muscles of palate

3. _____

4. _____

Inferior pharyngeal constrictor

5. _____

Cricothyroid

1. _____

6. _____

Grant's

9.11 SPINAL ACCESSORY NERVE (CN XI)

The spinal accessory nerve (CN XI) supplies the sternocleido-mastoid and trapezius muscles.

COLOR each of the following structures using a different color for each:

○ 1. **Spinal accessory nerve:** Arises from **posterior rootlets** of C1 to C6 spinal rootlets, ascends through the **foramen magnum**, and exits the cranium via the **jugular foramen** with the **vagus nerve (CN X)** and glossopharyngeal nerve (CN IX). Penetrates and innervates the **sternocleido-mastoid muscle**. Emerges along the posterior border of the sternocleidomastoid muscle crossing the lateral cervical region and passes deep to the superior border of the **trapezius**, innervating it. **Branches of cervical plexus (C2-C4)** join the spinal accessory nerve in the lateral cervical region, conveying proprioceptive fibers to the trapezius muscle.

CLINICAL NOTE: CN XI LESION

Damage to the spinal accessory nerve results in ipsilateral drooping of the shoulder with inability or significant weakness in raising the shoulder against resistance. If the damage is proximal to the sternocleidomastoid, the ability to turn the chin to the contralateral side against resistance may be compromised.

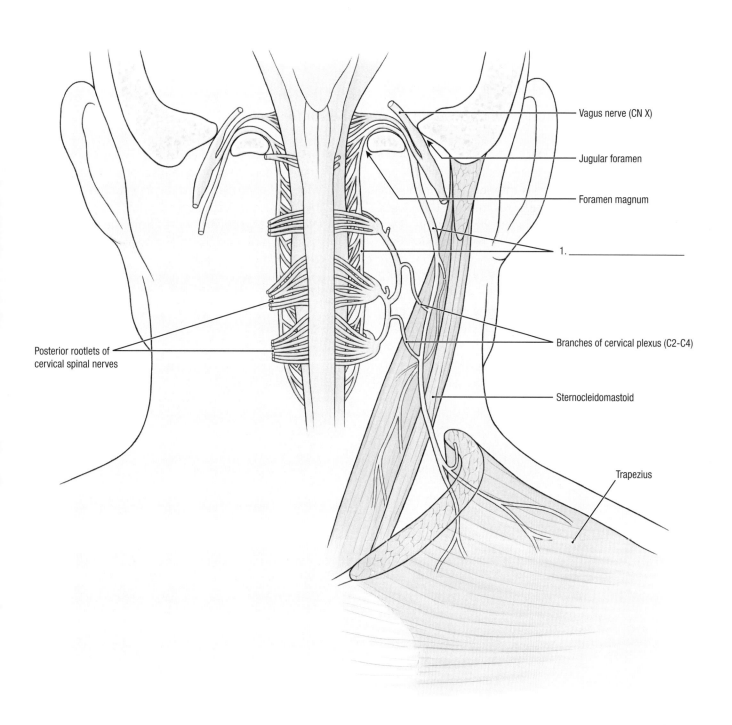

Vagus nerve (CN X)

Jugular foramen

Foramen magnum

1. _____

Branches of cervical plexus (C2-C4)

Sternocleidomastoid

Trapezius

Posterior rootlets of
cervical spinal nerves

Grant's

9.12 HYPOGLOSSAL NERVE (CN XII)

The hypoglossal nerve (CN XII) supplies the intrinsic and extrinsic muscles of the tongue except the palatoglossus muscle.

COLOR each of the following structures using a different color for each:

○ 1. **Hypoglossal nerve (CN XII):** Exits the cranium via the **hypoglossal canal** and descends until the level of the oral cavity where it turns to pass anteriorly. Enters the oral cavity lateral to the **hyoglossus** muscle supplying it along with the **styloglossus** and **genioglossus**. Then gives rise to **lingual branches** that supply the **intrinsic muscles of tongue**.

○ 2. **Superior root of ansa cervicalis:** Fibers from **C1 to C2** "hitch a ride" on the hypoglossal nerve as it courses lateral to the external and **internal carotid arteries** and exit to supply the **omohyoid**, **sternohyoid**, and **sternothyroid**

○ 3. **Inferior root of ansa cervicalis:** Fibers from **C2 to C3** travel independently forming a loop with the superior root and contributing to the innervation of the infrahyoid muscles except thyrohyoid

○ 4. **Nerve to thyrohyoid:** Arises from the **C1 to C2** fibers hitching a ride on the hypoglossal nerve to innervate the thyrohyoid muscle

CLINICAL NOTE: CN XII LESION

Damage to the hypoglossal nerve results in ipsilateral paralysis of the intrinsic and extrinsic muscles of the tongue. When a patient is asked to stick out the tongue, the intact muscles on the contralateral side push the tongue to the same side of the lesion.

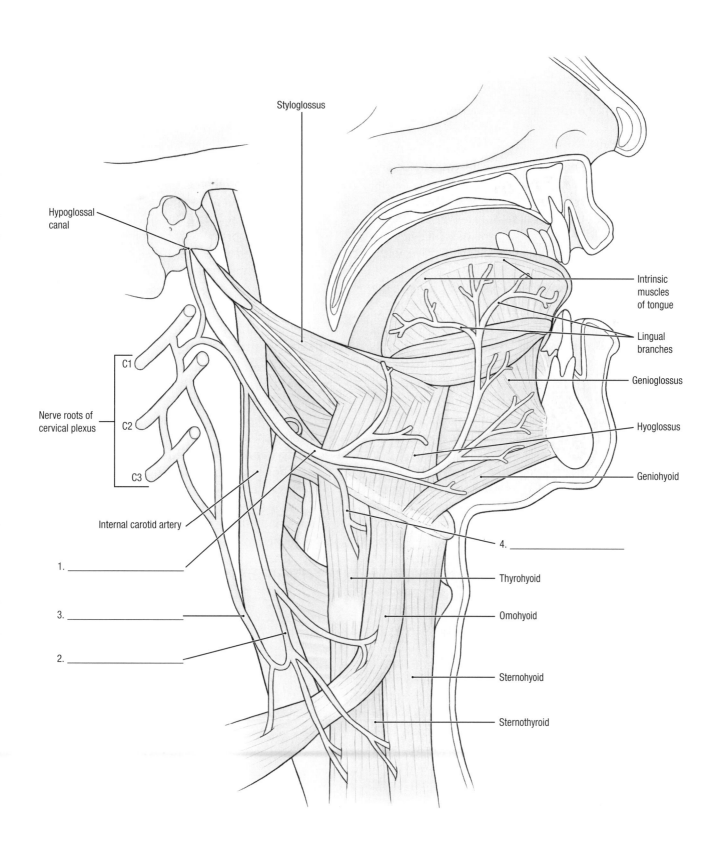

Styloglossus

Hypoglossal
canal

C1

Nerve roots of
cervical plexus

C2

C3

Internal carotid artery

1. _____

3. _____

2. _____

Intrinsic
muscles
of tongue

Lingual
branches

Genioglossus

Hyoglossus

Geniohyoid

4. _____

Thyrohyoid

Omohyoid

Sternohyoid

Sternothyroid

Grant's

9.13 SUMMARY OF AUTONOMIC INNERVATION TO THE HEAD

TRACE the lines of each of the following components (cell bodies and axons) using a different color for trigeminal, parasympathetic, and sympathetic:

Trigeminal Nerve

Almost all autonomic innervation, both parasympathetic and sympathetic, reach their target structures in the head by joining or "hitching a ride" on branches of the trigeminal nerve. Since the trigeminal nerve is the primary sensory nerve of the head, it has branches almost everywhere in the head, providing a framework of nerves for the autonomic fibers to travel with.

○ 1. *Cell bodies of primary sensory neurons:* Comprise the trigeminal ganglion. Peripheral processes travel through

$CN V_1$, $CN V_2$, and $CN V_3$ to reach their target structures. The central processes form the trigeminal nerve (*CN V*). The four parasympathetic ganglia, *ciliary*, *pterygopalatine*, *submandibular*, and *otic*, are suspended by branches of the divisions of the trigeminal nerve. Trigeminal branches pass through the parasympathetic ganglia without synapsing.

Parasympathetic Innervation

Parasympathetic innervation in the head begins in the nuclei of CN III, VII, and IX. Four parasympathetic ganglia composed of postsynaptic parasympathetic cell bodies are located in the head that project postsynaptic parasympathetic fibers. Postsynaptic fibers travel on branches of CN V to reach their target structures.

○ 2. *CN III:* Presynaptic parasympathetic fibers travel via the inferior division of CN III to reach the ciliary ganglion. Postsynaptic cell bodies within the ciliary ganglion project fibers that hitch a ride on short ciliary nerves of $CN V_1$ to pierce the posterior aspect of the eyeball to reach the sphincter pupillae and ciliary muscles.

○ 3. *CN IX:* Presynaptic parasympathetic fibers travel via the lesser petrosal nerve to reach the otic ganglion. Postsynaptic cell bodies within the otic ganglion project fibers that "hitch a ride" on auriculotemporal nerve to the *parotid gland*.

○ 4. *CN VII:* Presynaptic parasympathetic fibers travel via either the greater petrosal or the chorda tympani nerve. The greater petrosal nerve travels to the pterygopalatine ganglion. Postsynaptic cell bodies within the pterygopalatine ganglion project fibers that hitch a ride on branches of $CN V_2$ to reach the *lacrimal*, *nasal*, *palatine*, and *pharyngeal glands*. Chorda tympani travels to the submandibular ganglion. Postsynaptic cell bodies within the submandibular ganglion project fibers that hitch a ride on branches of lingual nerve to innervate the *submandibular* and *sublingual glands*.

Sympathetic Innervation

Preganglionic sympathetic fibers innervating the head originate in the upper thoracic levels (T1-T4) of the intermediolateral cell column of the spinal cord. Preganglionic sympathetic fibers ascend in the **sympathetic trunk** and terminate in the superior cervical ganglion.

○ 5. *Postsynaptic sympathetic cell bodies:* Comprise the superior cervical ganglion and project their fibers onto branches of the external and internal carotid arteries forming a **periarterial plexus**. Fibers then travel on the arterial branches or hitch a ride on trigeminal nerve branches to reach their target organs. Postsynaptic sympathetic fibers pass through parasympathetic ganglia of the head without synapsing.

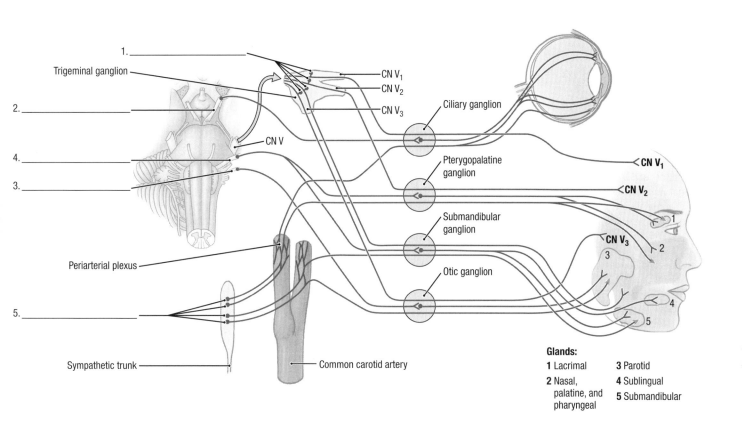

1. _____

Trigeminal ganglion _____

CN V₁

CN V₂

CN V₃

2. _____

CN V

4. _____

3. _____

Ciliary ganglion

Pterygopalatine ganglion

Submandibular ganglion

CN V₁

CN V₂

CN V₃

Periarterial plexus _____

Otic ganglion

1

2

3

5. _____

4

5

Sympathetic trunk _____

Common carotid artery

Glands:
1 Lacrimal
2 Nasal, palatine, and pharyngeal
3 Parotid
4 Sublingual
5 Submandibular

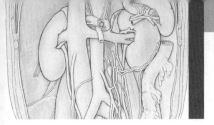

Index

Note: Page number followed by *f* and *t* indicates figures and tables.

RRS1802